Hearing Mechanisms and Speech

Psychologie Gießen Fachbereich 06 Bibliothek

AF804330

JUSTUS-LIEBIG-UNIVERSITÄT GIESSEN BIBLIOTHEKSSYSTEM
03/10 AUSGESONDERT W.W.

13.2
Inv. 17571
Sign. 13.2/C.1

Experimental Brain Research Supplementum 2

Hearing Mechanisms and Speech

EBBS-Workshop, Göttingen, April 26–28, 1979

Edited by
O. Creutzfeldt H. Scheich Chr. Schreiner

With 85 Figures and 12 Tables

Springer-Verlag Berlin Heidelberg New York 1979

Professor Dr. O. Creutzfeldt, Abt. Neurobiologie, Max-Planck-Institut für biophysikalische Chemie, Postfach 968, D-3400 Göttingen, FRG

Professor Dr. H. Scheich, Institut für Zoologie der Technischen Hochschule, Schnittspahnstraße 3, D-6100 Darmstadt, FRG

Dr. Chr. Schreiner, Abt. Neurobiologie, Max-Planck-Institut für biophysikalische Chemie, Postfach 968, D-3400 Göttingen, FRG

ISBN 3-540-09655-8 Springer-Verlag Berlin Heidelberg New York
ISBN 0-387-09655-8 Springer-Verlag New York Heidelberg Berlin

Library of Congress Cataloging in Publication Data.

This work is subject to copyright. All rights are reserved, whether the whole or part of the material is concerned specifically those of translation, reprinting, re-use of illustrations, broadcasting, reproduction by photocopying machine or similar means, and storage in data banks. Under § 54 of the German Copyright Law where copies are made for other than private use, a fee is payable to the publisher, the amount of the fee to be determined by agreement with the publisher.

© by Springer-Verlag Berlin Heidelberg 1979
Printed in Germany

The use of registered names, trademarks etc. in this publication does not imply even in the absence of a specific statement, that such names are exempt from the relevant protective laws and regulations and therefore free for general use.

Printing and Binding: J. Beltz, Hemsbach
2329/3321-543210

Contents

III) Brain mechanisms of speech perception and production.

List of Contributors

AERTSEN, A., Laboratorium voor medische fysica en biofysica Faculteit der Geneeskunde, Universiteit van Nijmegen, Geert Grooteplein Noord 21, Nijmegen, The Netherlands

AINSWORTH, W.A., Dept. of Communication and Neuroscience, University of Keele, Keele, Staffordshire, ST5 5BG, England

BAILEY, P., Dept. of Psychology, University of York, Heslington, York YO1 5DD, England

BRÜSER, E., Verhaltensforschung, Lehr- und Forschungsbereich der FU Berlin - FB 23 - WE 4, Haderslebener Straße 9, 1000 Berlin 41, FRG

CREUTZFELDT, O., Abt. Neurobiologie, Max-Planck-Institut für Biophysikalische Chemie, Postfach 968, 3400 Göttingen, FRG

DARWIN, C.J., Laboratory of Exp. Psychology, Sussex University, Brighton BN1 0QG, England

DE BOER, E., Academisch Ziekenhuis, Keel-, neus- en oorheelkundige Kliniek, Fysisch Laboratorium, Eerste Helmerstraat 104, Amsterdam - Oud west, The Netherlands

DEROUESNE, J., Clinique de Neurologie et de Neuropsychologie, Hôpital des la Salpêtrière, 47, Boulevard de L'Hôpital, F-75634 Paris Cedex 13, France

DROOGLEEVER FORTUYN, J., Kliniek voor Neurologie, Rijksuniversiteit, Oostersingel 59, Groningen, The Netherlands

DUIFHUIS, H., Institute for Perception Research, P. Box 513, den Dolech 2, Eindhoven 5612 AZ, The Netherlands

EHRENSTEIN, W., Universität Konstanz, Fachbereich Psychologie und Soziologie, Universitätsstr. 10, D-7750 Konstanz, FRG

FINKENZELLER, P., Institut für Physiologie und Biokybernetik, Universittät Erlangen-Nürnberg, Universitätsstr. 17, D-8250 Erlangen, FRG

GOLDBLUM, M.-C., U. 111 INSERM, 2TER, Rue d'Alêsia, F-75014 Paris, France

HAGGARD, M.P., Medical Research Council, Institute of Hearing Research, University of Nottingham, Nottingham NG7 2UH, England

HELLWEG, F.-C., Medizinische Hochschule Hannover, Hals-Nasen-Ohren-Klinik, Karl-Wiechert-Allee 9, D-3000 Hannover, FRG

HESS, W., Lehrstuhl für Datenverarbeitung, Technische Universität München, Postf. 202420, D-8000 München, FRG

HUBER, W., Abteilung Neurologie, Medizinische Fakultät, Techn. Hochschule Aachen, Goethestr. 27/29, D-5100 Aachen, FRG

JOHANNESMA, P.I.M., Laboratorium voor medische Fysica en Biofysica, Universiteit van Nijmegen, Geert Grooteplein Noord 21, Nijmegen, The Netherlands

JÜRGENS, U., Max-Planck-Institut für Psychiatrie, Kräpelinstraße 2, D-8000 München 40, FRG

KLINKE, R., Zentrum der Physiologie, J.-W.-Goethe-Universität, Theodor-Stern-Kai 7, D-6000 Frankfurt 71, FRG

KOCH, R., Tierärztliche Hochschule, Fachbereich Med. Physik, Bischofsholer Damm 15, 3000 Hannover, FRG

KORNHUBER, H.H., Abteilung Neurologie, Universität Ulm, Steinhövelstr. 9, D-7900 Ulm, FRG

LANGNER, G., Institut für Zoologie, Technische Hochschule, Schnittspahnstr. 3, D-6100 Darmstadt, FRG

LEHMANN, D., Universitätsspital Zürich, Neurologische Klinik und Poliklinik, Rämistr. 100, CH-8091 Zürich, Switzerland

LEPPELSACK, H.-J., Lehrstuhl für allgemeine Zoologie, Ruhruniversität, Postf. 102148, D-4630 Bochum 1, FRG

LONGUET-HIGGINS, C., Experimental Psychology, Sussex University, Brighton BN1 0QG, England

MARSLEN-WILSON, W., Max-Planck-Institut für Psycholinguistik, Berg en Dalseweg 79, Nijmegen,
The Netherlands

MEHRGARDT, S., III. Physikalisches Institut, Universität Göttingen, Bürgerstr. 42-44, D-3400 Göttingen, FRG

MEININGER, V., Laboratoire d'Anatomie, Faculté de Medecine, 45 Rue de St. Peres, F-75007 Paris Cedex 06, France

MERZENICH, M.M., Coleman Memorial Laboratory, School of Medicine, Dept. of Otolaryngology, San Francisco, Cal. 94143, USA

MICELI, G., Clinica Neurologica, Università Cattolica, Largo A. Gemelli 8, I-00168 Roma, Italy

MØLLER, A.R., University of Pittsburgh, Eye and Ear Hospital, 230 Lothrop, Pittsburgh, Pa. 15217, USA

MORATH, M., Verhaltensforschung, Lehr- und Forschungsbereich der FU Berlin - FB 23 - WE 4, Haderslebener Str. 9, D-1000 Berlin 41, FRG

MÜLLER-PREUSS, P., MPI für Psychiatrie, Dept. of Primate Behaviour, Kraepelinstr. 2, D-8000 München 40, FRG

NEWMAN, J.D., Dept. of Health, Education, and Welfare, Public Health Service, National Institutes of Health, Bethesda, Maryland 20014, USA

OJEMANN, G., Dept. of Neurological Surgery, School of Medicine, University of Washington, Seattle, Washington 98195, USA

OSEN, K., Anatomisk Institutet, Universitetet i Oslo, Karl Johans Gate 47 (Domus Media), N-Oslo 1, Norway

PALMER, A.R., Dept. of Communication and Neuroscience, Keele, Staffordshire, ST5 5BG, England

PERRET, E., Neuropsychologisches Laboratorium, Neurologische Univ.-Klinik, Vogelsangstr. 52, CH-8006 Zürich, Switzerland

PLOOG, D., MPI für Psychiatrie, Klinisches Institut, Kraepelinstr. 18, D-8000 München 40, FRG

POECK, K., Abt. Neurologie der Medizinischen Fakultät, Goethestr. 27/29, D-5100 Aachen, FRG

Saillant, B., Clinique de Neurologie et de Neuropsychologie, Hôpital de la Salpêtrière, 47, Boulevard de l'Hôpital, F-75634 Paris Cedex 13, France

SCHEICH, H., Institut für Zoologie der Technischen Hochschule, Schnittspahnstr. 3, D-6100 Darmstadt

SCHREINER, Chr., Abt. Neurobiologie, Max-Planck-Institut für biophysikalische Chemie, Postf. 968, D-3400 Göttingen, FRG

SCHROEDER, M.R., III. Physikalisches Institut, Bürgerstr. 42-44, D-3400 Göttingen, FRG

SYMMES, D., Dept. of Health, Education, and Welfare, Public Health Service, National Institutes of Health, Bethesda, Maryland 20014, USA

TERHARDT, E., Lehrstuhl für Elektroakustik, Technische Universität München, Arcisstr. 21, D-8000 München 2, FRG

WENIGER, D., Abt. Neurologie, Medizinische Fakultät, Techn. Hochschule Aachen, Goethestr. 27/29, D-5100 Aachen, FRG

WHITAKER, H., Dept. of Psychology, The University of Rochester, River Station, Rochester, N.Y. 14627, USA

Introduction

O. D. CREUTZFELDT, Max-Planck-Institut für Biophysikalische Chemie,
D-3400 Göttingen, FRG

In the name of the European Brain and Behaviour Society (EBBS) and the Max-Planck-Institute for Biophysical Chemistry, I welcome you to this workshop on Hearing Mechanisms and Speech.

It is the aim of EBBS, to tackle brain mechanisms of complex behavioral performances. Language is certainly a complex behaviour, and understanding of language as well. Through language an individual is able to express the internal processes within his brain in symbols of this experience and communicate them to others. This implies also the description of the world in which we live in as far as this world induces, through the sensory organs, activities in our brains. This symbolical representation of the world is, in itself, a real world to which our brain relates itself, in creating and in understanding it (Creutzfeldt, 1979). Therefore, any specific language influences thinking and broader aspects of behaviour, and this may explain some of the differences as found between language populations (Herder, 1772;Humboldt, 1836).

In as much as the function of language is a symbolical representation of reality, it must be able to describe this reality, sufficiently and generally. In so far, the rules to which any language is subjected, are dictated by the reality to which we relate ourself through language. These rules are general, and therefore general rules or a universal grammar may be generated, common to all languages (Chomsky, 1965). But at variance with the exclusive emphasis on grammatical structuralism, I tend to consider the universal properties of languages to follow from the fact that any language serves the same function, i.e. the representation of the (universal) world within and around us in linguistic symbols consistant with this internal representation of the world. The neurophysiological and anatomical constraints of speech production set the limits to such symbolic presentation, and these limits are closely linked with the cognitive constraints of our brains. Thus the rules of reality as it is represented in our brains determine the language rules which ought to be, therefore, universal.

Neurobiology can certainly not directly contribute to such philosophical considerations about language. On the other hand, neurobiologists may realize that their concepts about brain mechanisms are influenced by philosophical as well as by logical concepts about cognition, communication, thinking, and behaviour and even by naive reasoning about brain functions as derived from experience and introspection. In as much as classical aphasiology, which still dominates neurobiological concepts of language, represents philosophical concepts such as those expressed in association psychology, the search for a hierarchical structure of feature analysis in the brain reflects such naive logical concepts (Creutzfeldt, 1975).

Many concepts that guide certain approaches to the analysis of sensory cognition, including the understanding of language, are ultimately based on our naive reflection on cognition and understanding. Such reflection is, of course, only possible within the constraints of language, and it is thus trapped by the fact that it tries to explain its own explanation. It must not be and probably is not identical with the brain mechanisms of cognition and communication.

The information on any sensory signal, that is available to the brain, is contained in the neural signals that are elicited by it. All sensory systems are multichannel analysers, through which the original signal is dissected into smallest components such as points in space in the visual, points on the body surface in the somato-sensory and spectral loci in the auditory system. The spatial (or spectral) tuning of each channel (its receptive fields), the total range of the ensemble of available channels, and the available number of channels within that range determine the faithfulness of the neural representation of the signal in the brain. Kiang has called this neural representation of auditory signals in the auditory nerve the neurogram (Kiang et al., 1979).

At the peripheral level, this neural representation may still be quite faithful and essentially a linear transformation of the signal, but neuronal filtering mechanisms at each stage upwards reduce this representation further at the higher levels. These filtering mechanisms are largely based on lateral inhibition at each relais (Creutzfeldt, 1977). Consequently, only the transients within a complex stimulus (or signal) are represented in the primary sensory projection areas of the cortex, with preservation of the spatial (or spectral) location of the appearance of such transients relative to each other. In the visual system, this means a representation of contrasts or contours. In the auditory system, this reduction leads, at the cortical level, to the exclusive representation of transients within an auditory signal, i.e. sudden changes in power in the respective spectral regions (Creutzfeldt et al., 1979). A complex auditory signal will thus be dissected into frequency regions as well as into temporal sequences of transients. The completeness of this representation is the condition for identifying or recognizing it. In this sense one may say that the limits of the neural representation of sensory and, in our special case, of the auditory signals, at the higher levels of the brain are the limits for our understanding them.

Such a representation does not solve, of course, the problem of cognition of complex signals. Instead, we realize that the brain has to solve two tasks: First to read the message from the spatial distribution of spectral components from the many, spatially separate spectral channels and second to read the temporal sequence of transients which characterize the signal.

The time structure of temporal sequences of transients makes auditory signals, to some extent, invariant against spectral content. Maybe one could go so far as to consider the spectral components of auditory signals as carrier frequency and the actual modulation of this carrier as the real message. I admit that this is an oversimplification, but I may remarque here, that it is my feeling that the information contained in the sequences of transients in complex auditory signals including language appears to be underrepresented in neurophysiological considerations about hearing and speech. The shadow of Helmholtz and the fascination by spectral tuning curves and feature detection lie heavily over this field.

The problem of spatial, that is spectral, <u>and</u> of temporal integration is, of course, the major problem of what we may call higher order analysis of auditory signals. Physiologists, psychologists and neurologists tend to make big black boxes and call them "association" areas, or feature specific neuron sets. They assume, that there may be a next stage and that does it. It is true, and undisputed, that for higher order auditory cognition, there is more needed than just a primary auditory cortex with however vague a tonotopic frequency representation. But it is also true that frogs with no cortex can also correctly respond to at least a limited variety of auditory signals. The question is, are the additional cortical areas in the temporo-parietal lobe which are needed for language understanding as well as for cognition, just higher order analysers of what the primary cortex sends to them, or do they receive direct inputs from lower levels of the auditory pathways? The first possibility is, of course, the classical Wernicke-scheme of aphasia and might be called the hierarchical concept. But recent neurophysiological work on somatosensory and especially on visual association areas has taught us to be, at least, sceptical towards such models: neurons in for example area 21, a visual association area, respond as well and practically in the same way to visual stimuli with the primary and secondary visual areas intact or destroyed (Creutzfeldt and Watanabe, in prep.). All association cortex receives thalamic input, although mainly from intrinsic thalamic nuclei. It is therefore most probable, that the neuronal responses to auditory stimuli in association areas are not just a further filter stage behind the primary auditory cortex, but that they receive their own input and thus represent other aspects of the auditory signals as presented to them from their respective thalamic input (Creutzfeldt, 1977).

We are thus faced with the problem, that the brain has not only to deal with temporo-spatial integration across transient responses in the primary cortical area, but also across the different cortical areas, each representing possibly different transformations of the original peripheral neurogram, but each of them indisposable for the recognition of the signal. We are still far from understanding this integration capacity of the brain.

All we know about recognition and understanding is that the signal leads to a certain response of the subject. That means, that the sensory input leads to a related motor response. And only through this motor response we are able to judge whether the message has been understood or not. In the case of inter-individual communication this motor response maybe another signal. Are we justified, at this stage, to conclude that understanding and cognition means translation of the sensory input into the appropriate response, i.e. motor output? If this is so, than the motor and sensory sides of language and aphasia should be intricately linked with each other, as some presentations at this meeting indeed indicate. And if this is so, than the neurophysiologist should not expect to find the call detector or word detector neuron at some interim level between sensory input and motor output. As little as he might expect the specific command neuron for a call or a word. As much as any motor action including phonation and speech is dependant on the coordinated activation and inhibition of large neuronal assemblies across many cortical areas and subcortical structures, sensory signals may not be represented by single neuron sets at the receiving end of the brain, but by equally large assemblies, largely overlapping or even to some extent identical with the motor sets (Creutzfeldt, 1979). It is interesting to note, in this context, that a systematic analysis even of the phonetic aspects of the speech code may lead to the conclusion that the decoding mechanism identifies phonemes by referring them to motor command systems that produce such phonemes (Liberman et al., 1967). One may generalize here and consider language understanding and production as two aspects of the same phenomenon as they appear by looking at it from two different ends: the comprehension of language could then be the ability to transform the auditory input into a homologous linguistic output or, rather, to match the input with the available motor production mechanism that would be able to produce such outputs. More general, we can understand only what we can also reproduce.

But what are the physical properties of acoustic signals that match such output structures, and what are the minimal requirements for identification of a phoneme, a word or a sentence in terms of such a language production system? It appears, that both, spectral properties as well as the temporal sequence of sound segments and their relation to each other are important variables. Important progress might be expected, if the psycho-acoustic analysis of language could gear its approaches still further to neurophysiological mechanisms of encoding of auditory signals, and if neurophysiology would take more advantage of the progress of physical acoustics in dissecting the acoustical complexity into clearly defined phonemic elements and use them as probes for investigating neuronal codes for the internal representation of the complex auditory signals which constitute language.

I tried to communicate to you some of the thoughts which guided us in compiling this program. We are grateful, that you have all accepted this invitation of EBBS. Our intention was to bring together neurophysiologists, neurologists, psychologists and physicists, that is scientists whose activities center on the same problem, but which may not know of each other because the problem is so big that it obscures the view across to those, who approach it from the other side.

References:

1) Chomsky, N.: Aspects of the theory of syntax. The MIT Press, Cambridge, Mass. (1965).
2) Creutzfeldt, O.: Some problems of cortical organization in the light of ideas of the classical "Hirnpathologie" and of modern neurophysiology. An essay. In: Zülch, K.J.; O. Creutzfeldt and G.C. Galbraith (eds.): Cerebral localization. Springer Verlag, Berlin etc., 217-226 (1975).
3) Creutzfeldt, O.: The brain as a functional unity. In: M.A. Corner and D.F. Swaab (eds.): Perspectives in Brain Research. Progr. in Brain Res. 45, 451-462 (1976).

4) Creutzfeldt, O.: Generality of the functional structure of the neocortex. Naturwissensch. 64, 507-517 (1977).
5) Creutzfeldt, O.D.: Neurophysiological mechanisms and consciousness. Procl. of the Ciba-Symposion, in press (1979).
6) Creutzfeldt, O.; Hellweg, F.-C. and Schreiner, Chr.: Thalamo-cortical transformation of response to complex auditory stimuli. Exp. Brain Res., in press (1979).
7)Herder, J.G. von: Abhandlung über den Ursprung der Sprache. (1772).
8) Humboldt, W.v.: Über die Verschiedenheit des menschlichen Sprachbaus. Berlin (1836).
9) Kiang, N.Y.S.; Eddington, D.K. and Delgutte, B.: Fundamental considerations in designing auditory implants. Acta Otolaryngol. 87, 204-218 (1979).
10) Liberman, A.M.; Cooper, F.S.; Shankweiler, D.P.; Studdert-Kennedy, M.: Perception of the speech code. Psychological Review 74,6, 431-448 (1967).

Acknowledgements

After completetion of the meeting and of this volume, I should like to express my thanks to Prof. Henning Scheich and to Dr. Christoph Schreiner, with whom the scientific scope and the organization of this workshop were prepared.
The program was discussed also with Profs. K. Poeck, E. Perret and D. Ploog.

We express our sincere thanks to Mrs. Bärbel Bartsch, in whose hands the organization of the meeting and the publication of its proceedings in this volume have run as smoothly as the participants have experienced it and, as we hope, the reader of these proceedings will recognize.
We gratefully acknowledge the generous financial support from the Deutsche Forschungsgemeinschaft (DFG), the Max-Planck-Gesellschaft (MPG) and the Minister for Art and Sciences of the State of Niedersachsen.

I) Functional and Structural Conditions for Transmission of Auditory Signals in the Nervous System

Basic Mechanisms of Auditory Processing in the Cochlea

R. KLINKE, Zentrum der Physiologie, J. W. Goethe Universität,
D-6000 Frankfurt, Germany

For a meeting concerned with hearing mechanisms and speech it seems adequate to concentrate upon the neuronal message sent from the cochlea to the central nervous system. This seems particularly justified as an additional paper will deal with cochlear mechanisms (de Boer, this volume).
Any acoustic information available to the organism has to pass through the cochlea. It seems as if the signal is merely processed by a band of hundreds of parallel filters and that no particular feature extraction is performed at the level of the auditory nerve. It is assumed that data obtained from mammals (generally cats and guinea pigs) is applicable to humans.

The mammalian auditory nerve consists of some 30000 to 50000 afferent nerve fibres, 90 - 95% of which are radial fibres contacting the inner hair cells (Spoendlin, 1972). The remaining 5 - 10% are spiral fibres contacting the outer hair cells. Although much is known about the physiological properties of primary auditory fibres, they cannot yet be separated into two fibre populations corresponding to the radial and spiral fibres. This led Spoendlin (1979) even to the assumption that the central terminations of the spiral fibres do not transfer information to the central nervous system. Also many models of interactions between radial and spiral fibres or inner and outer hair cells respectively have been proposed, again they do not seem very probable. For review see Klinke (1978).

An exception to the previous statement that two fibre populations cannot be physiologically differentiated in the auditory nerve is found when spontaneous activity is considered. All afferents possess spontaneous activity between 1 and 120 spikes/s. Only occasionally are non-spontaneously active units found (Liberman, 1978). The spontaneous activity is bimodally distributed. About 20% of the fibres possess a rate below 20 imp/s. (Liberman, 1978; Kim and Molnar, 1979). It is unclear, whether or not low spontaneous activity is correlated with spiral fibres.

Each fibre responds best to a certain frequency, the characteristic frequency (CF) of the fibre (Kiang, 1965; see Evans, 1975 for review). This feature is illustrated in fig. 1. The orderly tonotopic arrangement of the fibres corresponds to the

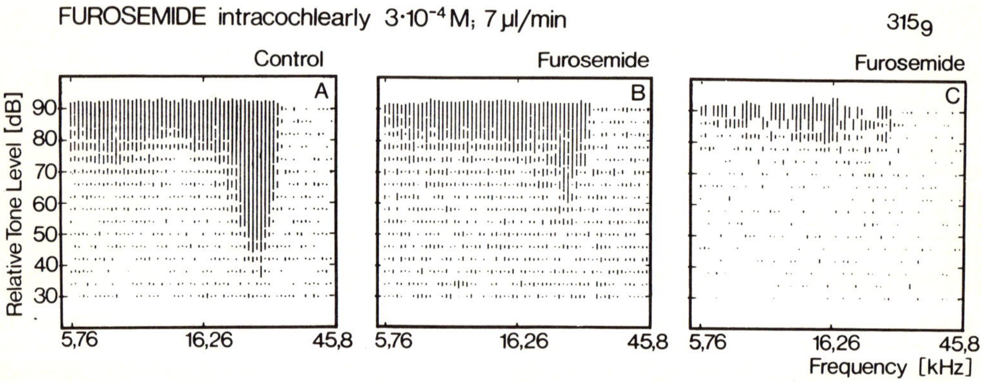

Fig. 1. Tuning curves of a cat primary afferent before (A) and after an intracochlear (B,C) instillation of Furosemide ($3 \cdot 10^{-4}$M at 7μl/min) into the scala tympani. Time between A and C about 14 min. At the end (see C) the unit was not responsive to its former CF. (Evans and Klinke, to be published)

place principle realized within the cochlea. Fibres of the same CF may possess different thresholds however, the possible spread amounting up to 50 dB. This spread is mainly brought about by fibres of low spontaneous activity whereas the thresholds of fibres with high spontaneous rate differ by only 5 dB (Kiang et al., 1976; Liberman, 1978). With high stimulus intensities the best excitatory frequencies of the fibres shift downwards with fibres of CF higher than 1 kHz and upwards below 1 kHz (Rose et al, 1971).

Frequency threshold curves (tuning curves) of the fibres show sharp tuning (slopes of up to 600 dB/oct. are possible). They also reveal that fibres of high CF additionally respond readily to low frequencies of sufficient intensity (so called low frequency tail, see fig. 1). This response is mainly caused by the low pass characteristics of the middle ear. The effective bandwidth of afferent fibres from the cat (Evans and Wilson, 1973) corresponds to the psychoacoustically determined critical bandwidth in man (Zwicker and Feldtkeller, 1967).
The high sensitivity and the frequency selectivity of the afferents are severely impaired by ototoxic drugs (Kiang et al., 1970; Evans and Klinke, 1974; Kiang et al., 1976; Dallos et al., 1977; Harrison and Evans, 1977; Klinke and Evans, 1977; Romahn and Boerger, 1977), disturbance of cochlear energy supply (Evans, 1974; Evans and Klinke, 1974; Robertson and Manley, 1974) or noise trauma (Kiang et al., 1976; Liberman and Kiang, 1978). An example is given in fig. 1, where Furosemide, an ototoxic diurectic was applied intracochlearly into the scala tympani. Common to most noxious influences upon the cochlea is

a threshold elevation and reduction of frequency selectivity of the fibre accompanied by an increase of its effective bandwidth (Evans and Klinke, to be published). These findings may be the basis of the reduced speech discrimination in patients with sensorineural hearing loss that cannot be compensated for by amplification of the acoustic signal. Recruitment can also be explained by these results.

The damage occurs prior to the auditory nerve fibres, as intoxication with tetrodotoxin (TTX) reduces afferent activity but leaves the shape of the tuning curve unaltered (Evans and Klinke, to be published). This is illustrated in fig. 2. TTX 10^{-6}M was applied intracochlearly (scala tympani) during recording of a high spontaneous unit. The responses of the unit prior to TTX are given in the left frame. Substraction of the mean spontaneous rate (3 spikes per stimulus interval) makes

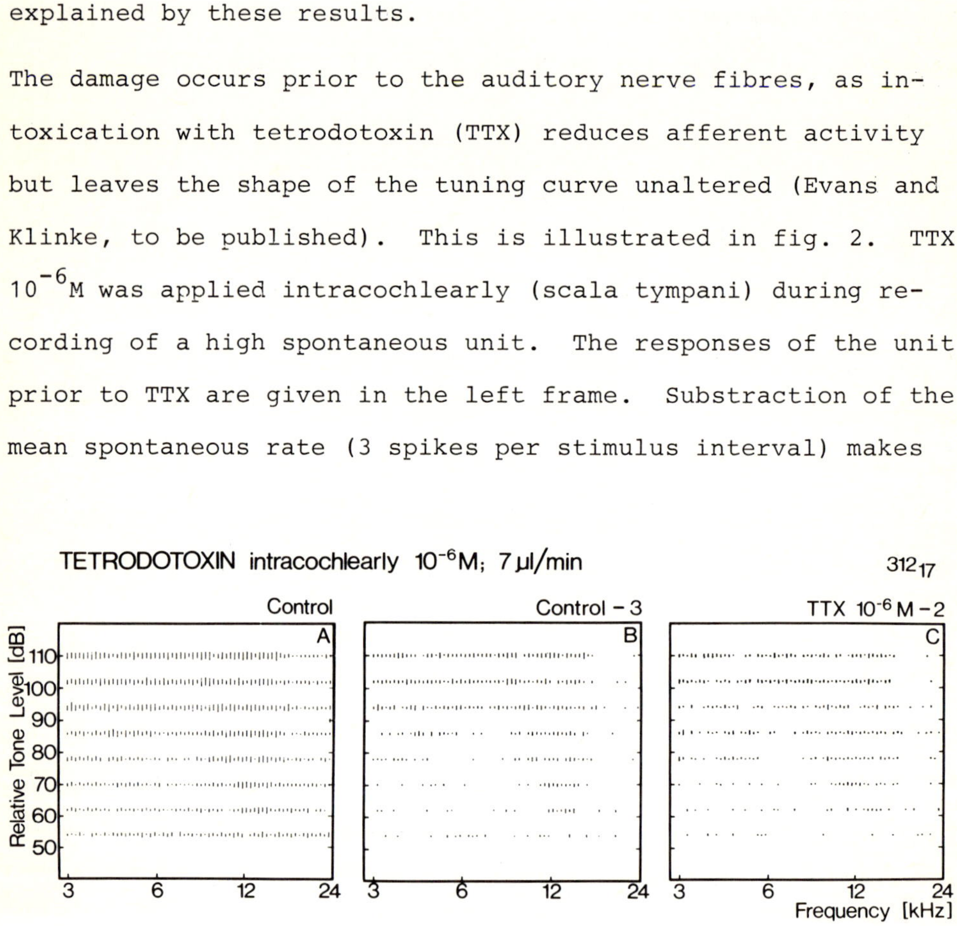

Fig. 2. Effect of tetrodotoxin 10^{-6}M intracochlearly upon the activity pattern of a cat primary auditory fibre. Because of high spontaneous activity (in the average 3 within a 60ms stimulus interval) the tuning curve is more prominent in frame B where the spontaneous rate has been substracted. In C the mean activity has been reduced after application of TTX but the tuning curve is not altered (Evans and Klinke, to be published) See text.

the tuning curve more evident. After TTX the activity is reduced. Substraction of the reduced spontaneous activity (2 spikes per stimulus interval) shows that the tuning properties have not changed by TTX. In other TTX experiments with low spontaneous units it could be shown that responses to tones in the tip region of the tuning curve were present until the very last seconds before the unit ceased discharging because of TTX poisoning. By this time spontaneous activity had virtually stopped.

As TTX blocks the quick sodium channels necessary for spike production this additionally seems to show that the sharpness of tuning cannot be brought about by a neuronal interaction between spiral and radial fibres at least as far as action potentials are involved in this interaction. Intracellular recordings from inner hair cells (Russell and Sellick, 1978) have shown that these cells are already sharply tuned, i.e. the filter characteristics of the cochlea are already present in the sensory cell.

The dynamic range of the human auditory system exceeds 120 dB. This probably also holds for other mammals. Neurophysiological data fail to explain this range. The dynamic range of a single fibre is in the order of 20-30 dB (Sachs and Abbas, 1976; Evans, 1975, 1978) for most fibres. In a caiman, a crocodile, which has an avian like cochlea, nonmonotonic intensity functions have also been found (Klinke and Pause, 1979). In some fibres in which the slope of the intensity function becomes less after the initial 20-30 dB the dynamic range is up to 40-60 dB (Sachs and Abbas, 1974), but these seem to be only a few fibres. So single primary afferents do not appear to cover the dynamic range of the auditory system. Of course there is a second possibility of intensity coding: The number of active fibres depends on stimulus intensity. Particularly fibres of high CF are affected. This follows from the shape of the tuning curve.

Therefore the number of active fibres might be used to code the intensity in these cells. Experimental results have failed, however, to support this view (Evans and Palmer, 1975), but nevertheless, these authors found cells in the dorsal cochlear nucleus that have a dynamic range of up to 110 dB under certain specific stimulus conditions. Also the primary fibres with exceptionally high threshold might feed into these cells. Yet it may be that intensity coding has to make use of a third unknown mechanism (Evans, 1978), based for example on phase-locked discharges. Phase-locking of spikes occurs for frequencies up to about 4 kHz (see Evans, 1975, for review). This means that during stimulation the probability of firing is maximal at certain phases of the stimulus. The phenomenon of phase-locking is a straightforward consequence of the assumption that a shearing movement of the cilia in one direction is the adequate stimulus for cochlear hair cells as it is in other hair cell receptors (Flock, 1971). It has long bee debated whether or not the organism may extract information from the time structure in the discharge pattern thus generated. (Place - versus periodicity - pitch, e.g., Whitfield, 1970). It was not until recently that with cochlear implants the existence of both place pitch and periodicity pitch could be directly demonstrated (Eddington et al., 1978a,b). These authors were able to show that multielectrode electrical stimulation of the cochlea leads to pitch sensations that are clearly related to the place of stimulation. The repetition rate of the stimulus, however, was important as well. For a certain place of stimulation the perceived pitch was higher with higher repetition rate of the electrical stimulus. The patient also reported that place could be traded against periodicity: If an electrode located at an apical place in the cochlea was stimulated with high repetition rate a similar pitch was percieved as if a more basal electrode was stimulated with a low repetition rate. This seems to indicate that both, place and periodicity pitch do exist independently from each other and that a central pitch processor exists that can trade place and periodicity.

Phase-locked discharges have been used to compute traveltime functions of the basilar membrane motion (Greenwood, 1977; Kim and Molnar, 1979a,b): There is no doubt about the existence of a travelling wave in the mammalian cochlea. There are doubts, however, whether the travelling wave is the only important mechanism of tuning. Initially the "second filter" concept was developed (Evans and Wilson, 1973). More recently it was found that tuning is temperature dependant in cold-blooded animals (Moffat and Capranica, 1976; Eatock and Manley, 1976; Smolders and Klinke, 1977). The shift of CF is downwards for about a third of an octave with a downward shift of 5°C. In mammals, however, hardly any influence of temperature can be seen (Smolder and Klinke, 1977; Emde and Klinke, 1977). One has to consider therefore that tuning may depend essentially on a different mechanism in cold-blooded animals (see Klinke,1978).

It is commonly accepted that the latency of the first peak in a click-evoked post stimulus time histogram (see later) correlates with the CF of the unit.
This is taken as indication of the travelling time along the cochlea. Is is interesting to note, however, that the respective latencies in caiman primary afferents are only slightly smaller (see fig. 3) or, in the low frequency range, identical to the mammalian values. The caiman papilla basilaris has a length of only 4 mm, and the spread of CFs is from 30 Hz to 2.8 kHz. Therefore the velocity of the travelling wave would have to be either considerably lower or the latencies of the first peak do merely reflect the response time of the auditory filters.

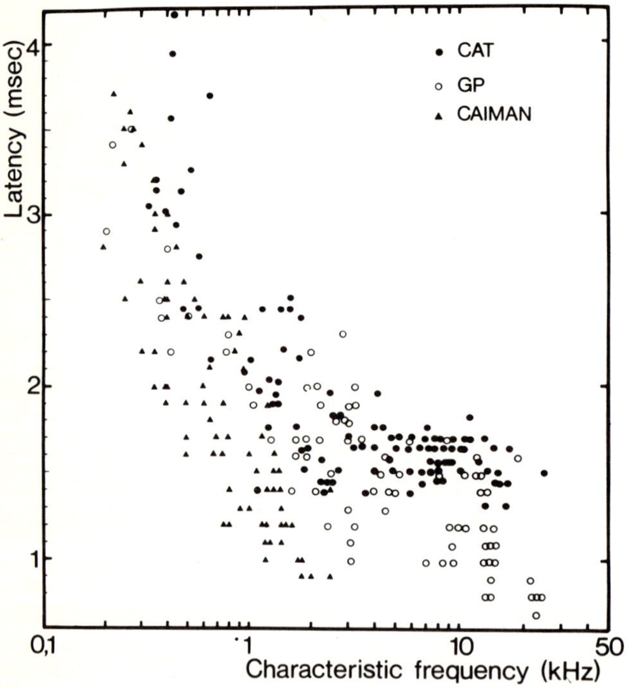

Fig. 3. Comparison of latencies of first peak in click PSTH in cat, guinea pig (GP) and caiman. Caiman data from Klinke and Pause (1979), mammalian data after Evans (1975).

Adaptation is another important feature of primary afferents. Although adaptation is very common in sensory systems, in the auditory system it has to be considered as an important factor in stimulus coding and decoding, particularly for speech sounds. It may be that transients are thus emphasized in the afferent discharge pattern.

Neuronal responses to multicomponent or broadband stimuli to a first approximation behave as predicted from linear filter characteristics of the afferent fibres. For example click stimuli, ideally having a uniform power spectrum over the interesting range, elicite some sort of ringing, multiple peaks in the post stimulus time histogram (Klinke et al, 1965), the interpeak distance being 1/CF. In the caiman the number of peaks is correlated with the sharpness of tuning (Klinke and Pause, 1979). This finding, although to be expected, has apparently not been reported yet from a mammal.

Similar to click stimuli any sharp transients as for example switching on or off of tone will produce widely distributed spectral components and therefore cause "ringing" in the afferent nerve fibres.

Discharge patterns following stimuli containing several spectral components in the range of the tuning curve contain responses to the individual components, as also to be expected from linear filters. This was shown by analysis of phase-locked responses (e.g. Rose et al., 1967; Brugge et al., 1969). Also reverse correlation techniques (de Boer and Kuyper, 1968) prove strong linear components in the cochlear information processing. There are, however, nonlinear components. These lead to phenomena like two tone suppression (Sachs and Kiang, 1968; Javel et al., 1978) and excitability by combination tones (Smoorenburg, 1972; Kim and Molnar, 1979b; see Evans, 1975).

Presentation of speech sounds means stimulation with multicomponent stimuli. Unfortunately there are only a few investigations of neuronal responses to speech sounds (Kiang and Moxon, 1972; Hashimoto et al., 1975; Sachs and Young, 1978; Kiang et al., 1979). These investigations mainly show that responses to speech sounds behave as to be expected. The fibres are activated if there is sound energy within the area of the tuning curve. Particularly fibres with high CF are activated by low and medium frequency components due to the low frequency tail. The fibres are easily saturated if there is energy in the CF region of the fibres. Responses are phase-locked to the different frequency components of the stimulus. This is of particular interest for the pitch frequency of a voiced sound. If the fibres are saturated for example by formant frequencies near their CF no fluctuations corresponding to the voice frequency can be detected in the neuronal pattern. The fibres do ring if sharp transients occur and two tone suppression can also be seen in responses to speech sounds.

It is yet unclear which of the features described are really of importance for speech processing. As speech is not easily masked by high-pass noise it may well be that excitation of the low frequency tail of high CF units by speech is not terribly important. In patients with hearing loss in high frequencies speech discrimination is poorer, however, with high intensities. It would be most useful to know the essential auditory nerve parameters necessary for speech intelligibility. In particular for the design of stimulus patterns for a cochlear prosthesis only necessary information should be fed into the electrode array (see Klinke and Hartmann, 1979). It certainly will be necessary to find the optimal code as the possibilities of a cochlear prosthesis will be limited anyhow. Any prosthesis conceivable will stimulate groups of nerve fibres rather than single fibres and stimulation will be performed in a deterministic rather than the natural probabilistic way. The number of channels will be limited whatever the final figure will be.

In this context it seems interesting to know what the information capacity of an auditory prosthesis might be, and whether this capacity might be sufficient for speech transmission. Such an estimate has to be based on psychoacoustic data. For the intact auditory system the capacity is in the order of 30000 - 40000 bit/s. This figure can be gained by the assumption that pitch and loudness are independent (which is not entirely correct), that there are 1000 different pitches perceivable, that, depending on frequency, 50 - 200 different intensity steps can be differentiated, that 25ms are sufficient to analyse one situation and that the probability of each combination is equal. Fack (1956) gives similar estimates using a more accurate measure. For comparison, in PCM transmission music transferred with 16 kHz bandwidth and 7 bit quantization needs 150000 bit/s. A speech channel, 3 kHz bandwidth, 6 bit quantization would acquire 36000 bit/s.

Assuming the above capacity of the auditory system the average capacity of one afferent nerve fibre would amount to about

1 bit/s. It is evident, that the capacity of a single fibre per se must be considerably higher, even if there is still controversy about the capacity of nerve fibres (see Eckhorn and Pöpel, 1974). Redundancy in the auditory system is high. As far as speech is concerned it seems that only some 1500 bit/s are the necessary minimum to produce intelligible speech, as can be concluded from vocoder techniques (Flanagan, 1972). This is still considerably more than the written equivalent (about 50 bit/s) but the important process of pattern recognition has not taken place yet in spoken language in contrast to the written equivalent. The question therefore is whether 1500 bit/s can be transferred through a prosthetic device.

If it is assumed that prosthetic channels should each cover a critical bandwidth then 15 parallel channels would be necessary in the speech region (250 Hz to 3.5 kHz). Introduced into the human cochlea this would mean that one channel would cover 1.2 mm of cochlear length (see Klinke and Hartmann, 1979, for detailled discussion). For the calculation the channels have to be independent. From cat data (Merzenich and White, 1977) on current spread in the cochlea it follows that only near threshold stimuli will not spread to neighbouring channels of 1.2 mm length. To maintain independency of the electrode channels for the purposes of this estimuate no variation of current strength will therefore be allowed and intensity should only be coded as increase of stimulation rate. To avoid periodicity pitch the stimuli should be delivered stochastically, so pure place pitch should result and the channels would also be independent in the pitch dimension.

Accepting all these restrictions which are necessary, however, to maintain independence the capacity of a prosthetic device can be estimated. If the mean stimulation rate is allowed to very between 60 and 240/s (1:4; electric stimulation lower than 60/s does not lead to a continuous percept), the jnd is accepted to be in the order of 4% (this for example is about the jnd for pure periodicity pitch, see Evans, 1978), and it is assumed that 50 ms are required to analyze one condition (10 to 20 phonemes/s are uttered during average speech) a capacity of 1,500 bit/s would result. A jnd of 2% would result in about 1800 bit/s (for more details see Klinke and Hartmann, 1979).

This estimation, though perhaps rather conservative as not to violate independence and partially based on assumptions not yet experimentally veryfied shows that a prosthetic device just could be capable of allowing the necessary data transfer. Whether realization will be possible is quite a different question, however.

Acknowledgements: The author's investigations mentioned here were supported by the Deutsche Forschungsgemeinschaft (Kl 219).

References:

1) De Boer, E.; Kuyper, P.: Triggered correlation. IEEE Transactions on Bio-Medical Engineering BME-15, 169-179 (1968).
2) Brugge, J.F.; Anderson, D.J:; Hind, J.E.; Rose, J.E.: Time structure of discharges in single auditory nerve fibres of the squirrel monkey in response to complex periodic sounds. J. Neurophysiol. 32, 386-401 (1969).
3) Dallos, P.; Ryan, A.; Harris, D.; McGee, T.; Özdamar, Ö.: Cochlear frequency selectivity in the presence of hair cell damage. In: Psyhchophysics and Physiology of Hearing. E.F. Evans and J.P. Wilson (eds.), London-New York, San Francisco, Academic Press, 249-258 (1977).
4) Eatock, R.A.; Manley, G.A.: Temperature effects on single auditory nerve fiber responses. J.Acoust.Soc.Am. 60, Suppl. 1, 80 (1976).

5) Eckhorn, R.; Pöpel, B.: Rigorous and extended application of information theory to the afferent visual system of the cat. I. Basic concepts. Kybernetik 16, 191-200 (1974).
6) Eddington, D.K.; Dobelle, Wm.H.; Brackmann, D.E.; Mladejovsky, M.G.; Parkin, J.L.: Auditory prostheses research with multiple channel intracochlear stimulation in man. Ann.Otol.Rhinol. Laryngol. 87, Suppl. 53, 5-39 (1978b).
7) Eddington, E.K.; Dobelle, Wm.H.; Brackmann, D.E.; Mladejovsky, M.G.; Parkin, J.: Place and periodicity pitch by stimulation of multiple scale tympani electrodes in deaf volunteers. Trans. Am.Soc.Artif.Intern.Orangs 24, 1-5 (1978a).
8) Emde, C.; Klinke, R.: Does absolute pitch depend on an internal clock? In: M. Portmann and J.M. Aran (eds.), Inner ear biology 68, 145-146, INSERM, Paris (1977).
9) Evans, E.F.: The effects of hypoxia on the tuning of single cochlear nerve fibres. J.Physiol. 238, 65-67 P (1974).
10) Evans, F.: Cochlear Nerve and Cochlear Nucleus. In: Handbook of Sensory Physiology, Vol. V/2, W.D. Keidel and W.D. Neff (eds.) Springer-Verlag Berlin-Heidelberg-New York, 1-108 (1975).
11) Evans, E.F.: Place and Time Coding of Frequency in the Peripheral Auditory System: Some Physiological Pros and Cons. Audiology 17, 369-420 (1978).
12) Evans, E.F.; Klinke, R.: Reversible effects of cyanide and furosemide on the tuning of single cochlear nerve fibres. J. Physiol. 242, 129P-130P (1974).
13) Evans, E.F.; Palmer, A.R.: Responses of units in the cochlear nerve and nucleus of the cat to signals in the presence of bandstop noise. J.Physiol., London 252, 60-62 P (1975).
14) Evans, E.F.; Wilson, J.P.: The frequency selectivity of the cochlea. In: Basic mechanisms of hearing, A.R. Møller (ed.) Acad. Press, N.Y., 519-551 (1973).
15) Fack, H.: Informationstheoretische Behandlung des Gehörs. In: Winckel, F. (Hrg.), Impulstechnik, Berlin, Spriner, 289-338 (1956).
16) Flanagan, J.L.: Speech analysis synthesis and perception. Springer Verlag, Berlin-Heidelberg-New York (1972).
17) Flock, A.: Sensory transduction in hair cells. In: Handbook of sensory physiology, V. I, Loewenstein, W.R. (ed.), Springer-Verlag, Berlin-Heidelberg-New York, 396-441 (1971).
18) Greenwood, D.D.: Empirical travel time functions on the basilar membrane. In: Psychophysics and Physiology of Hearing, E.F. Evans and J.P. Wilson (eds.) London-New York-San Francisco Academic Press, 43-55 (1977).
19) Harrison, R.V.; Evans, E.F.: The effects of hair cell loss (restricted to outer hair cells) on the threshold and tuning properties of cochlear fibres in the guinea pig. In: Inner Ear Biology, M. Portmann and J.M. Aran (eds.), INSERM, Paris, 68, 105-124 (1977).
20) Hashimoto, T.; Katayama, Y.; Murata, K.; Taniguchi, I.: Pitch-synchronous response of cat cochlear nerve fibers to speech sounds. Jap.J.Physiol. 25, 633-644 (1975).
21) Javel, E.; Geisler, C.D.; Ravindran, A.: Two-tone suppression in auditory nerve of the cat: Rate-intensity and temporal analyses. J.Acoust.Soc.Am. 63, 1093-1104 (1978).
22) Kiang, N.Y.S.; Eddington, D.K.; Delgutte, B.: Fundamental

considerations in designing auditory implants. Acta otolaryng. 87, 204-218 (1979).
23) Kiang, N.Y.S.; Liberman, M.Ch.; Levine, R.A.: Auditory-nerve activity in cats exposed to ototoxic drugs and high-intensity sounds. Annals of Otology, Rhinology and Laryngology 85, 752-769 (1976).
24) Kiang, N.Y.S., Moxon, E.C.: Physiological considerations in artificial stimulation of the inner ear. Ann.Otol. 81, 714-730 (1972).
25) Kiang, N.Y.S.; Moxon, E.C.: Tails of tuning curves of auditory-nerve fibers. J.Acoust.Soc.Am. 55, 620-630 (1974).
26) Kiang, N.Y.S.; Moxon, E.C.; Levine, R.A.: Auditory-nerve activity in cats with normal and abnormal cochleas. Sensori-neural Hearing Loss, G.E.W. Wolstenholme and Julie Knight (eds.) J. & A. Churchhill, London, 241-273 (1970).
27) Kiang, N.Y.S.; Watanabe, T.; Thomas, E.C.; Clark, L.F.: Discharge patterns of single fibers in the cat's auditory nerve. Research Monograph No. 35, M.I.T. Press, Cambridge, Mass., 1-154 (1965).
28) Kim, D.O.; Molnar, C.E.: A population study of cochlear nerve fibers: comparison of the spatial distributions of average-rate and phase-locking measures of responses to single tones. J.Neurophysiol. (1979, in press).
29) Kim, D.O.; Molnar, C.E.: Studies of cochlear nonlinearity. Workshop on models of the auditory system and related signal processing techniques, Münster (1979b, in press).
30) Klinke, R.: Frequency analysis in the inner ear of mammals in comparison to other vertebrates. Verh.Dtsch.Zool.Ges. 1978, Fischer, Stuttgart, 1-15 (1978).
31) Klinke, R.; Evans, E.F.: Evidence that Catecholamines are not the afferent transmitter in the cochlea. Exp.Brain Res. 28, 315-324 (1977).
32) Klinke, R., Hartmann, R.: Physiologische Grundlagen einer Hörprothese. Arch.Otolaryngol. 223, 77-137 (1979).
33) Klinke, R.; Pause, M.: Primary and auditory fibres in a crocodile (caiman crocodilus): Discharge properties and comparison to the mammalian auditory nerve. Submitted for publication (1979).
34) Liberman, M.Ch.: Auditory-nerve response from cats raised in a low-noise chamber. J.Acoust.Soc.Am. 63, 442-455 (1978).
35) Liberman, M.Chr.; Kiang, N.Y.S.: Acoustic trauma in cats (Cochlear Pathology and Auditory-nerve activity). Acta Otolaryngol., Suppl. 358, 1-63 (1978).
36) Merzenich, M.M.; White, M.W.: Cochlear implant. The interface problem. Biomedical Engineering and Instrumentation: Functional Electrical Stimulation 3, F.T. Hambrecht and J.B. Reswick (eds.) Dekker Inc., New York, 321-340 (1977).
37) Moffat, A.J.M.; Capranica, R.R.: Effects of temperature on the response properties of auditory nerve fibers in the american toad (Bufo americanus). J.Acoust.Soc.Am. 60, 80 (1976).
38) Robertson, D.; Manley, G.A.: Manipulation of frequency analysis in the cochlear ganglion of the guinea pig. J.comp. Physiol. 91, 363-375 (1974).
39) Romahn, G.; Boerger, G.: Filter function of the guinea pig cochlea after degeneration of outer hari cells. Arch. Oto-Rhino-Laryng. 215, 223-229 (1977).

40) Rose, J.E.; Hind, J.E.; Anderson, D.J.; Brugge, F.J.: Some effects of stimulus intensity on response of auditory nerve fibers in the squirrel monkey. J.Neurophysiol. 34, 685-699 (1971).
41) Russell, I.J.; Sellick, P.M.: Intracellular studies of hair cells in the mammalian cochlea. J.Physiol. 284, 261-290 (1978).
42) Sachs, M.B.; Abbas, P.J.: Rate versus level functions for auditory-nerve fibers in cats: tone-burst stimuli. J.Acoust. Soc.Am. 56, 1835-1847 (1974).
43) Sachs,M.B.; Kiang, N.Y.S.: Two-tone inhibition in auditory-nerve fibers. J.Acoust.Soc.Am. 43, 1120-1128 (1968).
44) Sachs, M.B.; Young, E.D.: Patterns of auditory-nerve fiber responses to steady-state wovels. J.Acoust.Soc.Am. 63, Suppl. No.1, S76 (1978).
45) Smolders, J.; Klinke, R.: Effect of temperature changes on tuning properties of primary auditory fibres in caiman and cat. In: Inner Ear Biology, M. Portmann and J.M. Aran (eds.), INSERM Paris, 68, 125-126 (1977).
46) Smoorenburg, G.G.: Combination tones and their origin. J. Acoust.Soc.Am. 52, 615-632 (1972).
47) Spoendlin, H.: Innervation densities of the cochlea. Acta Oto-Laryng. 73, 235-248 (1972).
48) Spoendlin, H.: Anatomisch-pathologische Aspekte der Elektrostimulation des ertaubten Innenohres. Arch. Otolaryngol. 223, 1-76 (1979).
49) Whitfield, I.C.: Central nervous processing in relation to spatio-temporal discrimination of auditory patterns. In: Frequency analysis and periodicity detection in hearing. R. Plomp; G.F. Smoorenburg (eds.) A.W. Sijthoff, Leiden, 136-152 (1970).
50) Zwicker, E.; Feldtkeller, R.: Das Ohr als Nachrichtenempfänger. S. Hirzel Verlag, Stuttgart (1967) 2. Auflage.

On the Peripheral Coding of the Level of Individual Frequency Components of Complex Sounds at High Sound Levels

A. R. PALMER, E. F. EVANS, Department of Communication and Neuroscience, University of Keele, Staffordshire ST5 5BG, England

'Place' theories, for the neural analysis of multi-component acoustic signals like speech, face a severe problem at high signal levels. The wide psychophysical dynamic range over which these signals are discriminated (e.g. Fletcher 1953, Fig. 239) contrasts with the restricted distribution of the thresholds of the majority of individual cochlear fibres (e.g. Kiang 1968, Evans 1972) and of their dynamic ranges, in terms of discharge rate (e.g. Galambos & Davis 1943, Kiang et al. 1965).

In order to deal with this problem, 'population' theories have been proposed, in which the frequency and intensity of single components are respectively signalled by the position and extent of activation across a neuronal array (e.g. Allanson & Whitfield 1955). However, these theories do not appear to be tenable at high levels in the speech context, where it is necessary to keep separate the information corresponding to *multiple closely spaced* components (see Evans 1978 for review). In any case, the dynamic range for intensity discrimination of a narrow band signal can be maintained in spite of simultaneous low and high pass (bandstop) masking (Viemeister 1974, Moore & Raab 1975), suggesting that information concerning the level of individual frequency components can be signalled by fibres of the appropriate characteristic frequency (CF) without the need for spread of activity to fibres of other CF.

We have in fact demonstrated, using two different experimental paradigms that, in the dorsal cochlear nucleus (DCN), a substantial proportion of cells are able to signal differences in the level of individual frequency components over a very wide dynamic range, at the appropriate "place". Evans and Palmer (1975) demonstrated that, *under bandstop noise masking conditions analogous to the psychophysical studies mentioned above* a substantial proportion of DCN neurones had dynamic ranges of up to 110dB. Evans (1977) showed that these DCN neurones were also capable of resolving the peaks and valleys in a comb-filtered noise signal over a similarly wide intensity range. However, neither of these studies were able to demonstrate responses over adequately wide dynamic ranges under similar conditions in the cochlear nerve, a finding confirmed by the study of Narins and Evans (1978).

The present experiments explore one possible means by which cochlear fibres might signal the level of individual components over an adequately wide dynamic range. Some authors (e.g. Nomoto, Suga and Katsuki 1964, Sachs and Abbas 1974) have reported cochlear fibres having dynamic ranges extending well beyond the range of the majority (20-60dB). The question is, how frequently are they found, and to what extent could they account for the coding of intensity differences at high stimulus levels?

Methods:

Recordings were made from as many single fibres as possible in the cochlear nerve of pentobarbitone anaesthetised cats using conventional methods (e.g. Evans 1972, Evans & Nelson 1973). Stimuli were presented in a closed system (bulla and septum intact but vented to atmosphere) and their intensities were corrected to dB SPL by means of a calibrated probe tube microphone at the tympanic membrane. A round window electrode enabled audio-visual thresholds of the compound action potential (CAP) in response to 4ms (2ms rise/fall) tone pips to be measured at different frequencies. The 'CAP audiogram' so obtained is a good predictor of single fibre thresholds and therefore of the state of the cochlea and was monitored periodically for signs of cochlear deterioration. Blood pressure and end-tidal CO_2 were monitored continuously and steps were taken to maintain these within normal limits for the several days duration of each experiment. Care was also taken to avoid over-stimulation in order to ensure stability of thresholds over the course of days. With these several precautions, the thresholds did not deteriorate by more than 8dB in any animal during the recording of the data presented, as judged by the CAP audiogram; in the case of the data of Fig. 1 no deterioration was detected.

Discharge rate versus intensity functions were obtained by using a computer to vary the level, over a 120dB range, of a 100ms tone (5ms rise/fall) presented at 3 per second at the CF of each fibre. The computer varied the level in a pseudo-random sequence with a resolution of 2dB and counted and stored the number of spikes elicited by each stimulus presentation. In cases of less than optimal stability, a resolution of 4dB was sometimes used.

For each fibre, the signal levels between which the discharge rate diverged significantly from spontaneous rate and from saturation rate were determined with the aid of plots of: the mean response and standard error; a mean response smoothed with a Hamming window of 16dB; and a plot of the probability that the slope of the linear regression through the data points in each 16dB interval differed from zero.

Results and Discussion:

Rate versus intensity functions were measured at CF for 333 fibres in six animals. Over 100 of these were obtained in a *single cochlear nerve*, and these data are representative of the total sample. The dynamic ranges in response to CF tones, of 121 cochlear fibres from this animal, are illustrated in Fig.1. For each fibre, the dynamic range is plotted as a vertical bar at the CF: each bar extends from the just subthreshold point in spontaneous activity up to the first level at which the discharge had saturated.

Irrespective of their threshold, the vast majority of the fibres in this nerve were completey saturated at a level of 80dB SPL. Those fibres which were not saturated at this level either had CFs located on the high or low frequency 'cut-offs' of the animal's audiogram or had relatively high thresholds and very wide dynamic ranges. Indeed as the arrowheads in Fig. 1 indicate, some fibres were not completely saturated at

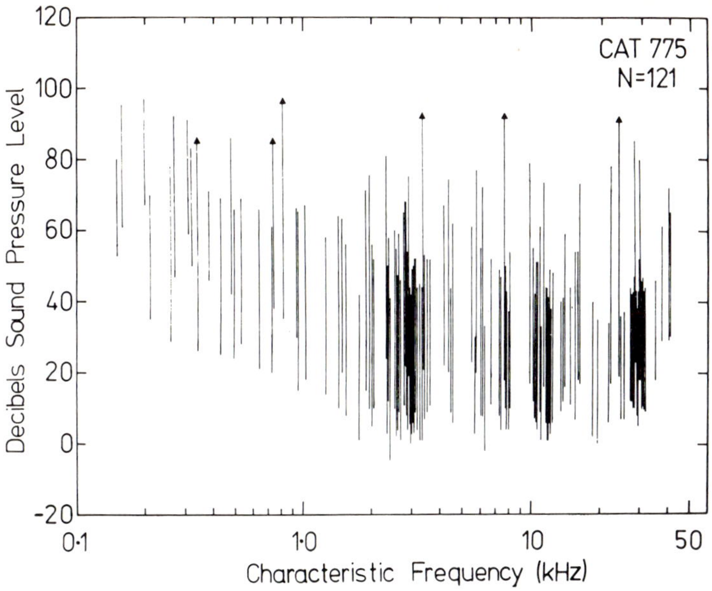

Fig. 1. The vertical bars represent the mean rate dynamic ranges, in response to a CF tone, of 121 individual fibres from one cochlear nerve plotted at their CF. The arrowheads indicate fibres which had not completely saturated at the highest levels presented, as in Fig. 2

the maximum stimulus level presented; their dynamic ranges therefore exceed the value indicated. The data for these 6 fibres are illustrated in Fig. 2, in which the smoothed rate versus intensity functions are shown. This figure indicates that although the functions do not saturate, they nevertheless show a very marked decrease in slope at about 30dB above threshold, and this divides the functions into an initial segment with steep slope and a final segment with shallower slope (see later).

For the data shown in Fig. 1, the distribution of dynamic ranges is unimodal, having a mean of 43.9dB (S.D. 10.3dB). Only 9% of the fibres from this animal had dynamic ranges in excess of 60dB and only 3% had dynamic ranges in excess of 70dB. In these and the following computations, fibres which did not completely saturate at the highest stimulus level used are included: thus, a fibre not saturated at 70dB above threshold is included as having a 70dB dynamic range.

In our pooled data (N=333) from 6 cochlear nerves, the mean dynamic range is 44.2dB (S.D. 11.7dB); 10% of the total exceeded 60dB and 5% exceeded 70dB.

It is therefore evident that at high signal levels, e.g. above 60dB SPL, there are still present in the cochlear nerve, fibres which are capable of indicating by their mean discharge rate, differences in the level of individual components of complex stimuli at the appropriate "place". However, the usefulness of these fibres in signalling intensity information may be doubted on two grounds.

First, as already shown, the proportion of fibres with very wide dynamic ranges (say 60dB) is small, about 10%. Secondly, if we consider the situation at SPLs exceeding say, 60dB SPL (of the order of mid frequency critical band levels in moderately loud conversational speech) it is clear that all the fibres having dynamic ranges extending beyond this *level* show a substantial reduction in the slope of their rate versus intensity functions, as illustrated for some of them in Fig. 2. Thus, the degree to which they could signal changes in stimulus level will be substantially attenuated above 60dB SPL compared with the situation at lower levels. To try to quantify this, the initial and final slopes for the fibres of Fig. 1 having CFs between 1 and 35 kHz, (corresponding to the relatively

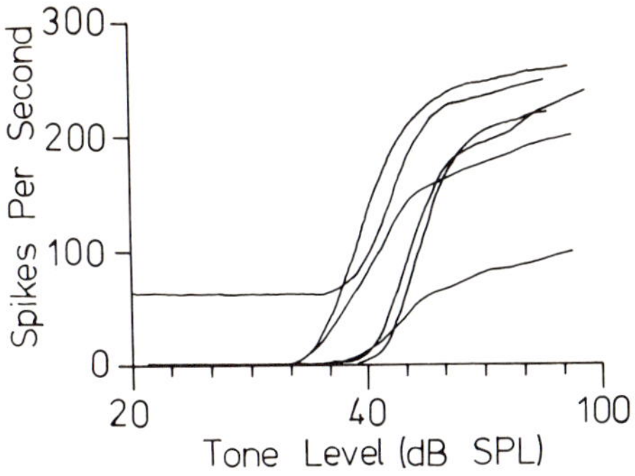

Fig. 2. Smoothed (Hamming window: 16dB) rate versus intensity functions corresponding to the six dynamic ranges marked with arrowheads in Figure 1

flat, low threshold region of the audiogram) were examined. 18 of these 99 fibres had rate functions with significant slopes extending above 60dB SPL (by a mean of 18dB). The mean slope of the final segment of these rate functions above 60dB SPL, was only 1.31 sp/sec/dB compared with a mean slope of 5.64 sp/sec/dB for their initial segments. There is no psychophysical evidence known to us for a deterioration in intensity difference limen corresponding to these levels in the bandstop noise masking situation. Furthermore, it is difficult to see how, at these levels the individual components of speech signals could be coded adequately by relatively few fibres with such attenuated responses.

References:

1) Allanson, J.T., Whitfield, I.C.: The cochlear nucleus and its relation to theories of hearing. In: Information theory 3rd London Symposium. London: Butterworths (1965).
2) Evans, E.F.: The frequency response and other properties of single fibres in the guinea pig cochlear nerve. J.Physiol. (Lond.) 226, 263-287 (1972).

3) Evans, E.F.: Frequency selectivity at high signal levels of single units in cochlear nerve and nucleus. In: Psychophysics and Physiology of Hearing. Academic Press eds. E.F. Evans & J.P. Wilson (1977).
4) Evans, E.F.: Place and time coding of frequency in the peripheral auditory system: some physiological pros and cons. Audiology 17, 5, 369-420 (1978).
5) Evans, E.F., Nelson, P.G.: The responses of single neurones in the cochlear nucleus of the cat as a function of their location and anaesthetic state. Exp. Brain Res. 17, 402-427 (1973).
6) Evans, E.F., Palmer, A.R.: Responses of units in the cochlear nerve and nucleus of the cat to signals in the presence of bandstop noise. J.Physiol. 252, 60-62P (1975).
7) Fletcher, H.: Speech and hearing in communication. Pp. 461. Princeton, New Jersey: Van Nostrand Co. (1953).
8) Galambos, R., Davis, H.: Responses of single auditory nerve fibres to acoustic stimulation. J.Neurophysiol. 6, 39-57 (1943).
9) Kiang, N.Y.-s: A survey of recent developments in the study of auditory physiology. Ann.Otol. (St. Louis) 77, 656-676 (1968).
10) Kiang, N.Y.-s, Watanabe, T., Thomas, E.C., Clark, L.F.: Discharge patterns of single fibres in the cat's auditory nerve. MIT Press, Cambridge, Mass. (1965).
11) Moore, B.C.J., Raab, D.H.: Intensity discrimination for noise bursts in the presence of a continuous, bandstop background: effects of level, width of bandstop and duration. J.Acoust.Soc.Amer. 57, 2, 400-405 (1975).
12) Narins, P.M., Evans, E.F.: The dynamic range of responses of single cochlear fibres in cat to individual spectral components of comb-filtered noise. J.Acoust.Soc.Amer. 64, Supp. 1, XX26 (1978).
13) Sachs, M.B., Abbas, P.: Rate versus level functions for auditory nerve fibres in cats: tone burst stimuli. J.Acoust. Soc.Amer. 56, 6, 1835-1847 (1974).
14) Viemeister, N.F.: Intensity discrimination of noise in the presence of band reject noise. J.Acoust.Soc.Amer. 56, 5, 1594-1600 (1974).

Universal Mechanical Response Curves for the Cochlea

E. DE BOER, Wilhelmina Gasthuis, Physics Lab/KNO (ENT),
Amsterdam, The Netherlands

Introduction

When the mechanics of the cochlea is operating in the way modern theorists envisage it - and there is little doubt it does - mechanical properties may set a limit to what can be achieved by physiological processes. To formulate these in the simplest way, a model of the cochlea is constructed that contains all the essential elements of the interaction of fluid motion and travelling waves along the cochlear partition. The mechanical problem can be put into mathematical terms and can be solved. The relevant relations can then be formulated.

Model

Fig. 1 shows the geometry of the simplified model of the cochlea: a fluid-filled box divided into two channels by the cochlear partition - the basilar membrane (BM). The fluid is,

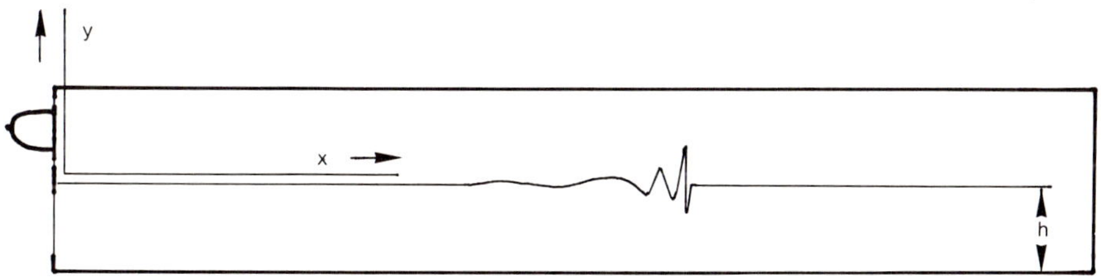

Fig. 1. Two-dimensional model of the cochlea

for simplicity, assumed to be incompressible, inviscid and linear. The mechanical properties of the BM are described by the (point) mechanical impedance function $z(x)$. In fact, for sinusoidal excitation $z(x)$ is just the complex quotient of the pressure difference $p(x)$ across the membrane and the vertical velocity $w(x)$ resulting from it; the magnitude of this quotient denotes the absolute value of this quotient and the argument angle denotes the phase difference between $p(x)$ and $w(x)$. The notion of impedance implies that the membrane is linear and that neighbouring points on the membrane do not interact directly with one another (in fact, they can only interact via the surrounding fluid).

Travelling waves

Cochlear mechanics is completey dominated by the course of the mechanical impedance of the BM $z(x)$ as a function of x. For excitation with a pure tone with a mid-range frequency the imaginary part of $z(x)$ is shown by Fig. 2. Near the windows the stiffness dominates, it is represented by an exponential function of x: $c(x)=C_o \cdot \exp(-\alpha x)$ where α is a constant (of the order of $3 cm^{-1}$). In this region a travelling wave is set up along the length of the BM. The associated fluid wave is nearly homogeneous across the channels and can be described by a so-called one-dimensional wave equation [1]. The rapid variation of stiffness causes the wave to have a propagation velocity that diminishes with increasing x, the wavelength $\lambda(x)$ diminishes at the same rate and the amplitude of the wave increases. In fact, for not too low frequencies (above 300 Hz), the wavelength decreases as $\lambda(x) = \lambda_o . \exp(-\alpha x/s)$ and the magnitude $|w(x)|$

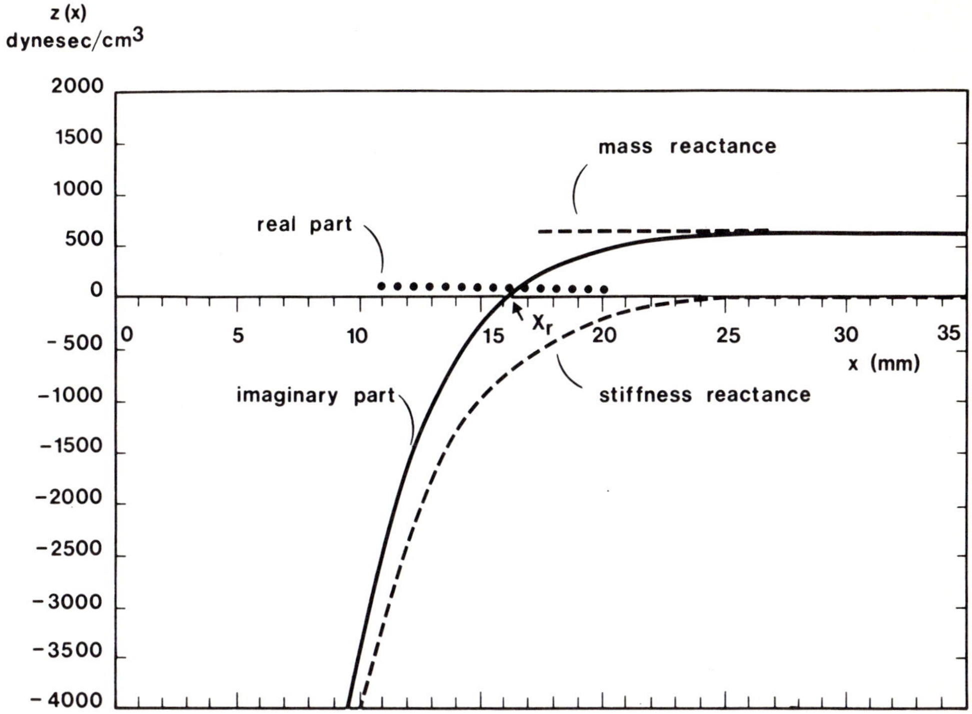

Fig. 2. Mechanical impedance of the cochlear partition (basilar membrane)

of BM velocity increases as $|w(x)| = w_o.\exp(3/4\alpha x)$. From the course of $\lambda(x)$ as a function of x the travel time $\tau(x)$ of the wave from the windows to the point x can be shown to be $\tau(x)=\tau_o\{\exp(\alpha x/2)-1\}$. These universal response functions for the region of the cochlea in which travelling waves arise are most useful for the interpretation of electrical responses of the cochlea, the cochlear microphonics (CM) and the compound action potential (AP). In particular, the latency of the experimental AP (which is used in the assessment of cochlear pathology in man) can readily be related to mechanical events in the cochlea and to sharpening effects associated with physiological functioning [2].

Resonance

For each frequency there is a location x_r in the cochlea where the imaginary part of the impedance is zero: the locus of resonance. In the vicinity of this point wave motion is radically different. Consensus has not yet been reached as to its true character in this region. To elucidate this point, the wave motion was calculated for the case where the impedance is proportional to $x-x_r$: $z(x)=i\beta(x-x_r)$. The coefficient β was chosen so that the simplified z(x)-function has the same slope as the actual one. This case lends itself to an analytical solution. The results show that (at least for low damping) in this region fluid motion is confined to a narrow layer on both sides of the BM and does not reach out to the walls. Accordingly, the height h of the channel may be taken as infinite and the resulting motion is found to have extremely interesting properties. For once, the behaviour of the pressure difference p(x) across the BM and the BM velocity w(x) is expressed by very simple formulae [3]:

$$p(x)=p_o\exp(\frac{i}{A}\ln x) \quad (1)$$

(x stands short for $x-x_r$)

$$w(x)=w_o\exp(\frac{i}{A}\ln x)/x \quad (2)$$

where A is a cochlear constant (for current values of the cochlear parameters A=0.075). These formulae hold true for the no-damping case. When damping is introduced via the familiar damping constant δ, the same formulae can be used with x replaced by the complex quantity $x-i\delta/\alpha$ [4]. The type of two-dimensional fluid motion for which h is essentially infinite is referred to as the *extreme two-dimensional case*. It is to be noted that A does not depend on frequency, this means that for this type of model the wave pattern is the same around the pertinent location of resonance - whatever is the frequency. Perhaps this is an oversimplification, but certainly in view of the other approximations involved. Anyway, it provides much insight [1].

Fig. 3 shows typical response curves, actually the derivative dw(x)/dx of w(x) as given by eq. (2). The parameter is the relative damping factor δ. All functions are computed for extreme two-dimensional fluid movements (h infinite). This

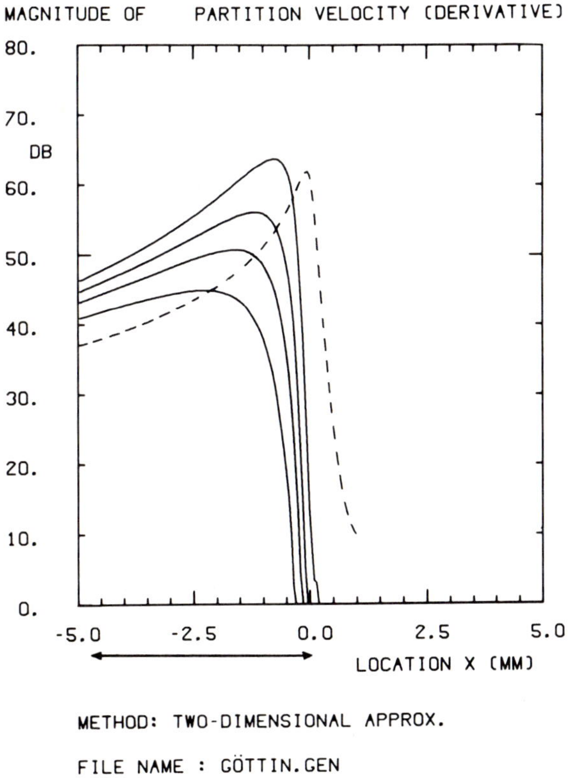

Fig. 3. Extreme two-dimensional solution (first spatial derivative of BM velocity). Abscissa: distance x from resonance location in mm. Damping factors: 0.03, 0.05, 0.07 and 0.1

result deviates significantly from that obtained from a one-dimensional approximation (see the dotted line for an example) for the same situation but it is certainly very close to the response for a more complete two-dimensional model.

Sharpening and nonlinearity

The simple analytical forms obtained for the resonance region in the extreme two-dimensional case provide facilities for further speculations. One problem that has been with us for over 30 years concerns sharpening. Neural (and microphonic) response curves [5,6] are like responses of band-pass filters

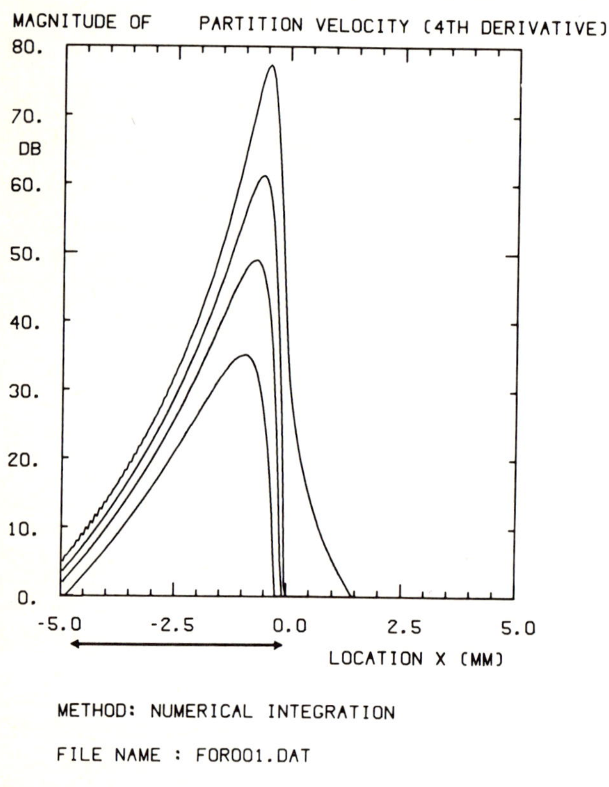

Fig. 4. Fourth spatial derivative of BM velocity. Damping factors 0.03, 0.05, 0.07 and 0.1. Abscissa in mm relative to resonance location. h=0.1 (cm). Double arrow: distance equivalent to one octave

whereas the mechanical response has essentially low-pass character. Possibly the effective filtering derives more from the slope or curvature of the mechanical response curve than from that response itself [7]. Pursuing this idea somewhat further, we show in Fig. 4 response curves for the fourth derivative $d^4w(x)/dx^4$. In contrast to Fig. 3, these curves have been computed for a *finite* value of the height h. Consequently, only the functions for the smallest values of δ show the true two-dimensional character where wave motion is confined to the immediate vicinity of the BM. Response functions for larger values of δ (0.07 and 0.1) reflect one-dimensional wave motion, where fluid motion occupies nearly the entire height h of the cochlear channels. The principal result is that the bandwidth of the response varies less than proportional to δ. Although the x-scale represents distances in the cochlea, the behaviour of the response at one location as a function of frequency is similar. For comparison the distance corresponding to one octave is indicated on the abscissa.

Two tendencies can be noted from this figure. With quite modest variations of damping the character of the fourth-derivative response changes from one with sharp resonance to that with a more pronounced low-pass character. This might parallel the change in neural and microphonic response properties when a cochlea becomes pathological [8]. A variation of effective damping may also be brought about in a normal cochlea by a change in level of excitation. Many nonlinear phenomena exhibited by the cochlea can be explained by such an intensity-dependent nonlinearity [9]. However, only the two-dimensional approach used in this paper can bring to light a response where the bandwidth of the response varies clearly less than the damping constant δ. Such a type of response is needed in view of the reported near-invariance of the (3 dB-) bandwidth of revcor spectra to variations in intensity [10].

Conclusions

Many features of cochlear mechanics, and, perhaps, of coupled physiological phenomena, can be described quite well on the basis of just a few simple mathematical functions. The properties formulated in section 3 for the stiffness-controlled region, all based on exponential functions, form the first example. They are useful for the interpretation of gross electrical responses from the cochlea. For the more intricate phenomena associated with resonance, the extreme two-dimensional approach leads to eqs 1 and 2. These serve to explain fundamental properties of fluid wave motion [3] but can also be used as a stepping-stone to the consideration of more involved phenomena such as the response of hair cells [5] or auditory nerve fibres [6]. In addition to sharpening, the functions can also be used to describe gross effects of nonlinearity [9] and cochlear pathology [8]. Further applications of these results have not yet been worked out completely.

References:

1) Boer, E. de: Auditory physics. Physical principles in hearing theory. Part I. (invited review paper, to be published in Physics Reports) (1979).
2) Boer, E. de: Travelling waves and cochlear resonance. (preprint for Proc.Münster Symp. on Models of the Auditory System and Related Signal Processing Techniques; to be published in Scandinavian Audiology) (1978).

3) Boer, E. de: Short-wave world revisited: Resonance in a two-dimensional cochlear model. (internal report) (1979).
Boer, E. de: Short-wave world revisited: Resonance in a two-dimensional cochlear model. (in preparation) (1979).
4) Boer, E. de and MacKay, R.: Reflections on reflections. (submitted for publication in J.Acoust.Soc.Amer.) (1979).
5) Russell, I.J. and Sellick, P.M.: Intracellular studies of hair cells in the mammalian cochlea. J.Physiol. 284, 261-290 (1978).
6) Evans, E.F.: Cochlear nerve and cochlear nucleus. In: Handbook of Sensory Physiology, vol. V, part 2. W.D. Keidel and W.D. Neff (eds.), Springer-Verlag, Berlin, 1-108 (1975).
7) Hall, J.L.: Spatial differentiation as an auditory "second filter": Assessment on a nonlinear model of the basilar membrane. J.Acoust.Soc.Am. 61, 520-524 (1977).
8) Evans, E.F.: The sharpening of cochlear frequency selectivity in the normal and abnormal cochlea. Audiology 14, 419-442 (1975).
9) Kim, D.O. and Molnar, C.E.: Cochlear mechanics: Measurements and models. In: The Nervous System, vol. 3. D.B. Tower (ed.), Raven Press, New York, 57-68 (1975).
10) Boer, E. de and Jongh, H.R. de: On cochlear encoding: Potentialities and limitations of the reverse-correlation technique. J.Acoust.Soc.Am. 63, 115-135 (1978).

The Human Cochlear Nuclei

J. K. MOORE, K. K. OSEN, Department of Neuroscience, University of California, San Diego, La Jolla, California 92093, USA
and Anatomical Institute, University of Oslo, Oslo 1, Norway

In man the central auditory pathway appears to be organized largely according to the same principles as in other mammals. Minor disparities exist, nevertheless, between many auditory centres in man and lower mammals. The structural species differences probably reflect differences in auditory function and therefore should be taken into account in comparative studies in hearing. The present paper will deal with the morphology of the human cochlear nuclei. As a basis for homologies and functional correlations the cat cochlear nuclei, which are relatively well known from previous cytoarchitectural, homological and electrophysiological investigations, will first be briefly considered. For a more complete description of the human cochlear nuclei, see Moore and Osen (1979).

Figure 1 demonstrates a simplified wiring-diagram of the cochlear nuclear complex and related brain stem centres, based on observations in the cat. In the cochlear nuclei of the cat, several different types of neurones can be identified in ordinary Nissl sections (Osen, 1969). Most of these are recognizable also in Golgi material (Lorente de Nó, 1933, 1976; Brawer et al., 1974). In our diagram the following types of cochlear nuclear neurones are illustrated: pyramidal cells, octopus

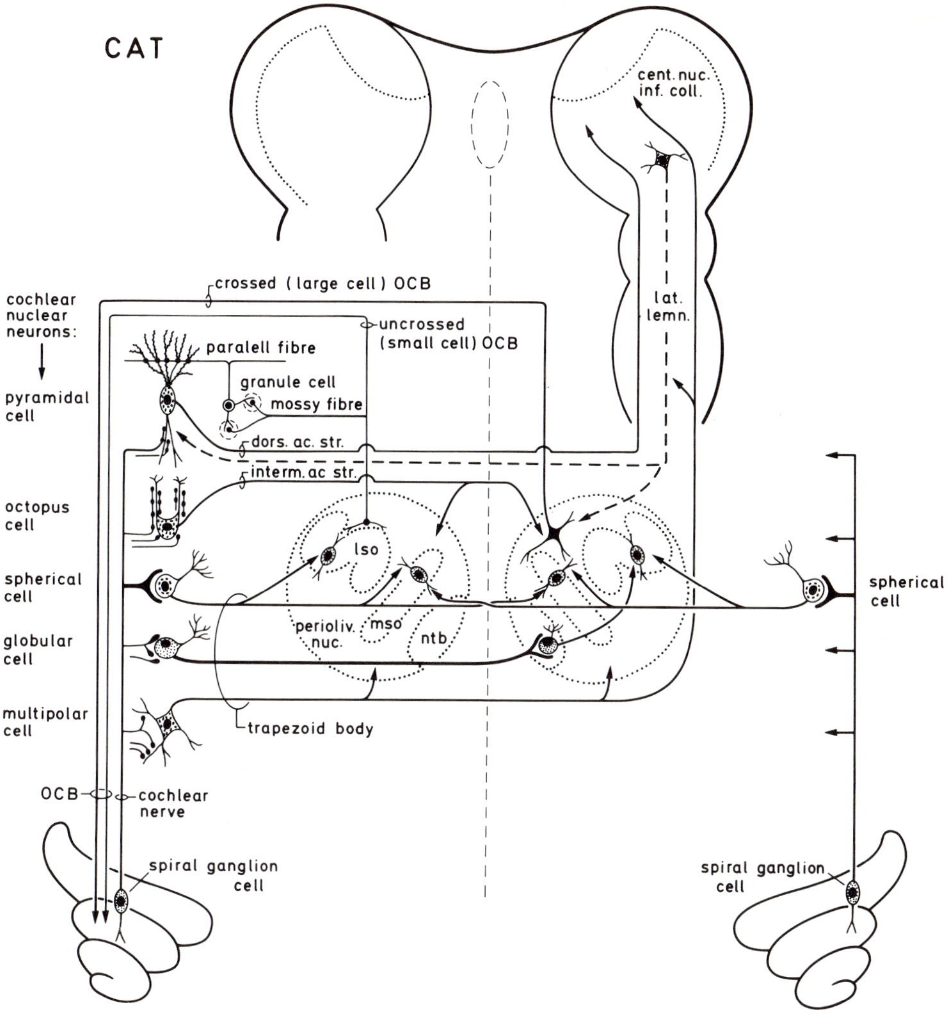

Fig. 1. A simplified wiring-diagram of the cochlear nuclear complex and related brain stem centres based on observations in the cat. For further explanation, see the text. Abbreviations: lso, lateral superior olive; mso, medial superior olive; ntb, nucleus of the trapezoid body; OCB, olivocochlear bundle

cells, spherical cells, globular cells, multipolar cells, and granule cells. With the exception of the latter type (Osen, 1970; Bird et al., 1978), these cells are supplied from the cochlear nerve by specific types of fibre terminals. The spherical cells and the globular cells receive a restricted number of large, axosomatic synaptic endings (bulbs of Held) which are larger on the former cells (Lorente de Nó, 1933). The pyramidal cells, octopus cells, and multipolar cells, in contrast, receive numerous small, mainly axodendritic boutons (Kane, 1974). Probably due in part to the different primary input, in part to differences in intrinsic and descending fibre connections (illustrated here only for the pyramidal cells), each cell type responds to auditory stimulation with a specific pattern of discharges (van Gisbergen et al., 1975).

In the cochlear nuclear complex, thus, the unichannel system of the cochlear nerve is converted into a multichannel system with different electrophysiological properties, different trajectories, and different targets for the various channels in the brain stem. The fibres which originate in the spherical cells and the globular cells make possible a binaural input to the medial and lateral superior olives, as indicated in Figure 1 (Harrison and Irving, 1966a,b; Warr, 1966). These neurones, therefore, are probably engaged, i.a., in localization of sound in space. The axons of the octopus cells, on the other hand, supply the peri-olivary nuclei (Warr, 1969) and may possibly be linked to the crossed olivocochlear bundle (OCB) which arises in this site (Rasmussen, 1946; Warr, 1975). The pyramidal cells, the multipolar cells, and the small cap cells (not illustrated) differ from the aforementioned types by projecting as far rostral as to the contra-lateral inferior colliculus (Adams, 1979), which is a link in the auditory projection to several regions of the brain, including the medial geniculate body, the midbrain tegmentum and the pontine nuclei.

The pyramidal cells of the cochlear nuclei in subprimates are unique among secondary, sensory neurones in being influenced, via the granule cells, by a local circuitry similar to that of the cerebellar cortex (Mugnaini et al., 1979). Like their counterparts in the cerebellum, the cochlear granule cells give rise to parallel fibres which, in the molecular layer of the dorsal cochlear nucleus (DCN), form synapses en passage with the apical dendrites of te pyramidal cells (Fig. 1, upper left). The latter cells thus have a position in the feline DCN which is similar in certain respects to that of the Purkinje cells in the cerebellum. In further analogy with the cerebellar cortex, the cochlear granule cells participate with their dendrites in glomerular synaptic arrays centred on large, mossy fibre terminals, some of which may originate in the OCB (McDonald and Rasmussen, 1971). On their basal dendrites, the pyramidal cells receive primary afferents and fibres descending from higher auditory centres including the inferior colliculus (van Noort, 1969; Kane, 1977).

In man, as in the cat, the cochlear nuclear complex is situated lateral to the restiform body in the floor of the lateral recess of the fourth ventricle. Due to the large size of the cerebellar peduncles in man, the cochlear nuclear complex is situated so far laterally in the brain stem that it is usually cut off with the cerebellum in routine postmortem examinations. For the same reason, the rostrocaudal axis of the complex is rotated with its anterior end pointing somewhat laterally (Fig. 2, upper right). In further contrast to the cat, the

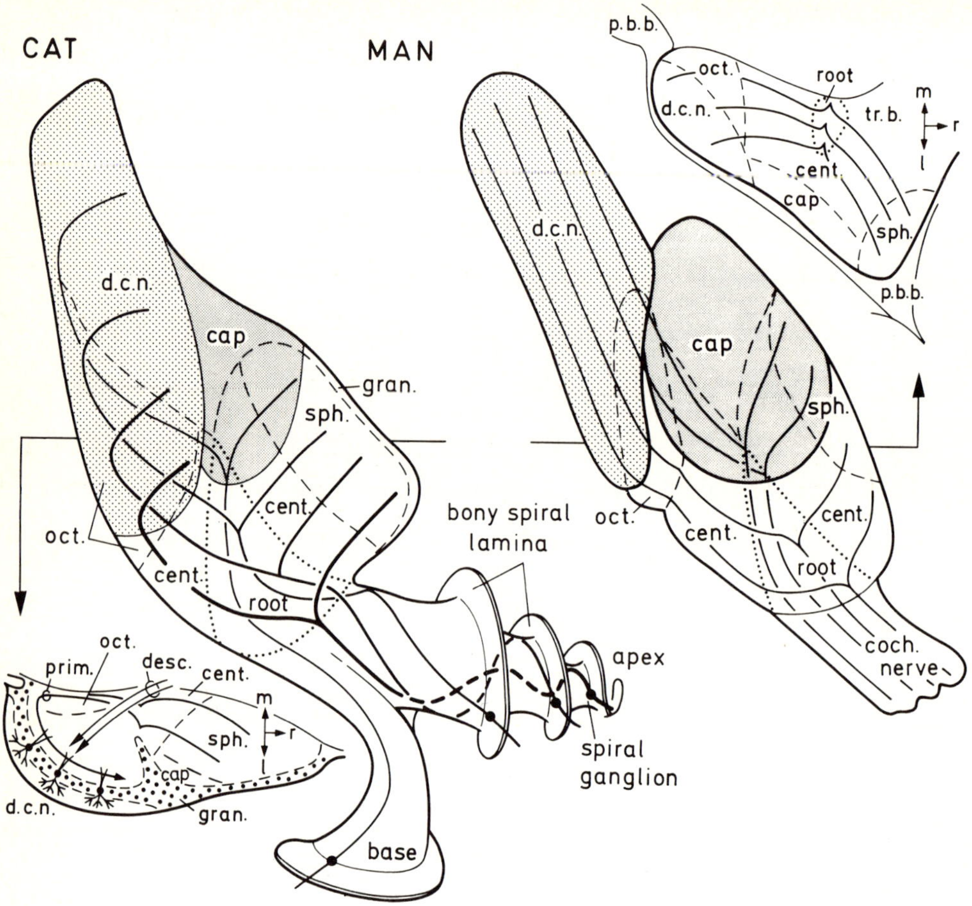

Fig. 2. Diagrams of the cochlear nuclear complex in man and the cat in lateral views (main diagrams) and in horizontal sections. For further explanation, see the text. The diagrams in the two species are of approximately the same magnification. Abbreviations: cap, cap of small cells; cent., central region of the ventral cochlear nucleus; coch.nerve, cochlear nerve; d.c.n., dorsal cochlear nucleus; desc., descending fibres; gran., granule cell layer; l, lateral; m, medial; oct., area of octopus cells; p.b.b., pontobulbar body; prim., primary afferent; r, rostral; root, cochlear nerve root; sph., area of spherical cells; tr.b., trapezoid body

cochlear nuclear complex in man is everywhere separated from the ependyma of the fourth ventricle by a fibrocellular capsule belonging to the large pontobulbar body.

Judged by myelin stained sections of the human brain stem, the distribution of the cochlear nerve fibres is about the same as in the cat, at least for the ventral cochlear nucleus (VCN) (Fig. 2). In the human VCN a similar tonotopical organization, therefore, is to be expected as in the cat, with high tonal frequencies represented dorsally and low frequencies ventrally (Rose et al., 1959). In the human DCN, however, the tonotopical organization may differ from the feline pattern since in man the primary afferents apparently do not make the typical, sharp turn on entering the DCN as seen in the cat and other subprimates (Osen, 1970).

In Nissl sections of the human VCN the same cell types are encountered as in the cat, although in somewhat different proportions (Moore and Osen, 1979). Only the granule cells are virtually absent. In man, as in the cat, the VCN proper may be divided into three subregions (Fig. 2), a rostral area of spherical cells (sph.), a caudal area of octopus cells (oct.), and an intervening central region (cent.) where globular cells, multipolar cells, and small cells are intermingled. Dorsolateral to the VCN proper is a cap of small cells (cap). While in the cat the VCN is covered superficially by a granule cell layer, this is missing in man in accordance with the general absence of cochlear granule cells. By a rough estimate the human VCN seems slightly smaller than that of the cat. This may be due in part to the absence of the granule cell layer, in part to a somewhat smaller size of the spherical and octopus cell areas in man. The larger part of the human VCN actually is made up of the central region which is populated mainly by multipolar cells. The cap of small cells is also relatively large in man.

The human DCN is of about the same size as in the cat, thus constituting a slightly larger proportion of the nuclear complex (for references, see Moore and Osen, 1979). The internal structure of the DCN, however, is strikingly different in man and the cat. In the cat, as in lower mammals in general, the DCN is distinctly stratified, consisting of a superficial molecular layer, an underlying layer of radially oriented pyramidal cells and granule cells (continuous with the granule cell layer of the VCN), and three deeper cellular layers which are less easily distinguished (Lorente de Nó, 1933) (Fig. 2, lower left). In sharp contrast to the cat, the DCN in man is unlaminated. The pyramidal cells may not be reduced in number, but they have lost their typical, radial orientation and only a vestige of a molecular layer is found. Virtually, the entire DCN in man consists of an area of cochlear fibre neuropile containing irregularly oriented pyramidal cells, small neurones, and occasional giant cells. These changes, which appear to be the end result of a phylogenetic process in primates (Moore, 1979), are probably secondary to the absence of a cochlear granule cell system in man. Since the functional significance of the DCN in lower mammals is completely unknown, there is also no easy explanation for its different structure in man. It is evident, however, that in man the DCN cannot be regarded as a structural analogue of the cerebellar cortex.

By rough estimate, thus, it seems that in man the multipolar cells, the cap cells, and the pyramidal cells, all of which project to the inferior colliculus, have increased their relative share in the cochlear nuclear complex. In contrast, the octopus cells, the spherical cells, and the globular cells, which have the superior olive as their main target, seem less numerous than in other mammals. This is in accordance with the relative smallness of the superior olivary complex in man. Furthermore, the modulation of the neuronal activity effected by local interneurones and descending fibres may be less elaborate in the primary auditory nuclei of man than of subprimates. In particular, the cochlear granule cell system is absent in man. These differences probably mean that in man the processing of auditory information takes place to a larger extent at the midbrain level or above.

References:

1) Adams, J.C.: Ascending projections to the inferior colliculus. J.comp.Neurol. 183, 519-538 (1979).
2) Bird, S.J.; Gulley, R.L.; Wenthold, R.J.; Fex, J.: Kainic acid injections result in degeneration of cochlear nucleus cells innervated by the auditory nerve. Science 202, 1087-1089 (1978).
3) Brawer, J.R.; Morest, D.K.; Kane, E.C.: The neuronal architecture of the cochlear nucleus of the cat. J.comp.Neurol. 155, 251-300 (1974).
4) van Gisberger, J.A.M.; Grashuis, J.L.; Johannesma, P.I.M.; Vendrik, A.J.H.: Statistical analysis and interpretation of the initial response of cochlear nucleus neurons to tone bursts. Exp. Brain Res. 23, 407-423 (1975).
5) Harrison, J.M.; Irving, R.: Ascending connections of the anterior ventral cochlear nucleus in the rat. J.comp.Neurol. 126, 51-64 (1966a).
6) Harrison, J.M.; Irving, R.: The organization of the posterior ventral cochlear nucleus in the rat. J.comp.Neurol. 126, 391-402 (1966b).
7) Kane, E.S.: Patterns of degeneration in the caudal cochlear nucleus of the cat. Anat.Rec. 179, 67-92 (1974).
8) Kane, E.S.: Descending inputs to the dorsal cochlear nucleus: An electron microscopic study. J.Neurocytol. 6, 583-605 (1977).
9) Lorente de Nó: Anatomy of the eigth nerve. III. General plan of structure. Laryngoscope (St. Louis) 43, 327-350 (1933).

10) Lorente de Nó: Some unresolved problems concerning the cochlear nerve. Ann.Otol.Rhinol.Laryngol. 85, Suppl. 34, 1-28 (1976).
11) McDonald, D.; Rasmussen, G.L.: Ultrastructural characteristics of synaptic endings in the cochlear nucleus having acetylcholinesterase activity. Brain Res. 28, 1-18 (1971).
12) Moore, J.K.: Loss of lamination as a phylogenetic process in the primate dorsal cochlear nucleus. (1979, in press).
13) Moore, J.K.; Osen, K.K.: The cochlear nuclei in man. Amer.J.Anat. 154, 393-418 (1979).
14) Mugnaini, E., Osen, K.K., Dahl, A.-L.; Friedrich Jr., V.L.; Korte, G.: Fine structure of granule cells and related interneurones (termed Golgi cells) in the cochlear nuclear complex of cat, rat and mouse. J.Neurocytol. (1979, in press).
15) van Noort, J.: The structure and connections of the inferior colliculus. Proefeschrift. Leiden: vna Gorcum & Comp. N.V. (1969).
16) Osen, K.K.: Cytoarchitecture of the cochlear nuclei in the cat. J.comp.Neurol. 136, 453-484 (1969).
17) Osen, K.K.: Course and termination of the primary afferents in the cochlear nuclei of the cat. An experimental anatomical study. Arch.ital.Biol. 108, 21-51 (1970).
18) Rasmussen, G.L.: The olivary peduncle and other fiber projections of the superior olivary complex. J.comp.Neurol. 84, 141-220 (1946).
19) Rose, J.E.; Galambos, R.; Hughes, J.R.: Microelectrode studies of the cochlear nuclei of the cat. Bull. Johns Hopk. Hosp. 104, 211-251 (1959).
20) Warr, W.B.: Fiber degeneration following lesions in the anterior ventral cochlear nucleus of the cat. Exp.Neurol. 14, 453-474 (1966).
21) Warr, W.B.: Fiber degeneration following lesions in the postero-ventral cochlear nucleus of the cat. Exp.Neurol. 23, 140-155 (1969).
22) Warr, W.B.: Olivocochlear and vestibular efferent neurons of the feline brain stem: Their location, morphology and number determined by retrograde axonal transports and acetylcholinesterase histochemistry. J.comp.Neurol. 161, 159-182 (1975).

Coding of Complex Sounds in the Auditory Nervous System

AAGE R. MØLLER, University of Pittsburgh, Department of Otolaryngology, Pittsburgh, PA 15213, USA

The great majority of studies of the coding of sound in single nerve fibers and cells in the auditory nervous system has so far been performed using simple sounds such as pure tones and click sounds as stimuli. However, the results of recent studies using more complex sounds indicate that it is not possible to deduce the response of single nerve fibers or nerve cells in the auditory periphery to complex stimuli on the basis of results obtained using simple stimuli such as pure tones and clicks. The present presentation concerns the responses of single auditory nerve fibers and single nerve cells in the cochlear nucleus to stimulation with a few types of complex sounds. The results are compared with those results obtained in response to pure tones and click sounds.

Auditory Nerve

Previously, it was assumed that the peripheral auditory analyzer could be regarded to function in the same way as a linear filter, and consequently, it was expected that the spectral filtering of complex sounds could be estimated on the basis of results obtained using pure tones. However, analysis of the discharge pattern in single auditory nerve fibers in response to pseudorandom noise shows a different spectral filtering than the frequency threshold curves obtained using pure tones, except for very low sound intensities. The results obtained using noise as stimulus reveals a spectral selectivity that decreases (bandwidth increases) with increasing sound intensity, as seen in Fig. 1. Also, the frequency where maximal response is obtained is seen to shift downward in frequency as the intensity of the noise stimulus is increased. The frequency threshold curve obtained using pure tones is shown for comparison (heavy line).

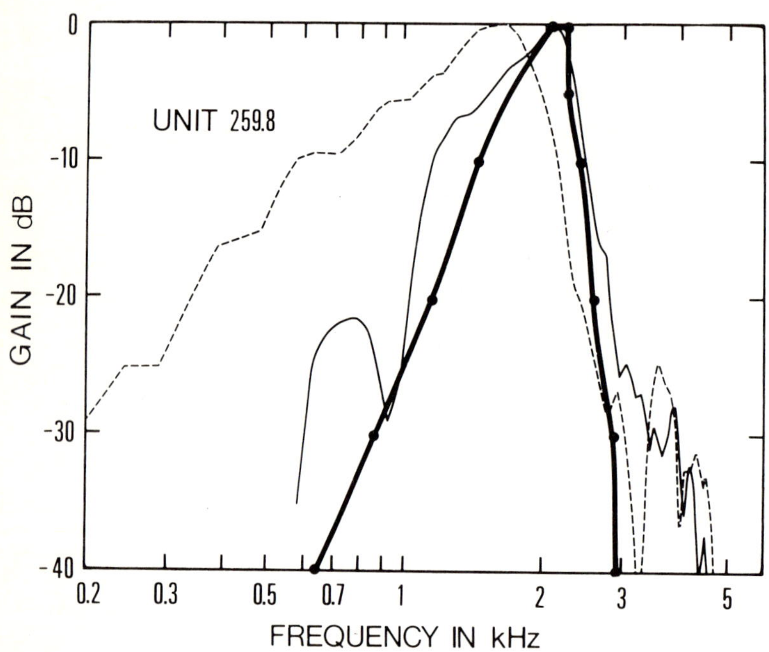

Fig. 1. Crosspectra (transfer functions) of the response of a single auditory nerve fiber in a rat when the ear was stimulated with pseudorandom noise (thin lines) compared with the frequency threshold curve of the same fiber obtained when stimulated with bursts of pure tones. The results shown by the dashed line were obtained at a level of the noise stimulus of 70dB above threshold and the thin solid line shows results obtained using noise at a level of 15 dB above threshold (From Møller, 1978a)

In these experiments, cross-correlation functions between the noise stimulus and a period histogram of the neural discharges were used as estimates of the impulse response function of the system under test. The results seen in Fig. 1 were obtained by Fourier transforming these cross-correlation functions to obtain the crosspectrum. These crosspectra are assumed to be valid estimates of the linear part of the frequency transfer function of the system under test (Møller, 1977a).

The cross-correlograms have the form of damped oscillations as expected, but when examined in detail, it emerges that the frequency of the damped oscillation is not constant but increases during the latter part of the damped oscillation as is illustrated in Fig. 2 (Møller and Nilsson, 1979).
This change in frequency is a result of the fact that the basilar membrane functions like a transmission line, and it implies that the filter function of a single point of the basilar membrane cannot be accurately mimicked by an ordinary bandpass filter made up of lumped components.

The results of these experiments emphasize the importance of phase-locking of the neural discharge as information carrying element (for frequencies below 4 - 5 kHz) contrary to the mean discharge rate. Thus, it emerges from these studies that the mean synchronized discharge rate reached a plateau only about 20 dB above threshold (Møller, 1977b, 1978a,b).

The great majority of experimental and theoretical work so far performed has concerned the frequency selectivity of a single point of the basilar membrane as it emerges when the vibration or the discharge rate of a single auditory nerve fiber was

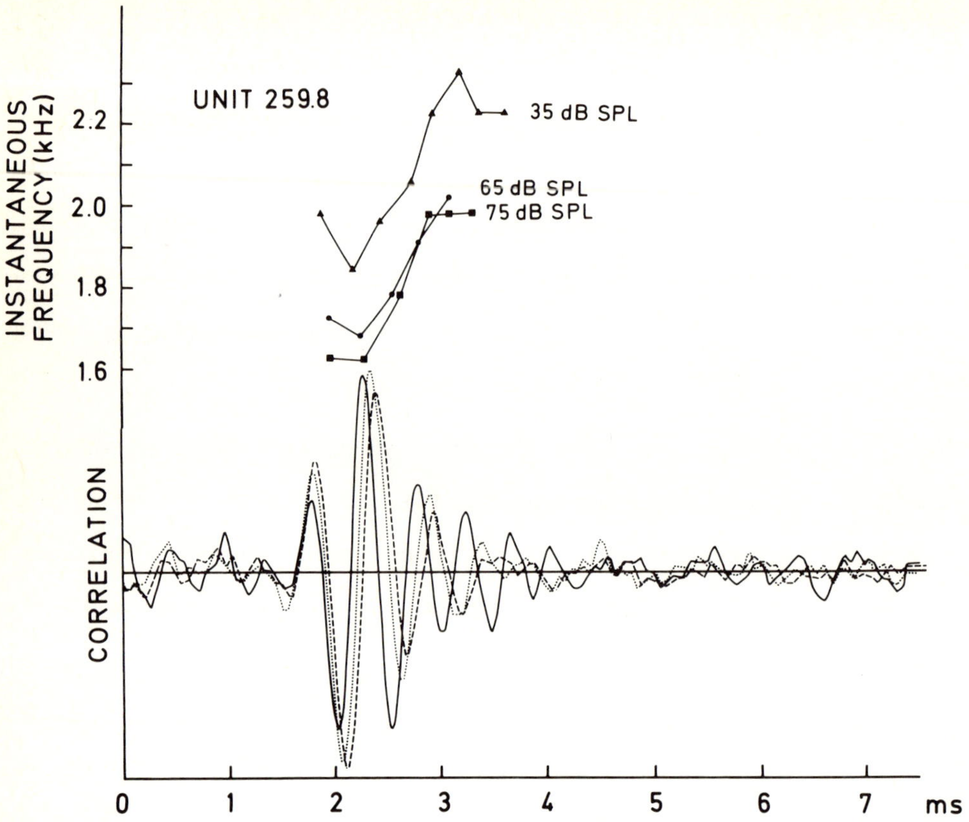

Fig. 2. Impulse response functions of a single auditory nerve fiber in a rat obtained using pseudorandom noise as stimulus. Solid lines: stimulus level 35 dB, dotted line 65 dB, and dashed line 75 dB (SPL measured over 1/3 octave band). Upper curves show the instantaneous frequency of the damped oscillation as a function of time (From Møller and Nilsson, 1979)

studied as a function of the frequency of a pure tone. It is, however, most likely that other features of the basilar membrane vibration are of physiological significance, namely, the distribution of vibration amplitude along the basilar membrane for complex sounds. This cannot be inferred from the above described experimental data since it depends on features of the cochlear hydrodynamics that influence little on the response of a single point, such as the change in wave velocity along the basilar membrane. Only a few experimental investigations have concerned that problem. In one such study, the discharge pattern in as many as several hundred single auditory nerve fibers was studied in a single animal (cat) using the same stimulus (pure tones) (Pfeiffer and Kim, 1975, Kim et al., 1979).

In a discussion of the frequency analysis in the auditory periphery, it may be of value to consider what information the inner ear may transmit to higher auditory centers in case of some basic types of sounds and see what a fundamental type of neural processing is taken into account; namely, integration of the activity of many nerve fibers by their convergence onto the same nerve cell in the cochlear nucleus:

A low frequency pure tone, well above threshold, will give rise to a phase-locking of the firing in many auditory nerve fibers. Since the firing in many fibers are phase-locked to the same frequency (i.e. the frequency of the tone), spatial neural integration will enhance the periodicity by the process of averaging of the discharges of many fibers. Another frequently used experimental sound, the click sound, gives rise to discharges that are phase-locked to the damped oscillation of the peripheral analyzer (Kiang et al., 1965; Møller, 1970) (Fig. 2). Since the frequency of the damped oscillation is equal to the CF of the fiber, it is different for different fibers. In that case, the discharge patterns of different individual fibers thus essentially tell the higher centers what the CF of the fibers are, and consequently, spatial integration of the activity of fibers with different CF results in an elimination of this periodicity, leaving only a brief excitation corresponding to the first part of the oscillation.

A broadband noise is assumed to be subjected to bandpass filtering in the peripheral spectral analyzer, and the excitation of different auditory nerve fibers (with low CF) will thus correspond to a bandpass filtered version of the stimulus noise. Such a signal is similar to an amplitude modulated sine wave, the frequency of which is equal to the CF, and the modulation being a low-pass filtered random signal. The discharge patterns of different low frequency auditory nerve fibers in response to such a signal can be assumed to be phase-locked to the periodicity of the excitation, i.e. a frequency equal to the CF of the fiber. Also in this case, it seems that the phase-locked discharge patterns in the various fibers mainly convey information to higher centers about their CF, and spatial integration of the activity of many nerve fibers with different CF seems to largely eliminate the phase-locking of the discharges in the individual fibers.

Cochlear Nucleus

We thus have to admit that our knowledge about the coding of complex sounds in single nerve cells in the auditory periphery is scarse, and we know practically nothing about how such information is processed at higher levels in the ascending auditory pathway. Almost all nerve cells in the cochlear nucleus respond to small changes in amplitude and frequency with a relatively large change in their discharge rate. That response to changes can be demonstrated in experiments where amplitude or frequency modulated tones are used. When sinusoidally amplitude (or frequency) modulated tones are used, the modulation is reproduced in the discharge pattern to a degree that depends on the modulation frequency (Møller, 1972). Between 50 and 200 Hz modulation frequency, most units respond with a large degree of modulation of their discharge rate. Thus, period histograms, locked to the modulation frequency, are often modulated as much as 50% in response to sounds, the amplitude of which is modulated only 1-2dB. This modulation of the discharge pattern takes place over a range of sound intensities that is much larger than that over which the mean discharge rate is a function of the sound intensity (Møller, 1974). It has been shown in other experiments that the reproduction of small changes in amplitude in the discharge pattern is enhanced by adding a second unmodulated tone to the modulated tone when the former has a frequency within the inhibitory range of the unit (Møller, 1975).

The response pattern of most units in the cochlear nucleus to a tone, the frequency of which is varied slowly across the unit's CF, is in accordance with the units response to steady tones of different frequencies presented one at a time. However, when the frequency of the same tone is varied rapidly, these units respond in a completely different fashion; namely, by discharging only within a narrow range of frequencies, that range being much narrower than that evoked by a tone with a slowly varying frequency (Møller, 1969, 1971, 1974b).

Many nerve cells in the cochlear nucleus respond poorly or not at all to bandpass filtered noise when the bandwidth is larger than a certain value (Greenwood and Goldberg, 1970). When, however, the center frequency of such a band of noise is varied rapidly, these nerve cells respond vigorously and show a pronounced frequency selectivity. That is so even for units that do not respond at all to the same noise when its center frequency is varied slowly (Møller, 1974a). This is illustrated in Fig. 3, that shows histograms of the responses of a typical neuron in the cochlear nucleus of a rat to a tone, the frequency of which is varied up and down over a large frequency range that covers and extends over the range where the unit responds to sound. The right hand part of the graph shows the response to a bandpass filtered noise. It is seen that there is almost no response when the center frequency is varied slowly; but when the center frequency is varied rapidly, the unit responds with a large number of discharges and the unit shows a pronounced degree of frequency (spectral) selectivity.

These results thus show that the response of single neurons in the cochlear nucleus to sounds, the spectrum of which changes cannot be deduced from knowledge about the response to static sounds, nor can the response to complex sounds such as bandpass filtered noise be deduced on the basis of knowledge about the response to pure tones.

The sounds used in the above described experiments have greater similarities with speech sounds than do pure tones, but they are anyhow much simpler, and it is therefore not obvious whether or not it is possible to draw conclusions about the response to speech sounds of single nerve cells in the auditory nerve and the cochlear nucleus. The above described results are the responses of single nerve elements at the very peri-

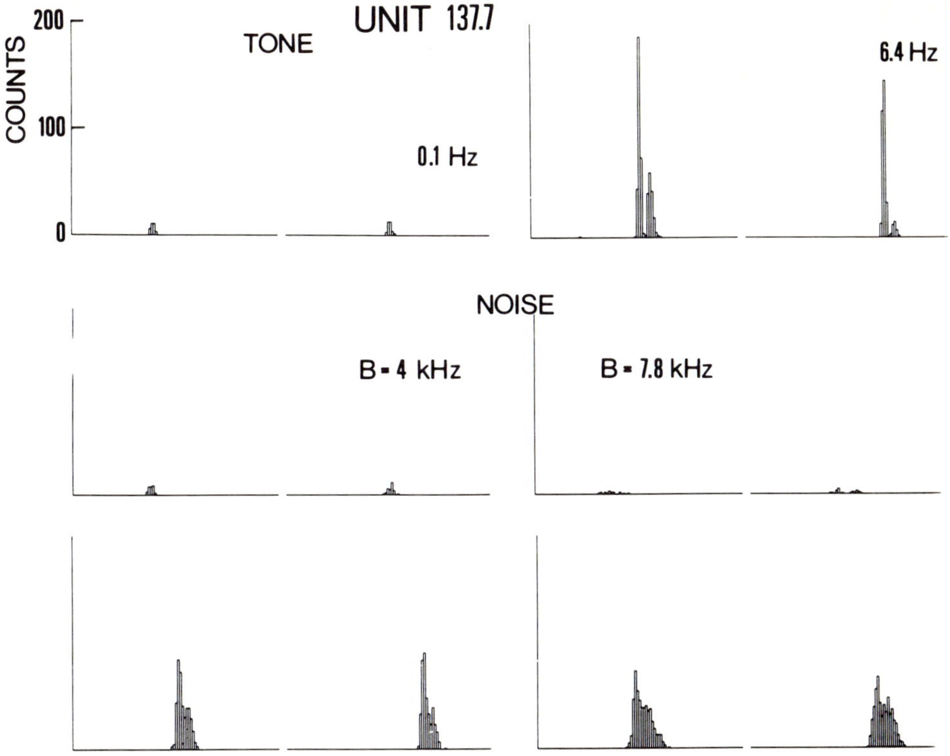

Fig. 3. Histograms of the responses of a single nerve cell in the cochlear nucleus in response to tones, the frequency of which was varied at different rates compared with responses to bandpass filtered noise, the center frequency of which was varied in a similar way. The bandwidth of the noise was 4 and 7.8 kHz. The frequency of the tones and the noise was varied trapezoidally up and down over a large range of frequencies, covering the response area of the cell with a rate of 0.1 Hz and 6.4 Hz.
The histograms show the distribution of nerve discharges as a function of frequency of the tone or noise (For details, see Møller, 1974)

pheral part of the ascending auditory pathway. Our knowledge about the processing at higher order nuclei of the ascending auditory pathway is extremely sparse, and we have practically no knowledge about how higher levels of the central nervous system make use of the information that reaches it from the auditory system.

References:

1) Greenwood, D.D. and Goldberg, J.M.: Responses of neurons in the cochlear nuclei to variations in noise bandwidth and to tone-noise combinations. J.Acoust.Soc.Am. 47, 1022-1040 (1970).
2) Kiang, N.Y.-S.; Watanabe, T.; Thomas, E.C.; and L.F. Clark: Discharge patterns of single fibers in the cat's auditory nerve. M.I.T. Press, Cambridge, Mass. (1965).
3) Kim, D.O. et al.: Cochlear nonlinear phenomena in two-tone responses. In Press: Scandinavian Audiology (1979).
4) Møller, A.R.: Unit responses in the cochlear nucleus of the rat to sweep tones. Acta Phys.Scand. 76, 503-512 (1969).
5) Møller, A.R.: Studies of the damped oscillatory response of the auditory frequency analyzer. Acta Phys.Scand. 78, 299-314 (1970).
6) Møller, A.R.: Unit responses in the rat cochlear nucleus to tones of rapidly varying frequency and amplitude. Acta Phys. Scand. 81, 540-556 (1971).
7) Møller, A.R.: coding of amplitude and frequency modulated sounds in the cochlear nucleus of the rat. Acta Phys.Scand. 86, 223-238 (1972).
8) Møller, A.R.: Coding of sounds with rapidly varying spectrum in the cochlear nucleus. J.Acoust.Soc.Am. 55, 631-640 (1974a).
9) Møller, A.R.: Responses of units in the cochlear units to sinusoidally amplitude modulated tones. Exp.Neurol. 45, 104-117 (1974b).
10) Møller, A.R.: Dynamic properties of excitation and inhibition in the cochlear nucleus. Acta Phys.Scand. 93, 442-454 (1975).
11) Møller, A.R.: Frequency selectivity of single auditory nerve fibers in response to broadband noise stimuli. J.Acoust. Soc.Am. 62, 135-142 (1977a).
12) Møller, A.R.: Frequency selectivity of the basilar membrane revealed from discharges in auditory nerve fibers. Psychophysics and Physiology of Hearing, E.F. Evans and J.P. Wilson (eds.) Academic Press, 197-206 (1977b).
13) Møller, A.R.: Frequency selectivity of the peripheral auditory analyzer studied using broad band noise. Acta Phys. Scan. 104, 24-32 (1978a).
14) Møller, A.R.: Responses of auditory nerve fibers to noise stimuli show cochlear nonlinearities. Acta Otolaryngol. (Stockholm) 86, 1-8 (1978b).
15) Møller, A.R. and Nilsson, H.G.: Inner ear impulse response and basilar membrane modelling. Acustica, 1979.
16) Pfeiffer, R.R. and Kim, D.O.: Cochlear nerve fiber responses: Distribution along the cochlear partition. J.Acoust. Soc.Am. 58, 867-869 (1975).

Embryological Evolution and Typology of Cells of the Inferior Colliculus

V. MEININGER, M. BAUDRIMONT, Laboratoire d'Anatomie, Faculté de Médicine, Paris, France

The inferior colliculus (I.C.) has a key importance in the auditory pathways. Among its connections it receives fibers from the cochlear nuclei (N.C.) and from the auditory cerebral cortex (A.C.C.). Physiological and anatomical data have established that the I.I. receives these fibers in at least two separate territories. Its dorso medial part receives fibers from the N.C., most of them from the controlateral side (1,2). As proposed (3,4,5) the ventral lateral division will be called the "central-nucleus" and the dorso medial division, the "dorso medial nucleus". The functional maturation of these two different systems arises at a different time (6,7). Therefore it is possible to test the consequences of the functional maturation of these different kinds of afferents on the post synaptic elements. Among the post synaptic elements, we focused our attention on the dendritic tree. A precise and quantitative analysis of the dendritic network was not feasible until recently due to the lack of an adequate quantitative methodology. As emphasized recently by Berry et al. (8) a methodology related to the graph theory has long been used in geography to describe and quantify different networks (rivers, roadways, lines of communication, 9). This methodology proved to be directly applicable to the study of the branching pattern of dendritic trees.

According to this methodology, the tree like pattern of the dendrites may be viewed as a non connective plane graph composed of points called "vertices" connected by lines or "arcs". In our study the arcs have been ordered according to the centripetal system of Strahler (9).

Such an ordering permits to calculate various parameters and to determine the mode of bifurcation cells, i.e. the pattern of growth of the dendritic tree (8).

Four adult cats (A.C.), four young cats (Y.C.) and fifteen female rats between the 15th and 23rd day post mating were sacrificed by perfusion. The inferior colliculi were impregnated by the Golgi method. Serial sections (90nm) were performed in the three plances of space. In each plane 50 almost complete cells were drawn in the central and in the dorso-medial nuclei. Various cell parameters were calculated and the topological analysis was performed as described by Berry and Bradley (8). The topological analysis permits to differentiate in the two nuclei of the I.C. of both young and adult cats two different cell types. The collaterally branched (or CB) cells are particular by a bifurcation ratio approximating the total number of pendant arcs, which defines a completely collateral system. The dichotomously branched (or D.R.) cells have a bifurcation ratio approximating 3, which defines a dichotomous branching on random terminal or pendant arcs (terminal mode of growth).

The proportion of these two cell types and of various cell parameters vary from young to adult cat. In the dorso-medial nucleus we observed a decrease of DR cells, similar in all planes of space, from YC to AC.

Such a variation was not observed in the central nucleus.

Dorso - Medial Nucleus						
Plane	VF		S		H	
cell type	DR	CB	DR	CB	DR	CB
YC	40	10	45	5	45	5
AC	37	16	34	16	33	17
Central Nucleus						
YC	42	8	43	7	42	8
AC	42	8	44	6	44	6

Other modifications may be described. In the dorso-medial nucleus comparison between the YC and the AC disclose some modifications of DR cells. The mean length of terminal segments increases inthe horizontal plane of the adult cat (47.4±, 11.9 in YC VS 60.7± 17.9 in AC, t = 3.8, P< 0.01). The number of spines/micron also slightly increases in the terminal segments.

In the central nucleus the number of terminal segments of DR cells of AC increases in the sagittal plane (17.9± 4.1 in YC vs 20.4± 5.9 in AC, t= 2.9, P< 0.01) and decreases in the vertico-frontal plane (22.8± 7.7 in YC vs 16.6± 2.8 in AC, t= 4.8, P< 0.01). These modifications are correlated with an increase of the mean length of the proximal segments of DR cells in the sagittal plane (39.1± 13.8 in YC vs 55.4± 16.9 in AC, t= 4.8, P< 0.01). So it is possible to suggest from YC to AC a reorientation of the dendritic tree or DR cells. In the dorso-medial nucleus it seems that the orientation plane is the horizontal one. In the central nucleus the orientation plane is the sagittal one. Such a modification fits well with pysiological (4) and anatomical (3) data which described laminae or isofrequency contours in the central nucleus of the AC and a spatial distribution of the cells mostly in the sagittal plane as suggested by the figure 3 of Rockel and Jones (10). We did not observe a spatial modification of the dendritic tree of the CB cells.

The embryological evolution of the rat's inferior colliculus may be divided in three stages.

Before the 16th day post mating (p.m.) most of the cells of the I.C. remains at the stage of the post migratory neuroblasts. In the external of the I.C. few axons are observed with some slightly differentiated cells. In the C.N. the cells are in a similar state of differentiation and remain at a stage of post migratory neuroblast. On the 17th day p.m., in the external part of the I.C. numerous cells differentiate and establish contacts with the axons of the cells of the C.N.. At the same stage it is possible to observe a differentiation of the cells of the C.N.. On the 18th day p.m. the internal part of the I.C. is invaded by axons. This phenomenon is correlated with a cell differentiation. The cell differentiation of the C.N. occurs at the same rate. After this stage the cells of both the I.C. and the C.N. continue to differentiate. Growth cones and filopodia are observed until the 4th postnatal week.

So it seems that at least the I.C. and the C.N. of the rat differentiate altogether at a critical period (17th and 18th day p.m.). We are not able to observe the successive stages of differentiation claimed by Morest (11), in his description of the "temporal sequence" of differentiation of the auditory nuclei. However, our data fit well those of Morest (11) in his assumption of the function of dendritic branches. The functional maturation of the afferents appears as a factor of stablization of the post synaptic elements and contribute to the definite remodelling of these elements in the post natal period. As suggested by Changeux et al. (12) in his "stabilization theory" it seems that the increase of specifity in a system is followed by the active stabilization of the post synaptic elements at critical periods of development.

(Partially supported by D.G.R.S.T. Grant 78.7.2766)

References:

1) Van Noort, J.: The structure and connections of the inferior colliculus. Van Gorcum, Leiden (1969).
2) Adams, J.C.: Ascending projections to the inferior colliculus. J.Comp.Neurol. 183, 519-538 (1979).
3) Geniec, M. and Morest, D.K.: The neuronal architecture of the human posterior colliculus. Acta oto-laryngol., Suppl. 295 (1971).
4) Merzenich, M.M. and Reid, M.D.: Representation of the cochlea within the inferior colliculus of the cat. Brain Res. 77, 397-415 (1974).
5) Meininger, V.; Baudrimont, M.: The cytoarchitecture of the inferior colliculus in the cat. J.Neurol.Sci. 34, 25-36 (1977).
6) Marty, R.: Maturation post natale du systême auditif. In: A. Minkowski (ed.): Regional development of the brain in early life. Oxford, Edinburgh, Blackwell (1967).
7) Shofer, R.J.; Sax, D.S.; Strom, M.G.: Analysis of auditory and cerebrocortically evoked activity in the immature and adult cat cerebellum. In: Llinas, R. (ed.): Neurobiology of cerebellar evolution and development. A.M.A. (1969).
8) Berry, M.; Bradley, M.M.: The application of network analysis to the study of branching patterns of large dendritic fields. Brain Res. 109, 11-132 (1976).

9) Haggett, P. and Chorley, R.J.: Network analysis in geography. In: E. Arnold (ed.), London (1974).
10) Rockel, A.J. and Jones, E.G.: The neuronal organization of the inferior colliculus of the adult cat. I. The central nucleus. J.Comp.Neurol. 147, 11-60 (1973).
11) Morest, D.K.: The growth of dendrites in the mammalian brain. J.Anat.Entwickl.Gesch. 128, 290-317 (1969).
12) Changeux, J.P.; Danchin, A.: The selective stabilization of developing synapses as a mechanism for the specification of neuronal network. Nature (London) 264, 705-712 (1976).

Functional and Topographic Organization of the Auditory Cortex

M. M. MERZENICH, R. A. ANDERSEN, J. H. MIDDLEBROOKS,
Coleman Laboratory, University of California at San Francisco, CA 94143, USA

1. Organization of Auditory Cortical Fields

a) Redefinition of field boundaries: Four cochleotopically organized fields have now been defined in the cat auditory cortex, on the basis of extensive microelectrode mapping studies within these fields (Figure 1). Al borders an anterior auditory field (AAF) rostrally[12,16] and a posterior auditory field (PAF) caudally.[16,21] There is a highly ordered representation of the cochlear sensory epithelium within Al, with the cochlear apex (lowest frequencies) represented rostrally. There is a reversal in the representational sequence across both the rostral and caudal borders of Al, i.e., highest frequencies are represented along the AAF-Al border; lowest frequencies are represented along the PAF-Al border; and the frequency sequences within AAF and PAF are in a reverse order to (mirrors) those in Al. Ventrally, the posterior field borders a fourth topographically organized field, the ventro-posterior field (VPAF). There is a reversal in representational sequence across the VPAF-PAF border, with highest frequencies represented along this border, and with the representational sequence in VPAF the reverse of that described for PAF.

As has been described earlier,[16,17,12] the boundaries of these identified fields are somewhat different from those of the earlier defined fields of Woolsey[26,27] (see Figure 1). This is at least principally because Woolsey always assigned large evoked response foci generated by apical or basal cochlear

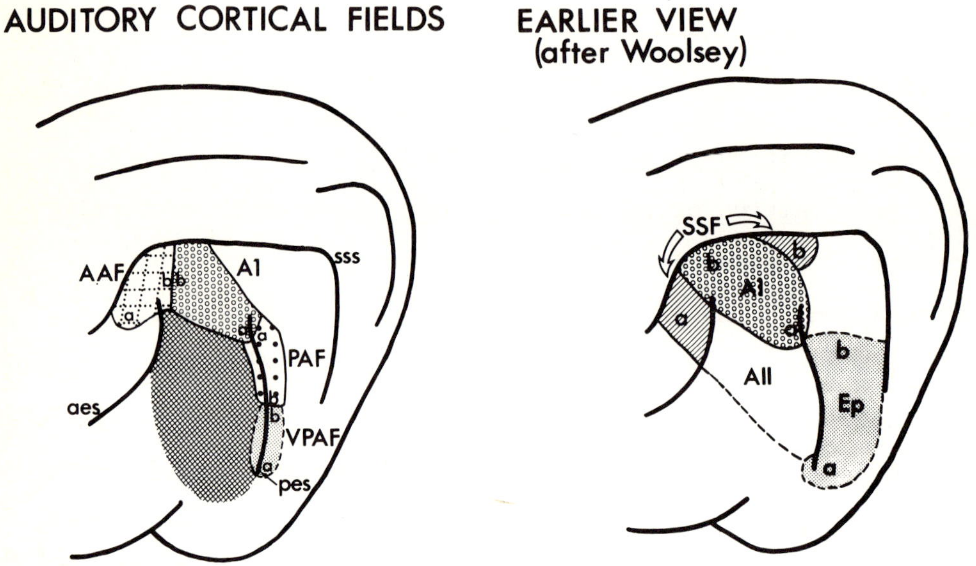

Fig. 1. LEFT: Schematic representation of the basic organization of auditory cortical fields in the cat. A1= primary auditory field; AAF=anterior auditory field; PAF=posterior auditory field; VPAF=ventroposterior auditory field. PAF and VPAF are largely buried within the posterior ectosylvian sulcus (pes). AAF is usually largely buried within the anterior ectosylvian sulcus (aes) and suprasylvian sulcus (sss); A1 almost always lies partly within the sss, pes, and less frequently, the aes. The region of representation of the cochlear apex (a) and cochlear base (b) is indicated for all four of these cochleotopically organized fields. A1, AAF, PAF and VPAF comprise four principle cortical divisions of the so-called "cochleotopic auditory system" (see text). AII and the so called temporal fields (collectively the area crosshatched in the figure) comprise the cortical fields of a parallel "diffuse auditory system". The number of these "non-topographic" cortical fields and their boundaries are not known; the cortical area that they occupy is very large. Note that the actual boundaries of these fields are very different in different cats. Therefore, this schematic drawing can not be taken as representing cortical field locations or boundaries in any given cat. RIGHT: Earlier view of cat auditory cortical fields, after Woolsey[26,27]. Ep=posterior ectosylvian field, SSF=suprasylvian fringe; other abbreviations as above.

stimulation and arising from regions of representational reversals to a single cortical "field". Recent microelectrode maps have revealed, again, that these response foci invariably arose from the bordering regions of two fields. Considered in this light, the experimental data of Woolsey and colleagues is wholly consistent with the results of contemporary microelectrode mapping studies. But: 1) AI is much smaller than as defined by Woolsey (see Figure 1); 2) there is a complete representation (AAF) just rostral to AI, i.e., this rostral representation does not extend caudally over the top of AI as a "suprasylvian fringe"; and 3) there are two complete fields in the classical "Ep" region.

It should also be emphasized that these fields have an inconstant location, when referenced to brain surface landmarks[27,16,17,12] which are themselves inconstant[23,11,16]. As a consequence of these factors, for example, in some cats most of AI is within or caudal to the posterior ectosylvian sulcus; while in other cats, most of AI is rostral to the posterior ectosylvian sulcus, and may lie partially within the anterior ectosylvian sulcus. Therefore the schematic drawing in Figure 1 represents the organization of fields in a hypothetical cat, not to be presumed to apply for any other.

The inconstancy of field location and redefinition of field boundaries in cats (and in monkeys[14,15]) raise serious problems for auditory cortical research. First, all earlier cortical ablation-behavioral, recording and anatomical studies have been conducted with reference to the earlier maps, and must be interpreted accordingly. But as cortical field locations are inconstant, those interpretations are invariably further clouded.

Thus, these factors necessitate definition of cortical field boundaries as a part of any experiment within specific auditory cortical fields. In actual practice neurophysiological controls (limited maps) are required, as the cytoarchitectonic boundaries of auditory cortical fields are difficult to define (especially in the cat, where the rostral and caudal borders of AI commonly fall within sulci).

b) Internal organization of the topographically organized cortical fields. "Cochleotopic" representation and binaural bands: One unique feature of the auditory nervous system is the representation of the sensory epithelium across one axis of the cochleotopically organized auditory fields. The auditory sensory epithelium is a line of cells, of insignificant width. In its representation in the cortex, any point along this line is itself represented along an a line (an "isofrequency contour") in AI. It was Woolsey and Walzl[28] who first appreciated a mediolateral extension of response in AI, consequent from stimulation of a point along the sensory epithelium. Tunturi[25] and Merzenich and colleagues[16] later emphasized this unique feature of organization of auditory cortical fields, and revealed in strychnine spike and unit mapping studies that any given sector of the auditory sensory epithelium occupied a band of cortex of constant width, that extended across AI from edge to edge. This basic organization is illustrated for AI and AAF in Figure 2A. All other defined cochleotopically organized fields appear to have this same basic organization (see Knight[12] and Imig, et al.[9]).

Recently, studies in Al have revealed a segregation of neurons with different binaural response properties into bands roughly orthogonal to isofrequency contours[18,19,6,7] (see Figure 2). In alternating bands in at least anesthetized cats (see Irvine and Phillips[20]), neurons are predominantly "excitatory-inhibitory" (driven by contralateral stimulation with driven responses inhibited by ipsilateral stimulation); or, in the second set of bands, "excitatory-excitatory" (driven by both contralateral and ipsilateral stimulation; or driven by one or the other ear, with the response strongly facilitated by stimulation of the other). There are probably three excitatory-inhibitory (EI) bands, and two or three excitatory-excitatory (EE) bands in Al (see Figure 2B for a schematic description of this organization).

There is anatomical evidence suggesting that the three other topographically organized fields in the cat also have alternating EE and EI binaural bands (see Andersen[1] and Imig and Reale[8]). Corresponding alternating EI and EE response sequences have recently been recorded in AAF[9].

It should be noted that there is also anatomical evidence for a banded organization of at least Al in primates, inherent in the classical cytoarchitectonic descriptions of the koniocortex in man especially by von Economo. He described auditory koniocortex as banded, with the koniocortical bands separated by less granular cortical strips. However, there is as yet no direct physiological demonstration of an alternating EE and EI banding in auditory cortical fields in primates.

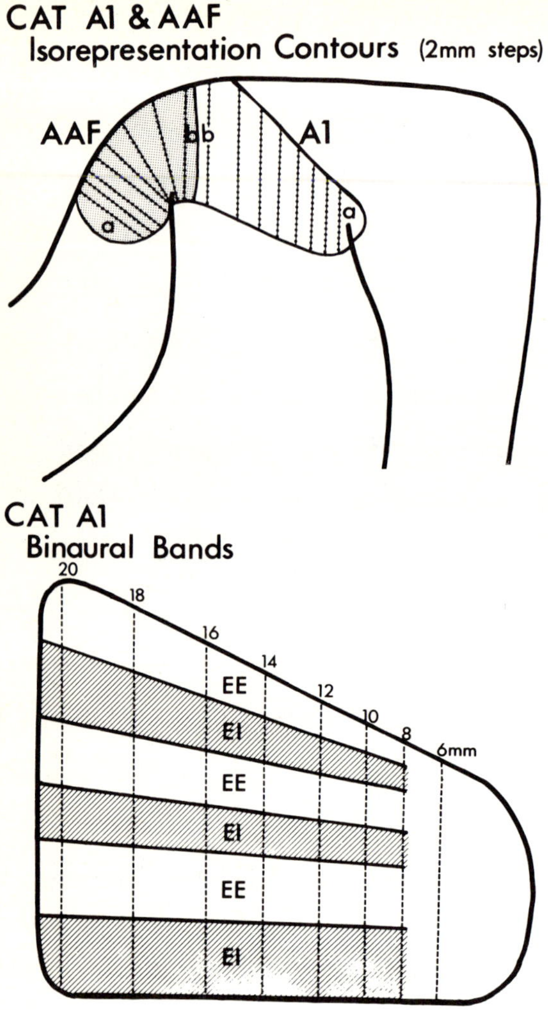

Fig. 2. Internal organization of cochleotopically auditory fields in the cat. TOP: Representation of the cochlea within two auditory fields, the "primary" field (A1) and the anterior field (AAF). Dotted lines are isorepresentational contours, indicating the lines over the cortical map over which points on the cochlear sensory epithelium about 2 mm apart are represented. The most apical isorepresentational contour represents a point on the cochlear 6 mm from the extreme apex. Note that any given sector of the cochlea (any given band of frequency) is represented across a band of cortex in A1 of approximately constant width, that extends across the field from edge to edge. This "rerepresentation" of the sensory epithelium across one axis of these fields is a unique feature of auditory cortical representations. Also note the disproportionately greater areal representation of the basal cochlea. Modified

c) "Non-topographic" auditory cortical fields: The auditory system is unique, in that there are cortical fields bordering the above defined topographically organized fields in which no clearly ordered representation of the cochlear sensory epithelium can be defined. By contrast to the topographically organized fields, tuning curves of neurons studied in these "non-topographic" cortical fields are characteristically very broad; and when best frequencies can be defined for these poorly tuned neurons, it is difficult to demonstrate an orderly representational sequence within these fields. The response characteristics of neurons within these "non-topographically" organized fields have been little studied. There are several such fields in cats, and at least one such field (the "caudomedial field") in primates[15].

d) The "cochleotopic" and "non-topographic" fields appear to constitute cortical processing regions for two largely segregated auditory projection systems: Recent neurophysiological and especially neuroanatomical studies[1-4] have led to the hypothesis that there are two large and largely segregated auditory projection systems in the cat. A "cochleotopic" sytem projects from the central nucleus of the inferior colliculus in the mid-

---

Cont. Fig. 2.
from Merzenich, et al.[17] and Knight[12]. BOTTOM: Schematic representation of the binaural bands of primary auditory cortex (Al) in the cat. Within this large cortical field, neurons within alternate bands orthogonal to the isopresentational (or isofrequency) contours (dashed lines) have predominantly excitatory-excitatory or excitatory-inhibitory (shaded) response. Contours representing points along the cochlear sensory epithelium 2 mm apart (6 to 20 mm) are illustrated schematically. There is actually very significant variability in the widths and exact position of these bands in different individual cats. Based on studies of Middlebrooks, et al.[19]

brain to the ventral division and deep part of the dorsal division in the auditory thalamus to the cochleotopically organized AI, AAF, PAF and VPAF; and a "diffuse" system, projects from the pericentral nucleus of the inferior colliculus *via* the caudal part of the dorsal nucleus and the ventrolateral nucleus in the thalamus to the non-cochleotopically organized auditory cortical fields (see Figure 1). Ascending and descending projections interconnecting the central nucleus of the inferior colliculus, component thalamic nuclei and the cochleotopically organized fields in the cochleotopic system are complex, but are all highly ordered. No clear order to the almost equally complex projections interconnecting the pericentral inferior colliculus with component thalamic nuclei and non-topographically organized cortical fields of the "diffuse" system can be discerned. Within the cochleotopic system, as reviewed before, neurons commonly have sharply defined best frequencies (sharply peaked tuning curves), and all component nuclei of the system can be demonstrated to be strictly cochleotopically organized. Within the diffuse system, tuning curves are characteristically very broad, and with the exception of the pericentral nucleus of the inferior colliculus, no topographic order has been demonstrated in any of its component nuclei or cortical fields.

2. There are Complex Convergent Projection Arrays from the Auditory Thalamus to Auditory Cortical Fields

Note that within the component nuclei of the cochleotopic projection system, there is a further dimension of the representation of the cochlea, i.e., within these nuclei, any point along the cochlear sensory epithelium is represented across a sheet of neurons that extends across these nuclei from edge to edge[17]. Retrograde injection (HRP) tracing studies have revealed that a restricted cortical locus less than 1 mm in diameter (i.e., extending across only a fraction of the length of an AI isofrequency contour) receives input from the topographically appropriate sheet of neurons, about 1 1/2 to 4 mm in length and 1-2 mm high in the ventral nucleus; as well as from a column of neurons several mm long, continuous from the medial division through the deep part of the dorsal division, and through the lateral part of the posterior group[5]. This basic neuronal array is seen to project to restricted cortical sites all along AI isofrequency contours, for injections that spread only 1/4-1/5 of the distance across the field. If multiple injections are made along isofrequency contours, this array does not change, i.e., the array projecting to 1/4 of the isofrequency contour is the same as that projecting to all of it. This suggests that there are spatially equivalent projections to repeating cortical subunits, e.g., to each of a set of adjacent EE and EI bands.

With still smaller injections, projection arrays in the ventral division are commonly seen to be discontinuous, i.e., there are columns of label within the framework of the overall projecting lateral neuronal sheet. From one to five columns of label have been seen in different projection cases, separated by columns or bands in which labelling is far lighter (or in which no labelling is recorded). We do not yet understand how this discontinuous labelling relates to the banded organization of the cochleotopically organized fields.

3. Response Characteristics of Cortical Neurons in A1; Specific Sources of Input to the Auditory Cortical Fields

The sources of input to the binaural bands of A1 have not been defined. A large number of auditory nuclei project to the central nucleus of the inferior colliculus, the source nucleus for the "cochleotopic" projection system. (Indeed, if response-specific neuronal populations of the cochlear nucleus complex are considered as separated sources, 13 major neuronal populations project to the central nucleus.) It has recently been demonstrated that these different inputs are processed at least largely in parallel in at least largely segregated regions of the ICC (see Roth et al.[22] and Jones[10]). Anatomical studies suggest that every source nucleus of the ICC of the cat has a different target region withing it[22], sometimes clearly overlapping with the target regions of other sources. Despite these apparently non-coincident target regions of different source nuclei, some sources of input to the ICC appear to be convergent on others. Thus, neurons in the ICC never respond as if they were deriving their input from at least two major anatomically-defined sources[22]. Finally, it is clear that input from these various sources all projects onto the same basic neural processing machinery, the cell laminae of the ICC.

This complex and largely segregated multisource projection to the midbrain is without parallel in other sensory systems. What neuronal processing could be performed in common by the ICC on its various binaural and monaural inputs? How is this multisource information processed separately or convergently in the complex divergent-convergent projections from ICC to cortical fields? And just what input in what form is actually delivered to the binaural bands of auditory cortical fields? These are now central questions for auditory anatomists and neurophysiologists. Embedded within these questions is a more elementary one, relevant to cortical field organization: Are the binaural bands of auditory cortical fields individual cortical processing units - e.g., terminal processing units of source-specific parts of the cochleotopic projection system? Or is AI the processing machine?

In the recent important studies of auditory cortex in the mustache bat, Suga and colleagues have demonstrated that sectors of a large cochleotopically organized cortical field spatially represent different aspects of this bat's behaviorally important echolocation signals, i.e., they have described a series of functional maps beyond the cochleotopic map in a large auditory cortical field (see reference 24, for an introduction to this important work). Are the binaural bands of AI in the cat singly or together (EE and EI pairs) equivalent subdivisions of the field, individually accounting for some aspect of auditory perception or behavior? Consistent with that possibility is the observation that the response properties of neurons in different binaural bands of like class are not identical. Against that conclusion is abundant anatomical evidence that different bands of the same class (i.e., all EE or all EI bands) receive input from the same thalamic neuronal arrays; and all appear to receive input from any single band of the same class in other cortical fields. As with the studies of Suga and colleagues, the practical question devolves to what is represented along isofrequency contours within the binaural bands of Al. That question is now being intensely investigated.

It should be noted that the several almost equal-sized cochleotopically organized fields in the cat are complexely, reciprocally interconnected[1,9]. The anatomical relationships, heavy direct thalamic inputs and physiological response properties strongly suggest that they should be regarded as parallel information processing areas, simultaneously activated and in operation for any auditory stimulus, i.e., Al has no obvious primacy over the other cochleotopic cortical fields.

The sources of input to the very large "diffuse" projection system are, astoundingly, not known, i.e., the sources of input to the pericentral nucleus of the inferior colliculus have still not been unequivocally determined. Note that the "non-topographic" fields of this system are only defined as such on the basis of their apparent lack of cochleotopic organization, i.e., there may be another basis for their topographic order. Thus, for example, Knudsen and Konishi[13] have recently described a systematic representation of sound space in an apparently non-cochleotopic region in the midbrain in the barn owl. Interestingly, this nucleus has a similar relationship to the apparent cochleotopically organized homologue of the mammalian central nucleus, as does the pericentral nucleus to the central nucleus of the cat.

From this brief summary of recent and ongoing work in the auditory forebrain, it should be evident that we are now beginning to understand the basic framework of the cortical processing machinery in the auditory system. The organization of projections to the system are more complex than in other sensory systems. We have seen interesting evidence for potentially very sophisticated spatial processing of information. We are uncertain as to how information from the many different brain stem sources are distributed to different cortical fields, or to the binaural bands within the cochleotopically organized fields. But we have made the essential step of defining large cortical processing subunits, so that a productive, directed search for how auditory perception and behavior are a product of the auditory forebrain can begin in earnest.

Acknowledgments: This work was supported by NIH Grant NS-10414, by the John C. and Edward Coleman Memorial Fund, and by Hearing Research, Inc. Described work from the Coleman Laboratory included the research contributions of many investigators as well as the authors, especially Drs. Linn Roth, Lindsay Aitkin, Robert Dykes, Steven Colwell, Paul Knight and Russell Snyder.

References:

1) Andersen, R.A.: Patterns of Connectivity of the Auditory Forebrain of the Cat. Thesis, University of California at San Francisco, San Francisco, CA. (1979).
2) Andersen, R.A., Snyder, R.L., and Merzenich, M.M.: Thalamocortical and corticothalamic connections of Al, AII and AAF in the cat. (Submitted for publication, J.Comp.Neurol.) (1979).
3) Andersen, M.M., Snyder, R.L., and Merzenich, M.M.: Corticotectal and other descending connections of Al, AII and AAF in the cat. (Submitted for publication, J.Comp.Neurol.) (1979).
4) Andersen, R.A., Roth, G.L., Aitkin, L.M., and Merzenich, M.M.: The topography of projection of the central nucleus of the inferior colliculus to the medial geniculate body of the cat. (Submitted for publication, J.Comp.Neurol.) (1979).
5) Colwell, S.A., and Merzenich, M.M.: Corticothalamic projections from physiologically defined loci in Al in the cat. J.Comp.Neurol. (in press) (1979).
6) Imig, T.J., and Adrian, H.O.: Binaural columns in the primary field (Al) of cat auditory cortex. Brain Res. 138, 241-257 (1978).
7) Imig, T.J., and Brugge, J.F.: Sources and terminations of callosal axons related to binaural and frequency maps in primary cortex of the cat. J.Comp.Neurol. 182, 637-660 (1978).

8) Imig, T.J., and Reale, R.A.: The origins and targets of corticocortical connections related to tonotopic maps of cat auditory cortex. Neuroscience Abstrs. 3, 8 (1977).
9) Imig, T.J., Reale, R.A., and Brugge, J.F.: Patterns of corticocortical projections related to physiological maps of cat auditory cortex. Federation Proceedings (in press) (1979).
10) Jones, D.: Ascending auditory pathways to inferior colliculus in the tree shrew. Neuroscience Abstrs. 2, 20 (1976).
11) Kawamura, K.: Variations of the cerebral sulci in the cat. Acta Anat. 80, 204-221 (1971).
12) Knight, P.L.: Representation of the cochlea within the anterior auditory field (AAF) of the cat. Brain Res. 130, 447-467 (1977).
13) Knudsen, E.I., and Konishi, M.: A neural map of auditory space in the owl. Science 200, 795-797 (1978).
14) Merzenich, M.M., and Brugge, J.F.: Representation of the cochlear partition on the superior temporal plane of the macaque monkey. Brain Res. 50, 275-296 (1973).
15) Merzenich, M.M., and Kaas, J.: Principles of organization of sensory-perceptual systems in mammals. In: Progress in Psychobiology and Physiological Psychology, Vol. IX, J.M. Sprague and A.N. Epstein, eds., Academic Press, N.Y. (in press) (1979).
16) Merzenich, M.M., Roth, R.A., Knight, P.L., and Colwell, S. A.: Some basic features of organization of the central auditory system. In: Psychophysics and Physiology of Hearing, E.F. Evans and J.P. Wilson, eds., Academic Press, London (1977).
17) Merzenich, M.M., Knight, P.L., and Roth, G.L.: Representation of cochlea within primary auditory cortex in the cat. J.Neurophysiol. 38, 231-249 (1975).
18) Middlebrooks, J.D., Dykes, R.W., and Merzenich, M.M.: Binaural responsespecific bands within Al in the cat: specialization within isofrequency contours. Neuroscience Abstr. 4, 8 (1978).
19) Middlebrooks, J.D., Dykes, R.W., and Merzenich, M.M.: Binaural responsespecific bands in primary cortex (Al) of the cat: Topographical organization orthogonal to isofrequency contours. (Submitted for publication) (1979).
20) Phillips, D.P., and Irvine, D.R.F.: Methodological considerations in mapping auditory cortex: Binaural columns in Al of cat. Brain Res. 161, 342-346 (1979).
21) Reale, R.A., and Imig, T.J.: An orderly frequency representation in the posterior ectosylvian sulcus of the cat. Neuroscience Abstr. 3, 10 (1977).
22) Roth, G.L., Aitkin, L.M., Andersen, R.A., and Merzenich, M.M.: Some features of the spatial organization of the central nucleus of the inferior colliculus of the cat. J.Comp.Neurol. 182, 661-680 (1978).
23) Rose, J.E.: The cellular structure of the auditory region of the cat. J.Comp.Neurol. 91, 409-440 (1949).
24) Suga, N., O'Neill, W.E., and Manabe, T.: Harmonic sensitive neurons in the auditory cortex of the mustache bat. Science 203 270-274 (1979).
25) Tunturi, A.R.: Physiological determination of the arrangement of the afferent connections to the middle ectosylvian area in the dog. Aerm.J.Physiol. 162, 489-502 (1950).

26) Woolsey, C.N.: Organization of cortical auditory system: A review and a synthesis. In: Neural Mechanisms of the Auditory and Vestibular Systems. G. Rasmussen and W. Windle, eds., C. Thomas, Springfield, Ill., 165-180 (1960).
27) Woolsey, C.N.: Organization of cortical system. In: Sensory Communication, W.A. Rosenblith, ed., MIT Press, Cambridge, Mass., 235-257 (1961).
28) Woolsey, C.N., and Walzl, E.M.: Topical projections of nerve fibers from local regions of the cochlea to the cerebral cortex of the cat. Bull. Johns Hopkins Hosp. 71, 315-344 (1942)

II) The Representation of Complex Natural Sounds in the Auditory System

Neural Image of Sound in the Grassfrog

PETER JOHANNESMA and AD AERTSEN, Workgroup Neurophysics, Dept. of Medical Physics and Biophysics, University of Nijmegen, Foundation for Biophysics, Organisation for the Advancement of Pure Research ZWO. The Netherlands.

Representation of simple elements of sound can be given either in temporal form by display of the waveform as function of time or in spectral form, either by real and imaginary part or by intensity and phase as function of frequency. For complex non-stationary sounds a combined spectro-temporal representation is better suited. This type of image is more directly related to auditory perception.

The spectro-temporal image of sound has a long tradition. For the notation of music notes on a staff display both frequency and temporal order. Intensity however has to be indicated in a separate form. In the musical notation timbre is missing altogether; only fundamental tones are represented, the higher harmonics are absent. Knowledge of the instrument on which the musical composition is performed is necessary to know the timbre. This lack of information has been overcome in the sonogram or dynamic spectrum which is widely used for the study of animal vocalisations and human speech (Potter et al., 1947; Singleton and Poulter, 1967). The sonogram displays the intensity of each spectral component as it increases and decreases in the course of time; as a consequence it includes both pitch and timbre as function of time.

In experimental practice the oscilloscope displays the acoustic waves as function of time, a digital computer supplies the spectral information while an analog or digital spectral analyser produces the combined spectro-temporal image of sound (Fig. C)..

The sonogram however has two drawbacks. The filters analysing different frequency components have to be chosen a priori with respect to both center of frequency and spectral width. This may be an absolute width e.g. 1, 10 or 100 Hz or a relative width e.g. 1/10 or 1/3 of an octave. The choice of spectral resolution also determines the temporal resolution, since one varies inversely with the other. A second limitation of a spectral analyser is the fact that each filter measures only the intensity of the sound for its own spectral region, other spectral regions are analysed independently. This implies that coherent aspects of sounds, phase-relations between different spectral components, will be absent in the sonogram. As a consequence it may be difficult or impossible to see in the sonogram the difference between a Gaussian process and a Poisson process with the same spectrum (wind and rain).

As a solution to these deficiencies of the sonogram we propose the <u>Complex Spectro-Temporal Intensity Density</u> (CoSTID) representation of a sound. Based on the work of Gabor (1946) and Ville (1948) on the complementarity of frequency and time this function has been introduced by Rihaczek (1968) under the name "complex energy density function". It is isomorphic, under double Fourier transformation, with the ambiguity function, which is used in the theory of radar signals (Woodward, 1953;

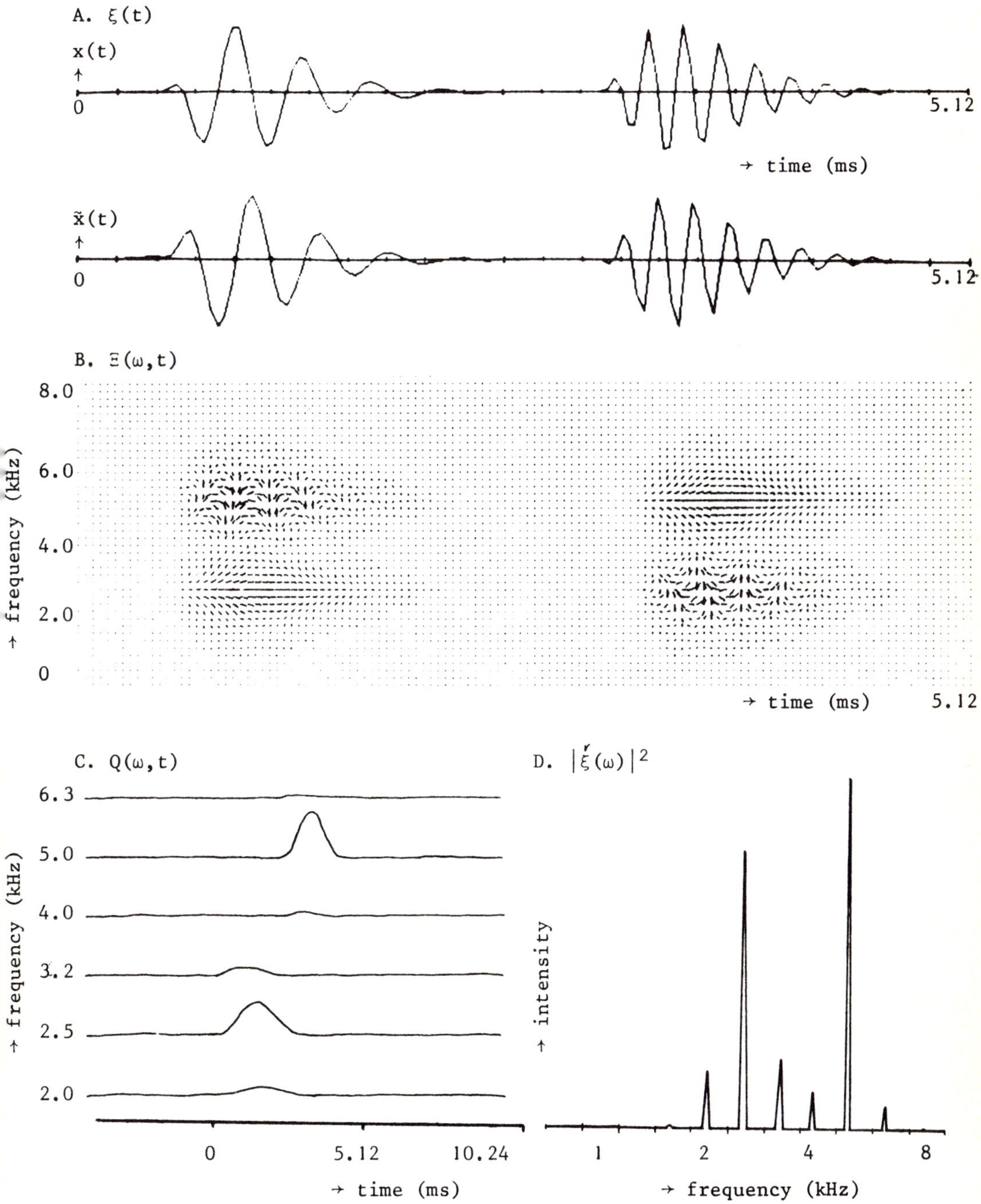

A. analytic signal $\xi(t)$: signal $x(t)$ and quadrature signal $\tilde{x}(t)$.

B. CoSTID-function $\Xi(\omega,t)$ of signal $x(t)$.

C. sonogram or dynamic spectrum $Q(\omega,t)$ of signal $x(t)$.

D. power spectrum $|\check{\xi}(\omega)|^2$ of signal $x(t)$.

Rihaczek, 1969) and in the study of echolocation in bats (Altes, 1973; Beuter, 1976).

The definition of the CoSTID-function is based on the concept of the analytic signal. If the real acoustic signal is given by x(t), then the analytic signal is a complex signal constructed by addition of the quadrature signal $\tilde{x}$ (t) as an imaginary part

$$\xi(t) = x(t) + i\tilde{x}(t) \tag{1}$$

where $\tilde{x}(t)$ = quadrature signal or Hilbert transformation of sound signal x(t) (Fig. A).

As a consequence the analytic signal has the same spectrum as x(t) for positive frequencies, but zero intensity at negative frequencies

$$\begin{aligned} \check{\xi}(\omega) &= 2\ \check{x}(\omega) && \omega > 0 \\ &= 0 && \omega < 0\ , \quad \omega = 2\pi f \end{aligned} \tag{2}$$

The intensity of the signal as function of times is then given by $|\check{\xi}(\omega)|^2$ (Fig. D).

The CoSTID function combines the temporal and the spectral form of the analytic signal. It is defined as

$$\Xi(\omega,t) = \check{\xi}^*(\omega)e^{-i\omega t}\xi(t) \tag{3}$$

where "*" denotes complex conjugation (Fig. B). It can easily be shown that the CoSTID is identical with the Fourier transform of the time dependent autocorrelation function of the analytic signal

$$\Xi(\omega,t) = \int d\tau\ e^{-i\omega t}\xi^*(t-\tau)\ \xi(t) \tag{4}$$

The CoSTID may be considered as the complex distribution of energy or intensity of the signal for all (ω,t)-values. Integration of the CoSTID leads to the usual expressions for the intensity. Spectral integration gives the temporal intensity

$$\int d\omega \quad \Xi(\omega,t) = \xi^*(t) \quad \xi(t) = |\xi(t)|^2 \tag{5}$$

whereas temporal integration leads to the spectral intensity

$$\int dt \quad \Xi(\omega,t) = \check{\xi}^*(\omega) \quad \check{\xi}(\omega) = |\check{\xi}(\omega)|^2 . \tag{6}$$

The CoSTID forms a generating function for all types of sonograms. Spectro-temporal integration with a weight-function which corresponds to the CoSTID of the impulse response f(t) of a linear filter gives a real and positive function which is equal to the temporal intensity of the output of that filter in response to the given sound. The mathematical equation reads

$$Q_f(t) = \frac{1}{8\pi} \int d\omega \int d\tau \quad \Phi(\omega,\tau) \quad \Xi(\omega,t-\tau) \tag{7}$$

where $\Xi(\omega,t)$ = CoSTID of signal x(t)

$\Phi(\omega,t)$ = CoSTID of filter impulse response f(t)

$Q_f(t)$ = intensity of output of filter.

Application of this procedure on a set of parallel bandpass filters generates the sonogram of a specific sound. The choice of different spectro-temporal weight-functions leads to a different type of sonogram. In this way all possible sonograms of a sound or vocalisation can be derived from the CoSTID function of this sound.

The distinctive property of the CoSTID is the preservation of phase relations of different tonal components in the spectro-temporal image. In this way coherent aspects of sound, vocalisation and speech can be evaluated.

Since the CoSTID is a complex function of two arguments, it can be regarded as vector field defined on two-dimensional (ω,t)-space. As such it can be represented by means of arrows located in the different spectro-temporal positions (Fig. B). A representation which is more suited to the characteristics of visual perception is based on the use of colour. Different colour aspects are used to indicate the components of a complex function: red and green for real and imaginary part, or hue and saturation for amplitude and phase of a complex variable for a given spectro-temporal position. In this way sound is represented by a two-dimensional colour image: the phonochrome. Examples of phonochromes, generated by a computer controlled colour display, will be shown for some artificial sounds.

Two applications of the CoSTID function will be presented. The first one is related to the study of animal vocalisation, in this case segments from the calls of Rana temporaria L. The question is considered if vocalisations of the grassfrog may be described as a sequence of invariant sound elements, only varying in amplitude and time of occurrence. An affirmative answer would then suggest the definition of phonemes as constitutive elements for the calls of a grassfrog; for some vocalisations this appears to be correct.

The second application is related to single unit recordings in the Torus semicircularis of the grassfrog (Aertsen and Johannesma, 1979b). A completely unstructured stimulus, Gaussian white noise, is presented to the animal. The segments of sounds preceding the occurrence of neural events are assembled in the Pre Event Stimulus Ensemble. For each of these sound segments the CoSTID-function is computed and then averaged over the Pre-Event Stimulus Ensemble (Johannesma, 1972; Aertsen et al.,1979a)

$$\langle \Xi(\omega,t) \rangle = \frac{1}{N} \sum_{n=1}^{N} \Xi_n(\omega,t) \tag{8}$$

In this way we have constructed the average spectro-temporal intensity of the sound elements eliciting the action potentials from this neuron. A representation in the form of a phonochrome then gives a clear impression of the auditory receptive field of the neuron.

The foregoing approach can be fitted in the framework of the nonlinear system theory of Volterra, Wiener and Lee. Since the CoSTID function is equal to the Fourier transform of the time-dependent autocorrelation function, it follows that the average CoSTID of the Pre-Event Stimulus Ensemble is equal to the Fourier transform of the complex second order cross-correlation function of auditory stimulus and neural events.

Finally we reach a double conclusion. The CoSTID function of the Pre Event Stimulus Ensemble corresponds with the intuitive notion of spectro-temporal receptive field of an auditory neuron. Moreover it supplies a firm connection between auditory neurophysiology and system theory.

Acknowledgement: Members of the workgroup Neurophysics who contributed to this work: Bert Cranen, Leon van Erning, Dik Hermes and Arnold Hoeks.

References:

1) Aertsen, A.M.H.J., Smolders, J.W.T., Johannesma, P.I.M.: Neural representation of the Acoustic Biotope: On the existence of stimulus-event relations for sensory neurons. Biol. Cybern. 32, 175-185 (1979a).

2) Aertsen, A.M.H.J., Johannesma, P.I.M.: Spectro-temporal analysis of auditory neurons in the grassfrog. EBBS-workshop "Hearing mechanisms and speech" Göttingen 1979b.

3) Altes, R.A.: Some invariance properties of the wide-band ambiguity function. J.Acoust.Soc.Am. 53, 1154-1160 (1973).

4) Beuter, K.J.: Systemtheoretische Untersuchungen zur Echoortung der Fledermäuse. Diss. Tübingen 1976.

5) Gabor, D.: Theory of communication. Journ.IEE (London), pt III, 93, 429-457 (1946).

6) Johannesma, P.I.M.: The pre-response stimulus ensemble of neurons in the cochlear nucleus. In: Proc. IPO Symp. on Hearing Theory pp. 58-69, Cardozo, B.L., ed. Eindhoven, the Netherlands (1972).

7) Potter, R.K., Kopp, G.A., Green, H.C.: Visible speech. New York: Van Nostrand (1947).

8) Rihaczek, A.W.: Signal energy distribution in time and frequency. IEEE Tr. on Inf. theory IT-14, 369-374 (1968).

9) Rihaczek, A.W.: Principles of high resolution radar. New York: McGraw-Hill (1969).

10) Singleton, R.C., Poulter, T.C.: Spectral analysis of the call of the male killer whale. IEEE Tr. on Audio and El.acoust. AU 15, 104-113 (1967).

11) Ville, J.: Théorie et applications de la notion de signal analytique. Cables et Transmission 2, 61-74 (1948).

12) Woodward, P.M.: Probability and information theory with applications to radar. London: Pergamon (1953).

Spectro-Temporal Analysis of Auditory Neurons in the Grassfrog

AD AERTSEN and PETER JOHANNESMA, Workgroup Neurophysics, Dept. of Medical Physics and Biophysics, University of Nijmegen.
Foundation for Biophysics, Organization for the Advancement of Pure Research ZWO, the Netherlands.

Area of Research: Perception

- Representation of sensory environment in patterns of neural activity in the brain.

Object of investigation: Auditory System

- It is easy to record and generate sounds.
- Formal methods of describing sound in time and frequency domain are available.
- Peripheral part of auditory system has been investigated extensively.

Stimulus ensemble: Technical and natural sounds

- Technical sounds: tones, clicks and noise are simple from a signal theoretical point of view, give clear information about simple systems; have proven to be effective and fruitful in the investigation of peripheral part of auditory system, less, however, in central parts.
- Natural sounds: environmental sounds and vocalizations constitute an embodiment of the acoustic biotope, in which the nervous system has evolved and normally functions; in this context vocalizations serve a.o. the purpose of recognition

of species and sex; have proven to be effective stimuli to study central parts of auditory system.

Subject of investigation: Frog (Capranica, 1976)

- First vertebrate in evolution which accomplishes sound perception by means of air pressure variation.
- Repertoire of vocalizations well defined, functionally known, relatively simple to describe and to synthesize.
- Grassfrog (Rana temporaria L.) is subject of ecological and ethological investigation at Univ. of Nijmegen (Van Gelder et al., 1978).

Brain area: Torus Semicircularis

- Central part, functionally interesting, simple experimental preparation.

Method of measurement: Extra-cellular single-unit recording, aimed at measuring action potentials

- Action potentials constitute elementary units of communication between neurons.
- Amplitude and duration ($\simeq$ 3ms) of action potentials are hardly variable, information is contained in the moment of occurrence: point process, consisting of neural events:

$$z(t) = \sum_n \delta(t-t_n).$$

- Relatively long recording times (1-60 minutes) in these measurements are possible.

Experimental method: Stimulus-event-registration

- Long and varied stimulus ensemble x(t), consisting of technical and natural sounds is presented at least twice and neural activity z(t) is recorded.

- Stimulus and neural activity are stored on analog tape and in a digital computer.

Question: Stimulus-event-relation

- Existence: does a relation exist between acoustic stimulus and simultaneously occurring action potentials?
- Nature: if so, what is the nature of this relation? Which stimulus properties determine the occurrence of neural events?
- Both existence and nature can depend on stimulation of other sensory modalities (visual, tactile) or external factors like attention, anaesthesia, hormonal condition.

Existence of stimulus-event-relation:

If first stimulus presentation results in $z_1(t)$ and second presentation gives $z_2(t)$, then the correlation function

$$R_{z_1 z_2}(\tau) = \frac{1}{T} \int_o^T dt\; z_1(t)\; z_2(t+\tau)$$

especially in the neighbourhood of $\tau = o$, gives an indication of the influence of the acoustic stimulus on the firing pattern of the neuron (Aertsen et al., 1979).

Investigation into the nature of the stimulus-event-relation

A. Definition of Pre-Event-Stimulus Ensemble PESE (Johannesma, 1972):

PRE EVENT STIMULUS ENSEMBLE (PESE)

$\stackrel{D}{=}$ ensemble of sensory stimuli which are followed by a neural event

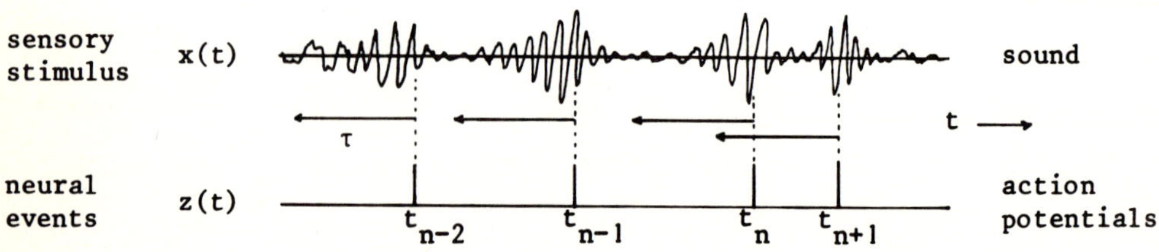

$$z(t) = \sum_{n=1}^{N} \delta(t-t_n)$$

t_n = moment of occurrence of action potential

N = number of events

PESE : $X_e = \{ x_n(\tau) = x(t_n-\tau) \; ; \; n = 1,\ldots,N \}$

B. Properties of PESE describe the relation between sensory stimulus and neural events.

1. <u>average</u> value of PESE (first order moment function)

$$r_e(\tau) = \frac{1}{N} \sum_{n=1}^{N} x_n(\tau) = \frac{1}{N} \sum_{n=1}^{N} x(t_n-\tau) = \frac{T}{N} \frac{1}{T} \int_{o}^{T} dt \; x(t-\tau).z(t)$$

so: average of stimuli preceding a neural event is proportional to first order cross correlation function of input- and output-signal. (De Boer and Kuyper, 1968; Johannesma, 1972; Grashuis, 1974; De Boer and De Jongh, 1978).

2. <u>second order moment function</u> of PESE

$$q_e(\sigma,\tau) = \frac{1}{N} \sum_{n=1}^{N} x_n(\sigma) \; x_n(\tau) = \frac{1}{N} \sum_{n=1}^{N} x(t_n-\sigma)x(t_n-\tau) =$$

$$= \frac{T}{N} \frac{1}{T} \int_{o}^{T} dt \; x(t-\sigma)x(t-\tau).z(t)$$

so: second order advantage of stimuli preceding a neural event is proportional to the second order cross correlation function of input- and outputsignal.

A related approach, which appears to be suited better to the characteristics of the auditory system can be based on a description of sound as a function of both <u>frequency</u> and <u>time</u>: the average pre event dynamic power spectrum $Q_e(\omega,\tau)$.

This function describes the average spectro-temporal structure of stimuli, preceding an action potential.

3. <u>Parametric description</u> of tonal part of PESE.

Tonal components in the Stimulus Ensemble can be characterized by instantaneous amplitude (= envelope) and frequency, both as functions of time.

Hence also the tonal part of the PESE can be completely described in terms of frequency and amplitude as function of time

AVERAGE PRE EVENT STIMULUS $r_e(\tau)$

UNIT 26-6 N-557-440

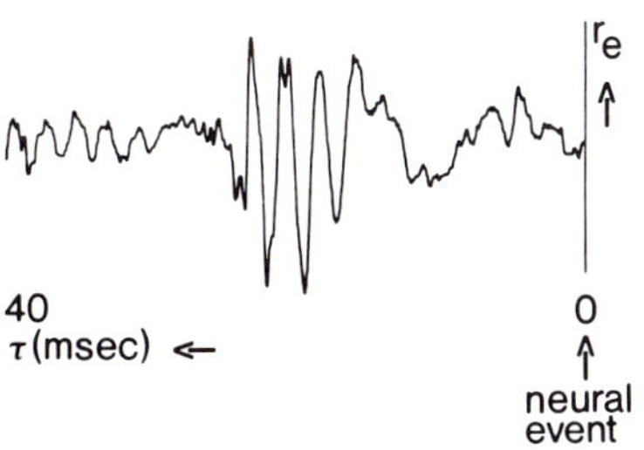

AVERAGE PRE EVENT DYNAMIC SPECTRUM $Q_e(\omega,\tau)$ divided by stimulus spectrum $I(\omega)$

UNIT 26-6 N-557-539

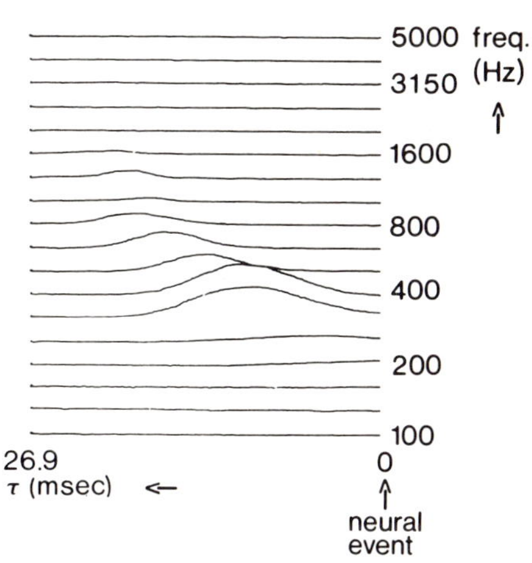

before the occurrence of neural events. This method of analysis results in an Amplitude Frequency Time-display: <u>AFT-cube</u>.

Quadratic averaging over different amplitude values then gives the average Intensity of tones as a function of Frequency and Time before occurrence of a neural event: <u>average IFT</u>.
The average IFT is related to the average pre event dynamic power spectrum $Q_e(\omega,\tau)$ for natural sounds. After proper normalization a comparison of quantitative results from approach 1 to those from approach 3 provide an indication to what extent the stimulus-event relation is invariant with respect to the choice of the stimulus ensemble.

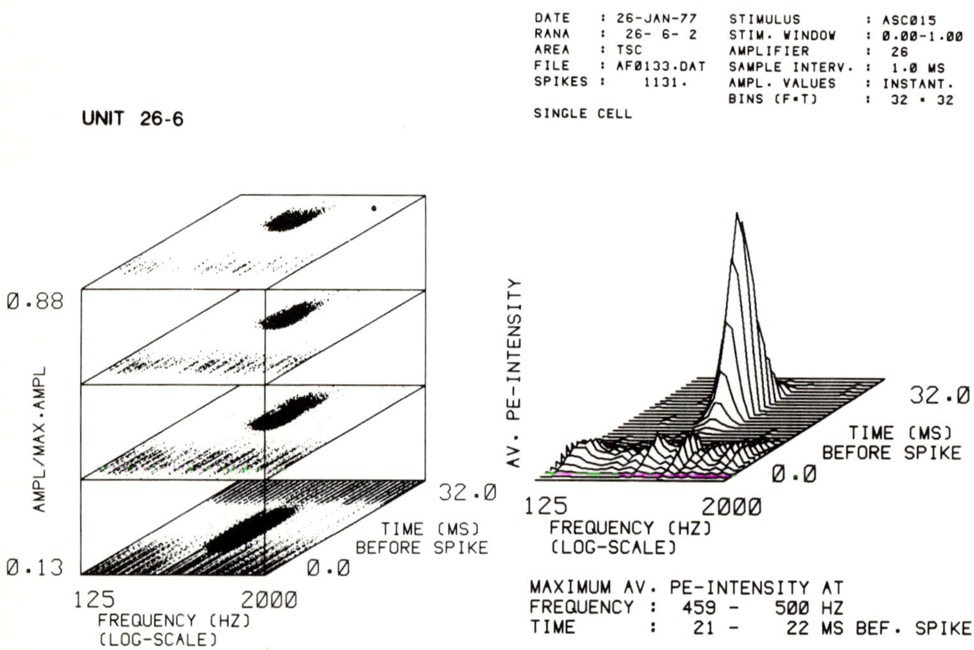

AFT-cube average IFT

The relation between average IFT and average pre event dynamic power spectrum can be given a formal basis by introduction of the Complex Spectro-Temporal Intensity Density function (CoSTID) (Johannesma and Aertsen, contribution to this Workshop).

Acknowledgement: Members of the workgroup Neurophysics who contributed to this work: Dik Hermes, Arnold Hoeks and Jos Olders.

References:

1) Aertsen, A.M.H.J.; Smolders, J.W.T., Johannesma, P.I.M.: Neural representation of the Acoustic Biotope: On the existence of stimulus-event relations for sensory neurons. Biol. Cybern. 32, 175-185 (1979).
2) Boer, E. de, Kuyper, P.: Triggered correlation. IEEE Tr. on Biomed. Eng. BME-15, 169-179 (1968).
3) Boer, E. de; Jongh, H.R. de: On cochlear encoding: potentialities and limitations of the reverse correlation technique. J.Acoust.Soc.Am. 63, 115-135 (1978).
4) Capranica, R.R.: Morphology and Physiology of the Auditory System. In: Frog Neurobiology, a Handbook, pp. 551-575. Llinas R., Precht, W. (eds.) Berlin: Springer (1976).
5) Gelder, J.J. van; Evers, P.M.G.; Maagnus, G.J.M.: Calling and associated behaviour of the common frog, Rana temporaria L. during breeding activity. J.Anim.Ecology 47, 667-676 (1978).
6) Grashuis, J.L.: The pre-event stimulus ensemble: an analysis of the stimulus response relation for complex stimuli applied to auditory neurons. Ph.D. Thesis, Nijmegen, the Netherlands (1974).
7) Johannesma, P.I.M.: The pre-response stimulus ensemble of neurons in the cochlear nucleus. In: Proc. of the IPO Symp. on Hearing Theory, Cardozo, B.L. (ed.), Einhoven, 58-69 (1972).
8) Johannesma, P.I.M., Aertsen, A.M.H.J.: Neural image of sound in the grassfrog. EBBS-workshop, Göttingen (1979).

Tonotopy and Analysis of Wide-Band Calls in Field L of the Guinea Fowl

H. SCHEICH, D. BONKE and G. LANGNER, Institut für Zoologie der Technischen Hochschule Darmstadt, Schnittspahnstr. 3, 6100 Darmstadt, West Germany
(Supported by the Deutsche Forschungsgemeinschaft Sche 132/4.)

There is considerable interest in understanding basic organizational principles of auditory fields in the forebrain of vertebrates in conjunction to the processing of species-specific and other complex sounds by neurons in these structures. Birds lacking a cortex may nervertheless be highly suitable objects for such investigations. They have a cochlea functionally comparable to that of mammals (Takasaka and Smith, 1971; Manley, 1971) with an orderly representation of frequencies on the cochlear partition and tonotopy in the primay auditory projection field of the forebrain. This area, field L of the neostriatum, is a laminated structure. Two complex layers are separated by a more simple input layer. As indicated by the capability of many birds to imitate sounds the bird auditory system in principle must be a superb analyser for complex acoustic patterns.

In our investigations in the Guinea Fowl we were interested in the question where within the tonotopic map of field L species-specific calls with a wide-band spectrum are analysed. In other words: How does tonotopy relate to wide-band analysis? The recognition of calls with multiple spectral components requires convergence of several frequency channels at the level of central neurons. Knowing the response topology to wide-band sounds in an auditory structure appears to be relevant in view of the universal use of wide-band sounds in communication. There may also be some bearing on the analysis of speech sounds: all elements of human speech have a wide-band spectrum.

Organization of field L:

The neostriatal field L in the bird forebrain receives the primary input from the auditory nucleus ovoidalis in the diencephalon, an analogue to the medial geniculate body (Karten, 1968). It is an area larger and with more complex organization than has been previously assumed. Injections of tritiated aminoacids of nucleus ovoidalis produce an autorradiographic pattern of field L with two layers of moderate terminal labelling (L_1 and L_3) separated by the heavily labelled lamina L_2 (Fig. 1A), which receives the main input (Bonke, B. et al., 1979).

As has been discovered by Bonke, D. et al. (1979) field L is tonotopically organized in such a way that isofrequency contours can be drawn in two directions: in the horizontal plane parallel to the three layers from lateral-rostral to medial-caudal (Fig. 1C) and in the frontal plane perpendicularly across L_1, L_2 and L_3. Thus, there are sheets across field L in which neurons receive their strongest input from one place on the cochlear partition.

A new way to visualize the distribution of neurons which have strong input from a particular frequency channel is provided

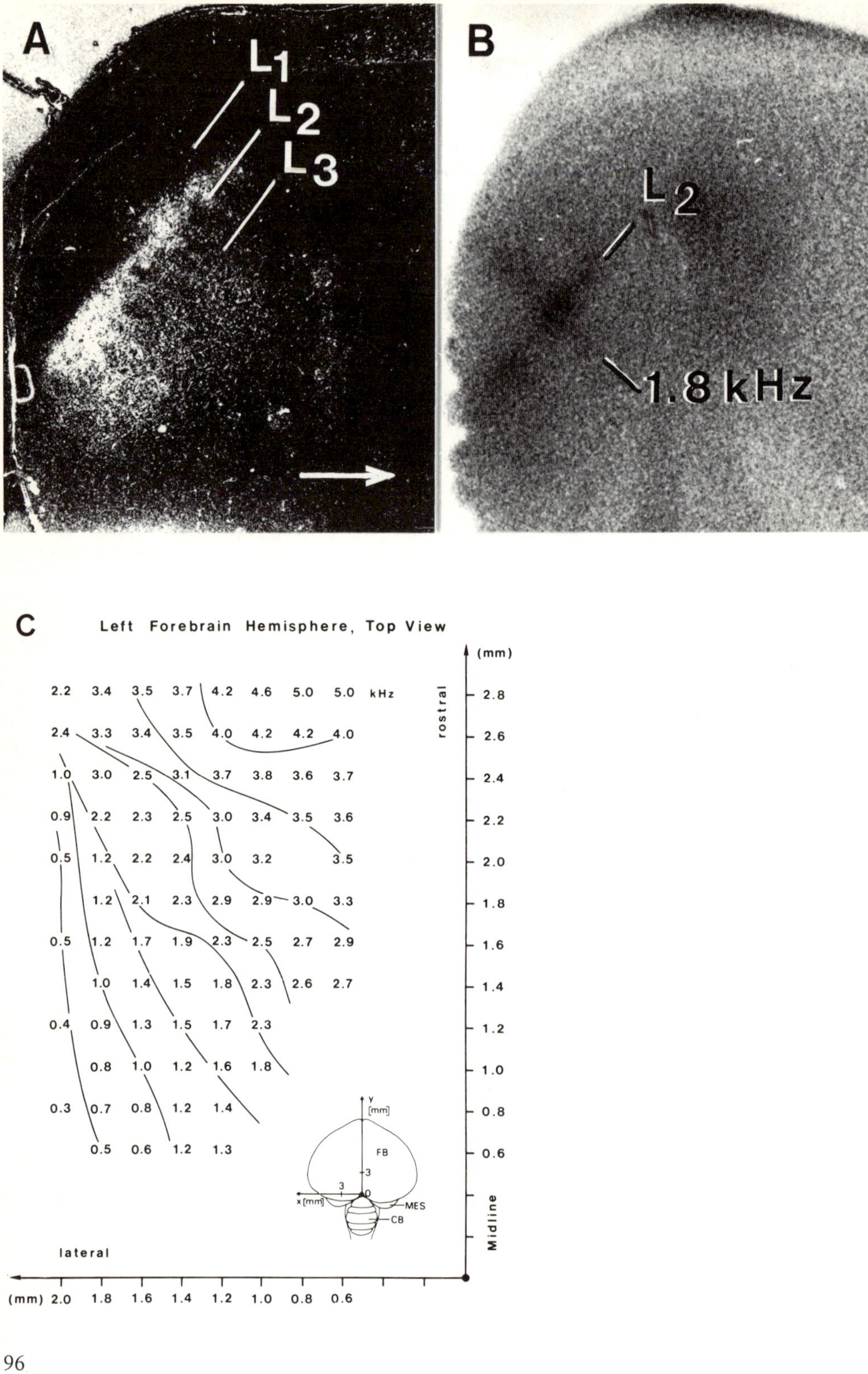
A
L1
L2
L3
B
L2
1.8 kHz
C
Left Forebrain Hemisphere, Top View
2.2 3.4 3.5 3.7 4.2 4.6 5.0 5.0 kHz
2.4 3.3 3.4 3.5 4.0 4.2 4.2 4.0
1.0 3.0 2.5 3.1 3.7 3.8 3.6 3.7
0.9 2.2 2.3 2.5 3.0 3.4 3.5 3.6
0.5 1.2 2.2 2.4 3.0 3.2 3.5
1.2 2.1 2.3 2.9 2.9 3.0 3.3
0.5 1.2 1.7 1.9 2.3 2.5 2.7 2.9
1.0 1.4 1.5 1.8 2.3 2.6 2.7
0.4 0.9 1.3 1.5 1.7 2.3
0.8 1.0 1.2 1.6 1.8
0.3 0.7 0.8 1.2 1.4
0.5 0.6 1.2 1.3
(mm)
2.8 2.6 2.4 2.2 2.0 1.8 1.6 1.4 1.2 1.0 0.8 0.6
rostral
Midline
lateral
(mm) 2.0 1.8 1.6 1.4 1.2 1.0 0.8 0.6
y [mm]
FB
3
3
0
x [mm]
MES
CB

by autoradiography with labelled 2-deoxyglucose (Sokoloff et al., 1974). Units which received prolongued acoustic stimulation show levels of radioactivity well above background.

Fig. 1B illustrates the result of an experiment in which a Guinea Fowl was stimulated with tone bursts of 1.8 kHz for 45 min. (1 s duration, 1 s pause). Activated neurons in a transverse section lie within a narrow strip which runs perpendicularly through all three layers of field L. In this plane also L_2, the main input layer, shows labelling (presumably of fibers) throughout its extent so that a cross pattern is formed together with the perpendicular strip.

The deoxyglucose experiments confirm the results on tonotopic organization of field L obtained with micro-electrode recordings namely that neurons in a sheet of tissue perpendicular to the lamination have their strongest input from one frequency channel. The complementary information, e.g. whether neurons beside one main input receive input from other frequency channels is only available from micro-electrode recordings (see below).

Fig. 1. Basic Organization of field L in the Guinea Fowl.
A. Autoradiography of field L in a frontal plane as obtained by injecting tritiated aminoacids into n. ovoidalis. Darkfield microphotograph developed for maximal contrast of L_2. Terminal labelling in L_3 is not visible (after Bonke, B. et al., 1979).
B. Deoxyglucose-autoradiography of field L in the same plane as A. The animal was stimulated with tone pips of 1.8 kHz. The micrograph shows L_2 and a stripe at right angle which corresponds to maximal excitation of neurons by 1.8 kHz.
C. Tonotopic map of field L in a dorsal view (from Bonke, D. et al., 1979)

Tonotopy and formant frequencies of calls:

Tonotopy in the forebrain of the Guinea Fowl provides some explanation for the responsiveness and selectivity of units to species-specific calls. There is an obvious connection between the spectral content of a wide-band call and the locus within field L where units are responsive or nonresponsive to this call. This would be a trivial matter if among such responsive units there were not units which show a strong preference for this call in comparison to other calls with energy in the same frequency band (selective units).

Species-specific calls can be thought of as a complex of several independent acoustic dimensions. The Iambus call of the Guinea Fowl, for instance, consists of a short followed by a long note (Fig. 2A). It has a harmonic spectrum with a fundamental which varies somewhat about 1 kHz (Fig. 2B). The second dimension is an amplitude modulation of the periodic (harmonic) signal which varies somewhat about 300 Hz. This

---

Fig. 2.

A. High resolution serial power spectra of a Iambus call. The epoch of each spectrum is 30 ms with 15 ms overlap of adjacent spectra. The time runs from bottom to top.

B. Power spectrum of a 30 ms epoch from another Iambus. Harmonic lines, sidebands, and the formant are visible. The oscillogram of this epoch is shown below. It has a distinct amplitude modulation.

C. Average Power Spectra of Iambi and of 7 Potpourri Calls used as stimuli. The sequence of the Potpourri Calls on the stimulus tape was from Chirp (1) to Tremolo (7). The Iambus spectrum represents the average of 16 Iambus spectra, variations of the one shown in Fig. 2. Dotted lines indicate 1, 1.8 and 2 kHz. Note that the energy peak in the Iambus spectrum is between 1.7 and 1.8 kHz (formant frequency). This is similar in the Tremolo front where the 2 kHz band dominates. In the Rhythmic Cry 1 and 2 kHz and the sidebands in between dominate. All other calls have formant frequencies above 2 kHz

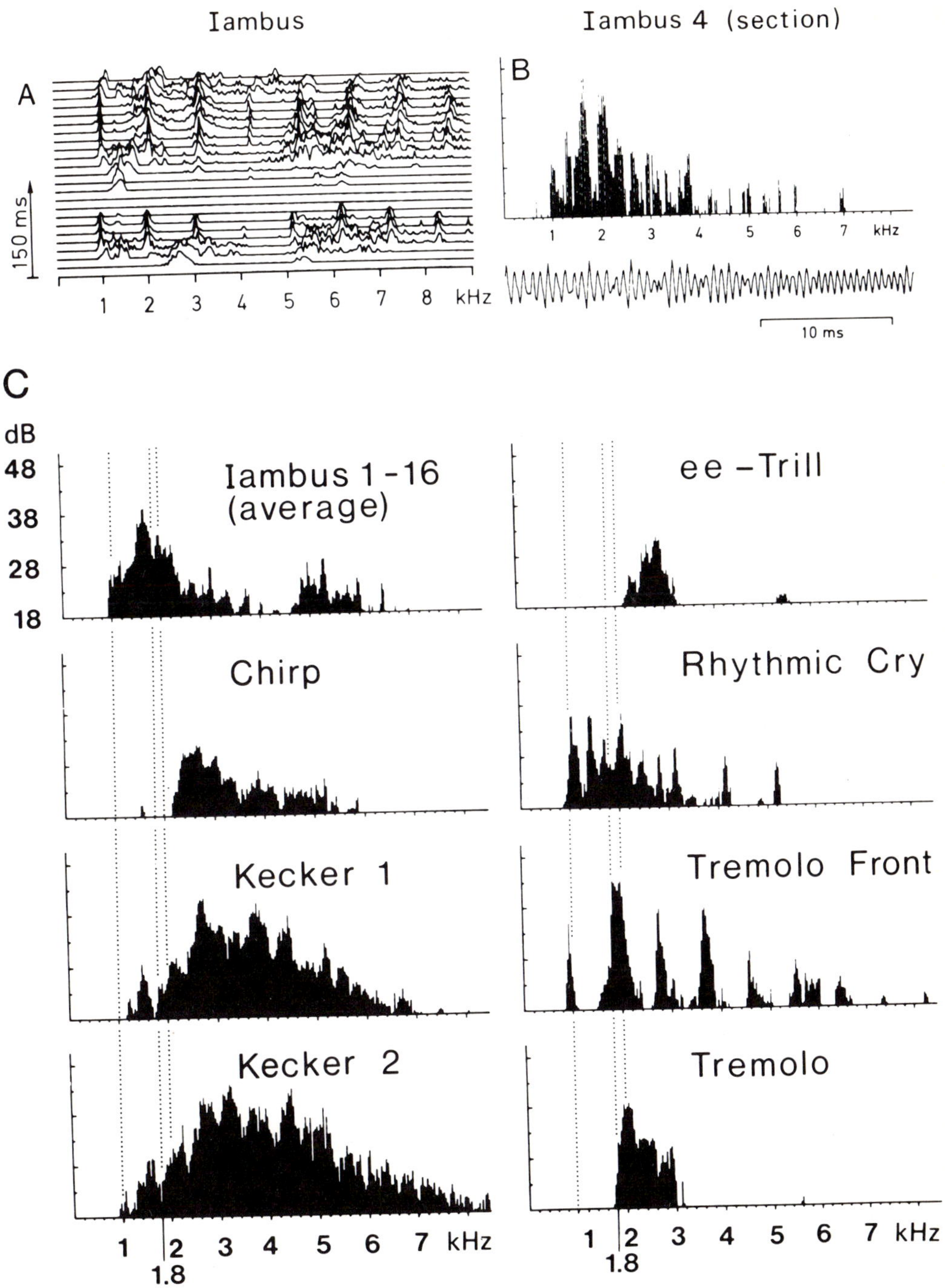

Iambus
Iambus 4 (section)
A
B
150 ms
1 2 3 4 5 6 7 8 kHz
1 2 3 4 5 6 7 kHz
10 ms
C
dB
48
38
28
18
Iambus 1-16
(average)
ee -Trill
Chirp
Rhythmic Cry
Kecker 1
Tremolo Front
Kecker 2
Tremolo
1 2 3 4 5 6 7 kHz
1.8

modulation produces sidebands 300 Hz above and below each harmonic line in the spectrum. A third spectral dimension is the frequency of the formants, i.e. of the energy peaks in the wide-band spectrum. There are usually two formants in Iambus, a stronger one between 1.7 and 2 kHz (average maximum 1.7 - 1.8 kHz) and a weaker and more inconsistent one between 5 and 6 kHz. These spectral dimensions combined are found in each of the two notes of the Iambus.

Other wide-band calls of the Guinea Fowl besides having different acoustic dimensions like frequency modulations, noise or different fundamental frequencies, exhibit formant frequencies different from Iambus calls. Average spectra of these calls which were used in a stimulus ensemble, called "Potpourri", are shown in Fig. 2C.

Our results indicate that the formant frequencies of calls are a mayor cue for the neuronal distinction of wide-band calls. The formant frequencies relate to the locus in the tonotopic map of field L where a call excites a high proportion of neurons. Among them are neurons which respond selectively to this call.

Fig. 3 shows neurons which were recorded in electrode penetrations approximately perpendicular through the layers 1, 2, and 3 of field L. The penetrations were made at three loci 1, 2, and 3, as indicated by the encircled number above each penetration. The depth of each recorded neuron was measured stereotaxically and related to electrolytic iron deposits. The neurons were stimulated with 8 natural variations of the Iambus call.

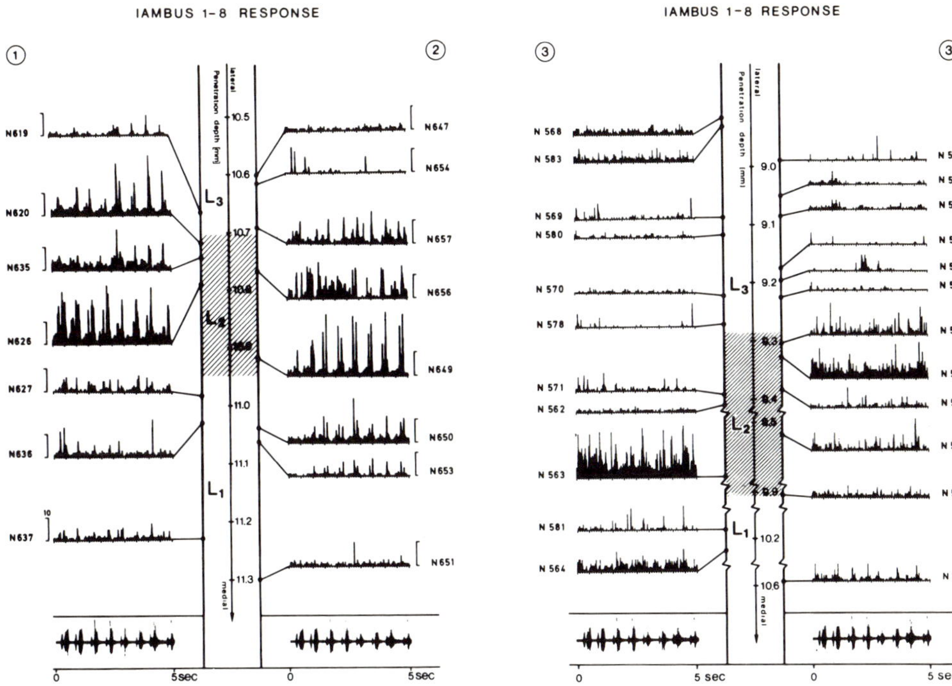

Fig. 3. Responses of locus 1, 2, and 3 units to 8 natural Iambus variations. The depth position of each unit in field L in the latero-medial penetrations is given by a scale in the middle. The hatched region indicates L_2. The PSTHs with 5 ms bin-width represent responses to 20 repetitions of the calls (vertical bar: 10 spikes/bin). The oscillograms of the calls and a time scale are given below

Units recorded in loci 1 and 2 (two left columns in fig. 3) show reliable responses to a high proportion of the eight Iambus calls. Units recorded in locus 3 (two right columns) show only few responses, except for some units in layer L_2 which harbours unselective units (N 563, N 575, N 576). Unselective units in layer L_2 have the highest response score in loci 1, 2, and 3. They are characterized by high general activity in the histogram.

Loci 1 and 2 correspond to places within the tonotopic map of field L where best frequencies of units (if they had best frequencies) were between 1.8 and 2 kHz. Expecially in locus 1 units showed prominent response peaks to pure tones between 1.7 and 2 kHz. Locus 3 had best frequencies between 2 and 4 kHz. The best frequencies of neurons in loci 1 and 2 thus corresponded to the formant frequency of Iambus calls. This appears to be a particularly relevant result with respect to the low Iambus-responsiveness and different best frequency of units in locus 3. It is noteworthy since Iambus calls have energy between 2 and 4 kHz (Fig. 2C) and could therefore excite units in locus C.

Selective neurons:

Among 360 neurons analysed in the 1 - 2 kHz area of field L 56 clearly preferred Iambus-like calls over other wide-band calls with different formant frequencies but with spectral overlap in the 1.7 - 2 kHz and other frequency bands (Fig. 2C). The analysis of the 56 selective responders with synthetic stimuli revealed more complex spectral preferences, beside tuning to tone frequencies which are relevant in the Iambus

---

Fig. 4. Frequency distribution of response maxiam of selective units.

A. Stimulation with pure tones. A high proportion of units respond to 1 kHz and to 1.8 - 1.9 kHz which are prominent bands in the Iambus spectra. Many additional responses are seen to frequencies below 600 Hz.

B. Stimulation of the same neurons with harmonic spectra of varying fundamental frequency. A distribution of response maxima is obtained similar to A.

C. Distribution of response peaks to modulation frequencies of amplitude modulated harmonic tones. There is tuning to low and to high modulation frequencies (from Scheich et al., 1979)

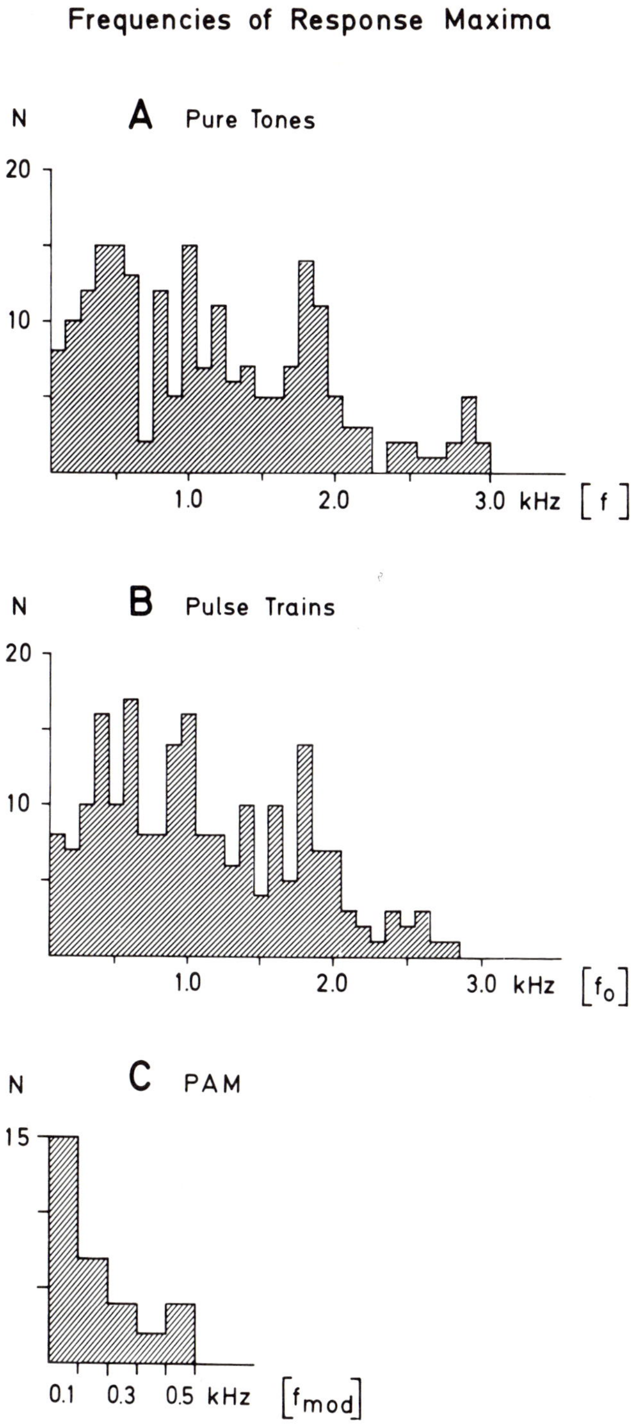
Frequencies of Response Maxima
N
A Pure Tones
20
10
1.0
2.0
3.0 kHz [f]
N
B Pulse Trains
20
10
1.0
2.0
3.0 kHz [f₀]
N
C PAM
15
0.1
0.3
0.5 kHz
[f mod]

spectra. Fig. 4A illustrates the tuning of the population of selective neurons to pure tones at 65 dB SPL. Since more than 20 of these neurons showed response peaks at several frequencies (multi-peak neurons) the distribution is broad. There are, however, two maxima: one at 1 kHz which is the fundamental of the Iambus spectrum and one at 1.8 kHz, the formant frequency to the Iambus.

Among complex preferences tuning to harmonic tones with fundamentals around 900 Hz and 1.8 kHz was found. Since the preference of the neuronal population has shifted from 1 kHz (pure tone response) to 900 Hz fundamental frequency when tested with harmonic tones (Fig. 4B), this may be some indication that the combination of the formant frequency with the fundamental frequency is important for these neurons. For many neurons with a pure tone response maximum at 1 kHz, 900 Hz as the fundamental of a harmonic tone would be still with the response range and its second harmonic would then correspond to the formant frequency of the Iambus.

Among selective neurons some were found which did not respond to pure tones but only to harmonic tones. Response maxima in these cases were seen around 1 kHz. Iambus spectra show sidebands above and below each harmonic line. These sidebands are due to an amplitude modulation of the harmonic carrier. Selective neurons responded to synthetic stimuli with the same spectral composition. Fig. 4C illustrates which modulation frequencies of an harmonic carrier around 1 kHz fundamental frequency were preferred by selective units. The strongest preference was around 120 Hz modulation frequency but also tuning to higher modulation frequencies occurred.

Selectivity for calls and intensity of stimuli

The analysis of selective units with calls played at various intensities yielded different results. Some units lost their responsiveness to certain calls when the intensity was low or lost their preference for certain calls when the intensity of other calls was very high. A shift of preference from certain natural variations of the Iambus to other variations was seen in some cases.

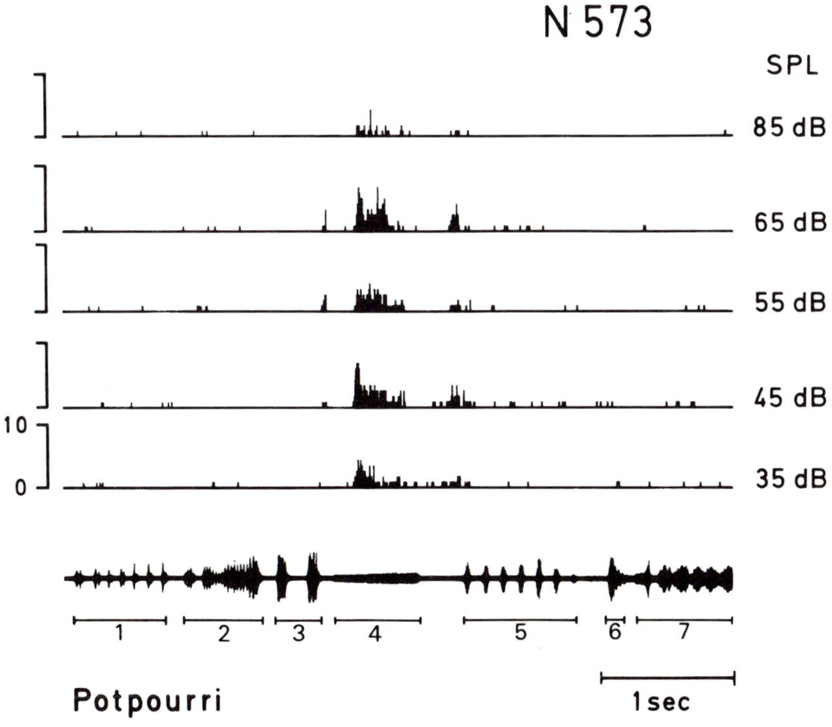

Fig. 5. Selective response of a unit to the ee-trill (no. 4) in the potpourri (Fig. 3). Selectivity is preserved over 50 dB intensity variation

A significant support for the concept of call selectivity of neurons in field L are those units which preserved their selectivity over a large range of intensities. Fig. 5 shows the responses of a unit which preferred the ee-trill no. 4 in the potpourri stimulus ensemble (a type of "warning call"). The response selectivity is essentially unchanged over 50 dB.

Discussion:

The concept of neurons in the central auditory pathway of vertebrates which are specialized to recognize species-specific calls has originally been proposed by Frishkopf, Capranica and Goldstein (1968) for the bullfrog system. Meanwhile, it has gained support from a number of studies in anurans (Mudry et al., 1977; Capranica, 1977) in birds (Leppelsack and Vogt, 1976; Scheich, 1977; Bonke, D. et al., 1979; Scheich et al., 1979); primates (Winter and Funkenstein, 1973; Newman and Wollberg, 1973) and in bats (Suga, 1973; Suga and Jen, 1976; Suga, 1977). Reviews of this topic have been provided by Scheich (1977) and by Newman et al. (1977).

The present account, based partly on data from Bonke, D. et al. (1979) and Scheich et al. (1979), is an attempt to relate the concept of vocalization-selective neurons to tonotopy in a primary projection area of a vertebrate forebrain. Suga and Jen (1976), Suga (1977), and Suga et al. (1978) have provided a convincing picture of processing of bat orientation sounds in specialized areas of the bat auditory cortex. Our work, far from giving final answers, aims at two different aspects. Firstly, neural responsiveness and selectivity for calls was analysed within a "regular" tonotopic map which does not show gross distortions or large specialized areas. With this statement we do not mean to exclude the possibility of small specialized networks for call analysis (Focal Zones) within this map (see Scheich, 1977). Given some twenty call types in the repertoire of the Guinea Fowl (Maier, 1977) the analysis of these calls probably takes place within one map. The tonotopic range covers the formants of all call types. Secondly the calls which are the object of the present investigation are spectrally more complex than bat orientation calls and are wide-band so that there is spectral overlap of different call types, a condition which is found in the repertoire of many species.

The presented results suggest some principles how wide-band calls are analysed within the tonotopic map of field L. There is a high proportion of units which respond to a particular call in loci where the best frequency corresponds to the formant frequency of the call. Due to lamination with units having more simple or more selective properties in the three layers the neuronal population in one locus is non-homogeneous in terms of the responsiveness to the complex call. Even adjacent neurons may differ in their preference for one or another Iambus variation (Bonke, D. et al., 1979; Scheich et al., 1979). Spatial axes along which additional stimulus parameters determine this relative heterogineity of neuronal properties have not been discovered. In the above-cited work there was no indication of call detectors i.e. units which would respond to any call of the Iambus type. If such units exist they must be a small minority. However, among units which only responded to Iambus calls there was a gradient of preference from units which only responded to few Iambus calls (individualizers) to units which responded to many Iambus variations (categorizers).

There are indications that excitatory and inhibitory convergence of several frequency channels occurs at the single neuron level in field L. Pure tone and harmonic tone stimuli revealed response peaks in several frequency bands (multi-peak neurons) and often several bands of suppression (Scheich et al., 1979; Scheich, 1979). One of the excitatory peaks often corresponded to the best frequency of other neurons in a given locus. It may be that units in a locus receive a common main input which corresponds to the formant frequency of a call together with various inputs which correspond to other relevant spectral bands of the call. If these secondary inputs were somewhat different among units in a locus this would explain general preference of neurons for calls of a given type on the one hand and individual preference for different samples of a type on the other hand.

References:

1) Bonke, D.; Scheich, H.; Langner, G.: Responsiveness of units in the auditory neostriatum of the Guinea Fowl (Numida meleagris) to species-specific calls and synthetic stimuli. I Tonotopy and functional zones. J.Comp.Physiol. (in press).
2) Bonke, B.A.; Bonke, D.; Scheich, H.: Connectivity of the auditory forebrain nuclei in the Guinea Fowl (Numida meleagris) Cell tissue Res. (in press).
3) Capranica, R.R.: Auditory processing of vocal signals in anurans. In: Taylor, D.H.; Guttman, S.I. (eds.): The reproductive biology of amphibians. Plenum Publishing Corp., 337-353 (1977).
4) Frishkopf, L.S.; Capranica, R.R.; Goldstein, M.R. jr.: Neural coding in the bullfrog's auditory system. A teleological approach. Proc. JEEE 56, 969-980 (1968).

5) Karten, H.J.: The ascending auditory pathway in the pigeon (Columba livia). II. Telencephalic projections of the nucleus ovoidalis thalami. Brain Res. 11, 134-153 (1968).
6) Leppelsack, H.J.; Vogt, M.: Responses of auditory neurons in the forebrain of a songbird to stimulation with species-specific sounds. J.Comp.Physiol. 107, 263-274 (1976).
7) Maier, V.: Vocal communication in the Guinea Fowl (numida meleagris). Proc. XVth int. Ethological Conference, Bielefeld, Section II, 48 (1977).
8) Manley, G.A.: Some aspects of evolution of hearing in vertebrates. Nature 230, 506-509 (1971).
9) Mudry, K.M.; Constantine-Paton, M.; Capranica, R.R.: Auditory sensitivity of the diencephalon of the leopard frog Rana p. pipiens. J.Comp.Physiol. 114, 1-13 (1977).
10) Newman, J.D.; Wollberg, Z.: Multiple coding of species-specific vocalizations in the auditory cortex of the squirrel monkey. Brain Res. 54, 287-304 (1973).
11) Newman, J.D. (Rapporteur), Bodenstein, G.; Bullock, T.H.; Capranica, R.R.; Ehret, G.; Evans, E.F., Goldstein, J.L.; Hellweg, F.C.; Huber, F.; Kalmring, K.; Langner, G.; Leppelsack, J.L.; Müller-Preuss, P.; Neff, W.D.; Scheich, H.; Sovijärvi, A.R.A.; Suga, N.; Worden, F.G.: Biological filtering and neural mechanisms. Group report. In: Bullock, T.H. (ed.): Dahlem workshop on recognition of complex acoustic signals. Berlin: Dahlem Konferenzen, 280-306 (1977).
12) Scheich, H.: Central processing of complex sounds and feature analysis. In: Bullock, T.H. (ed.): Dahlem workshop on recognition of complex acoustic signals. Berlin: Dahlem Konferenzen, 161-182 (1977).
13) Scheich, H.: Common principles of organization in the central auditory pathway of vertebrates. Verh.Dtsch.Zool. Ges. 1979 (in press).
14) Scheich, H.; Langner, G.; Bonke, D.: Responsiveness of units in the auditory neostriatum of the Guinea Fowl (Numida meleagris) to species-specific calls and synthetic stimuli. II Discrimination of Iambus-like calls. J.Comp.Physiol. (in press).
15) Sokoloff, L.; Reivich, M.; Patlak, C.S.; Pettigrew, K.D.; Des Rosiers, M.; Kennedy, C.: The (^{14}C) deoxyglucose method for quantitative determination of local cerebral glucose consumption. Trans.Am.Soc.Neurochem. 5, 85 (1974).
16) Suga, N.; O'Neill, W.E.; Manabe, T.: Cortical neurons sensitive to combinations of information-bearing elements of biosonar signals in the mustache bat. Science 200, 778-781 (1978).
17) Takasaka, T.; Smith, C.A.: The structure and innervation of the pigeon's basilar papilla. J. ultrastructure Res. 35, 20-65 (1971).
18) Winter, P.A.; Funkenstein, H.H.: The effect of species-specific vocalizations on the discharge of auditory cortical cells in the awake squirrel monkey (Saimiri sciureus). Exp. Brain Res. 18, 489-504 (1973).

Selective Responses of Neurons to Vowel Sounds in the Auditory Neostriatum of the Mynah Bird

G. LANGNER, D. BONKE and H. SCHEICH, Institut für Zoologie der Technischen Hochschule Darmstadt, Schnittspahnstr. 3, 6100 Darmstadt, West Germany
(Supported by the Deutsche Forschungsgemeinschaft Sche 132/4.)

There is some recent evidence that animals possess the ability to categorize certain classes of speech sounds in a way similar to man (Miller, 1977). This holds for temporal as well as spectral aspects of speech (Kuhl and Miller, 1975; Burdick and Miller, 1975). These findings suggest that categorization of speech-like sounds may be a basic functional principle of auditory systems of vertebrates, at least of mammals and birds which have functionally similar cochleae and tonotopically organized central auditory systems. Further evidence for accurate processing of speech signals is provided by the ability of certain birds, notably parrots and mynahs, to imitate human voices. The aim of this investigation was to analyse neuronal mechanisms in the auditory neostriatum of "talking" mynah birds pertaining to the processing of vowels. The auditory neostriatum (Field L) of birds is a laminated primary auditory projection area in the forebrain (Bonke, B. et al., 1979).

Single units were recorded in 7 adult mynahs which were awake and had chambers implanted in the skull for stereotaxic recording. Methods for the implant and for closed-field acoustic stimulation were as described for another bird (Scheich et al., 1977). For acoustic stimulation we used 9 natural vowels from a male speaker (fundamental frequency $f_o \simeq 140$ Hz) and 5 synthetic vowels with altogether 600 variations of f_o and intensity of the formants F_1 and F_2.

Each synthetic vowel consisted of 2 formants with 3 harmonics each of which, for a given vowel, were always multiples of f_o varying from 120 Hz to 220 Hz in steps of 20 Hz. These simplified vowels were, for the human ear, good approximations of /a:/, /æ:/, /e:/, /i:/ and /o:/. The overall sound pressure level was kept at 65 dB SPL or was lower when the relative intensity of F_1 versus F_2 was varied. Vowels and constant amplitude with a rise and decay time of 5 ms and a total duration of 200 ms.

About 50% of 250 analysed units were responsive to natural vowels. Some 20% may be considered selective because they responded to only 1 or 2 out of 9 vowels. About 12% gave a response to only 1 vowel. Many units could distinguish between two vowels which shared one formant. Stimulation of these units with synthetic vowels showed that the frequencies of the second formants which were not shared provided the cues for the neuronal distinction. The second formant of the response eliciting vowel was either excitatory or neutral while that of the other vowel was inhibitory. This integrational effect occurred as well even in the responses to vowels in which F_1 and F_2 are widely separated in frequency as in /æ:/, /e:/ and /i:/.

Neurons of this type are illustrated in Fig. 1. Unit N 181 responded to the complete vowel /a:/ but not to /æ:/. N 164 gave the reverse response. Obviously in both units F_2 of the

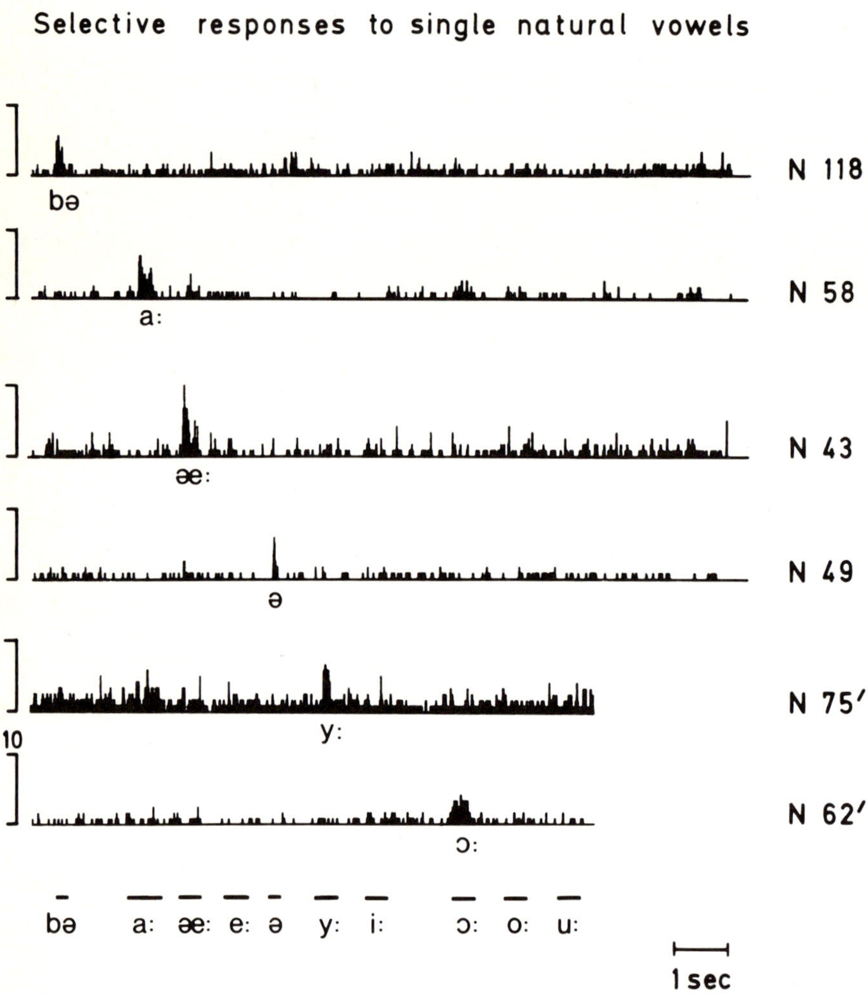

Fig. 1. Each PSTH (bin width 15 ms) shows the response of one unit to a distinct synthetic vowel (F_1 + F_2) and to either formant alone (F_1), (F_2). The number of stimulus repetitions was 10. The sound pressure level was 65 dB SPL. For the isointensity tone response (IR) the number of repetition was 3, the sound pressure level was 50 dB SPL, and the duration was 200 ms. Below the IR histograms the positions of the formant frequencies F_1 and F_2 of several synthetic vowels are marked along the frequency scale

non-excitatory vowel suppressed the response to F_1 which was identical for these vowels. As can be seen from the supra-threshold response to pure tones (isointensity response: IR) F_2 of the non-excitatory vowel was outside the main excitatory frequency band.

Unit N 123 gave a selective response to /e:/ and N 125 to /i:/, vowels with a wide separation of F_1 and F_2. Unit N 123 also responded to F_2 of /æ:/ and /i:/ which are roughly the same as in /e:/. However, F_1 suppressed these responses to F_2 so that the complete vowels /æ:/ and /i:/ did not yield a response. The same suppression effect of F_1 on F_2 in /æ:/ and /e:/ is illustrated for unit N 125.

The selective response of a unit for a distinct vowel may be explained by one excitatory input at one formant frequency and one or several inhibitory inputs which are way off the frequency of the second formant. In some cases we could demonstrate combinations of two excitatory inputs corresponding to F_1 and F_2. These units preferred certain amplitude ratios of the formants. Most units did not reveal their complexity in the IR which mostly showed simple excitatory inputs and sometimes weak bands of suppression.

Fig. 2 shows selective response of several units to single natural vowels. Although most units in our material responded to several vowels, some of them strongly preferred one distinct vowel. The same mechanisms as suggested for synthetic vowel responses may be responsible for the distinction of natural vowels.

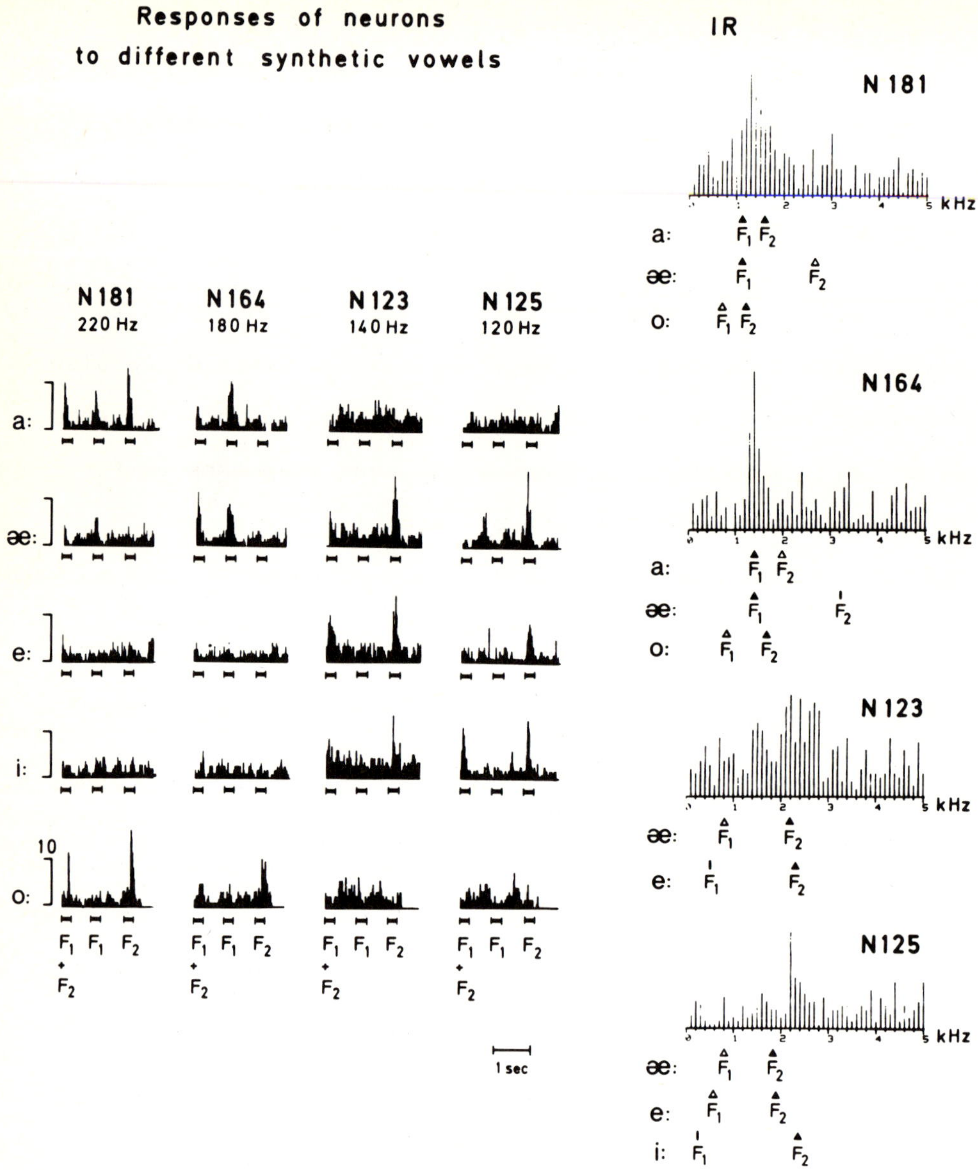

Fig. 2. Each PSTH (bin width 10 ms) (for N 118 : 15 ms) shows the selective response of a unit to one natural vowel. The number of stimulus repetitions was 10, the sound pressure level was 65 dB SPL. The duration of the natural vowels is marked below the PSTHs by a bar

As we could recently show in the Guinea Fowl field L may be subdivided into three layers (Bonke, B. et al., 1979; Bonke, D. et al., 1979; Scheich, H. et al., 1979). Units selective for species-specific vocalizations are mainly found in layers L_1 and L_3 and not in the input layer of L_2. The same distribution of selectivity could be demonstrated for the vowel responses of units in field L of the Mynah bird.

References:

1) Bonke, B.A.; Bonke, D.; Scheich, H.: Connectivity of the auditory forebrain nuclei in the Guinea fowl (Numida meleagris). Cell tissue Res. (in press)

2) Bonke, D.; Scheich, H.; Langner, G.: Responsiveness of units in the auditory neostriatum of the Guinea Fowl (Numida meleagris) to species-specific calls and synthetic stimuli. I Tonotopy and functional zones. J.Comp.Physiol. (in press).

3) Burdick, C.K.; Miller, J.D.: Speech perception by the chinchilla: Discrimination of sustained /a/ and /i/. J.Acoust. Soc.Am. 58, 415-427 (1975).

4) Kuhl, P.K.; Miller, J.D.: Speech perception by the chinchilla: voiced - voiceless distinction in alveolar plosive consonants. Science 190, 69-72 (1975).

5) Miller, J.D.: Perception of speech sounds in animals: Evidence for speech processing by mammalian auditory mechanisms. In: T.H. Bullock (ed.): Dahlem Workshop on recognition of complex acoustic signals. Berlin - Dahlem Konferenzen, 49-58 (1977).

6) Scheich, H.; Langner, G.; Koch, R.: Coding of narrow-band and wide-band vocalizations in the auditory midbrain nucleus (MLD) of the Guinea Fowl (Numida meleagris). J.Comp.Physiol. 117, 245-265 (1977).

7) Scheich, H.; Langner, G.; Bonke, D.: Responsiveness of units in the auditory neostriatum of the Guinea Fowl (Numida meleagris) tospecies-specific calls and synthetic stimuli. II Discrimination of Iambus-like calls. J.Comp.Physiol. (in press).

The Increase of Response Selectivity within the Avian Auditory Pathway

HANS-J. LEPPELSACK, Lehrstuhl für Allg. Zoologie, Ruhr-Universität, Bochum, West-Germany

By exploring the response properties of neurons in single brain centers and the demonstration of the structural organisation of these centers, comparison of differences in response or organisation between different levels of the auditory pathway is of great help for the understanding of their function. For such differences must necessarily be produced by the processing of the central nervous system. Thus they allow some important insights into the principles of analysis within the information processing system of the auditory pathway.

It is already known that in the auditory pathway acoustical information is represented at the level of the inner ear in a crudely processed manner (Leppelsack and Manley, 1978). During the course of the pathway the information represented by the responses of single neurons becomes increasingly refined. As a consequence there are units in the forebrain auditory center which respond only to specific acoustic combinations embedded in complex sounds (Leppelsack, 1978). Quantitative comparisons between neurons in the periphery and higher centers will give some indication of the processing mechanisms that lead to these complex response properties. A general problem appearing during the investigation of these phenomena is that certain neurons within higher centers do not respond to simple stimuli like pure tones, which are usually the standard stimulus used in the analysis of the auditory system. For this reason it seems to be necessary to use species-specific sounds as a basis for such a comparison (Watanabe and Katsuki, 1974).

The two extreme levels within the avian auditory pathway have been chosen to investigate these differences. These are the inner ear and the forebrain. Neuronal response of the cochlear ganglion (Manley and Leppelsack, 1977) and of the neostriatum caudale, an area that includes Field L (Leppelsack and Vogt, 1977) were recorded extracellularly by glass capillary micropipets in the starling. Besides pure tones and white noise, other stimuli used were sounds out of the vocal repertoire of the starling. A stimulus program was composed from social communication calls and elements of the song. For this investigation 80 distinct sounds were chosen as representative of the starling's vocal repertoire. These sounds were presented and the responses to them were analysed.

Based on this stimulus program a quantitative measure for the selectivity of a neuron was developed. Accordingly, we describe a neuron as less selective the more types of stimulus sounds it responds to.

The selectivity of both centers investigated in this way is shown in fig. 1. The results obtained from each neuronal population are quite different. More than 50 per cent of the neurons in the cochlear ganglion respond to between 30 and 45 out of the 80 sounds. There are neurons that respond to less than 16 or more than 55 sounds. This limited range of selecti-

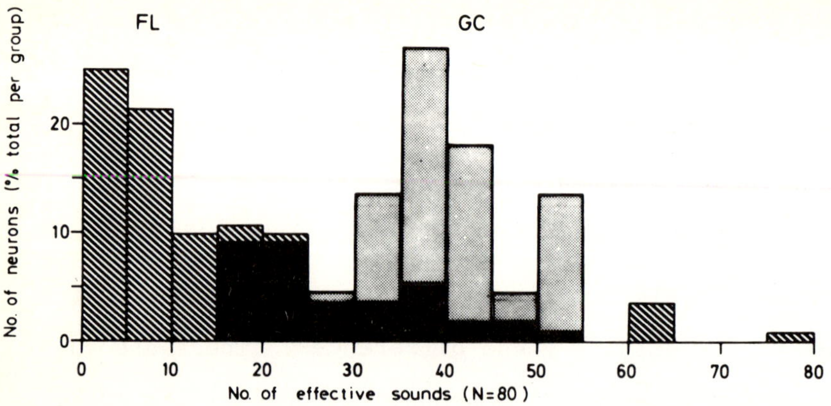

Fig. 1. Selectivity of auditory units in the Neostriatum caudale (FL) and the cochlear ganglion (GC). Bins represent numbers of units that respond to a certain number out of 80 sounds of the starling, used as a stimulus. Forebrain units show a higher selectivity

vity values among chochlear ganglion neurons has to be explained by the matching of frequency bands in the stimulus sounds to neuronal tuning curves, as most of these neurons respond like simple frequency filters.

In the Neostriatum caudale more than 50% of the neurons respond to between 1 to 15 out of the 50 sounds. The total range of selectivity within this neuronal population includes neurons that respond to only one or nearly all 80 of the sounds. These results indicate that as an effect of central nervous processing the average neuronal selectivity increases significantly from the periphery to the center. All neurons do not simply become more selective; there are also neurons found at the forebrain level that have a lower selectivity than any neuron in the inner ear.

There is a certain number of neostriatal neurons with a clear interdependency between their response to complex sounds and the responses to pure tones and thus to the tuning curve of the unit (Leppelsack, 1978). So it is of interest to look at how the tuning curves change from lower to higher centers. Such a comparison shows a change in the bandwidths of the tuning curves (measured at 70 dB SPL) parallel to the development of selectivity. The bandwidths of neurons in the forebrain, measured in octaves, extend over a wider range of values than in neurons of the inner ear. There is also a shift of the maximum of the distribution to a smaller bandwidth. Thus arises the question as to how this increasing acuity of the frequency response can explain the increase of neuronal selectivity along the auditory pathway.

A direct correlation between the bandwidth of the tuning curve and the selectivity of a neuron can contribute an answer to this question. The distribution of neurons in the coordinate systems of bandwidth-selectivity clearly indicates a higher representation of cochlear ganglion units in the range of lower selectivity (Fig. 2). That becomes obvious by a higher number of responses in GC-neurons. The linear regressions' relationship between bandwidth and selectivity in both groups of neurons shows that among units with the same bandwidth of tuning there is a higher selectivity among forebrain units.

These results show that

1) during the course of the pathway the average selectivity of neurons is increasing and that the range of selectivity is expanding from the inner ear to the forebrain.

2) an increase in selectivity is accompanied by a decrease in the bandwidth of the tuning curves.

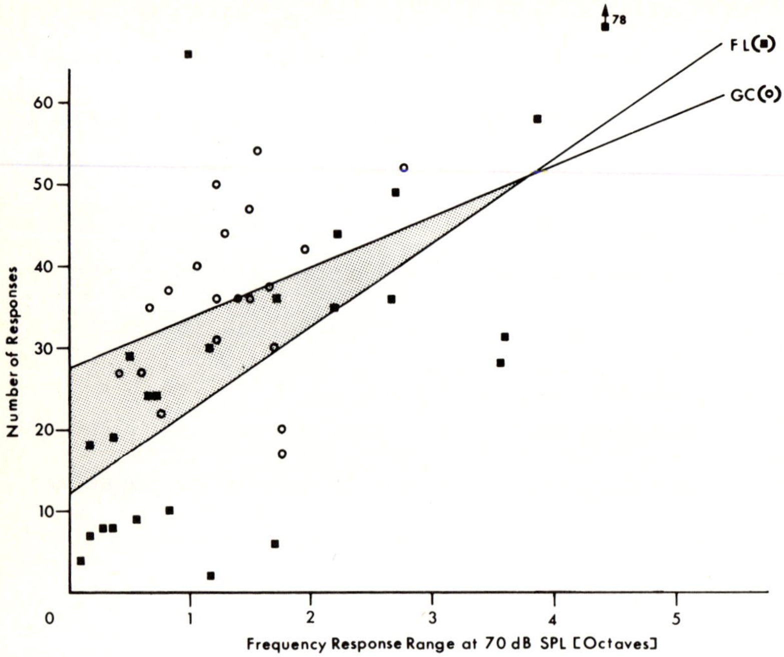

Fig. 2. Correlation between frequency response and selectivity of single units in the Neostriatum caudale (FL) and the cochlear ganglion (GC). Lines represent the linear regression of both groups of neurons. Neurons with the same frequency response bandwidth show a higher selectivity in forebrain units

3) the sharpening of tuning is not able to completely explain the increase in selectivity.

This implies that there must be additional processing mechanisms responsible for this increase. This is especially true for those highly selective units that respond to only a very few sounds and show no frequency response at all. Such units could not be dealt with in these considerations at all.

Part of the program of the Sonderforschungsbereich 114 (Bionach). The investigations of GC-neurons were done in cooperation with Dr. G.A. Manley.

References:

1) Leppelsack, H.-J.: Unit responses to species-specific sounds in the auditory forebrain center of birds. Fed.Proc. 37, 2236-2341 (1978).
2) Leppelsack, H.-J., Manley, G.A.: Reaktionen akustischer Neuronen im Ganglion cochleare des Staren auf arteigene Laute. Verhdl.deutsche Zool.Ges. 71, 192 (1978).
3) Leppelsack, J.-J., Vogt, M.: Responses of auditory neurons in the forebrain of a songbird during stimulation with species-specific sounds. J.comp.Physiol. 107, 263-274 (1976).
4) Manley, G.A., Leppelsack, H.-J.: Preliminary data on activity patterns of cochlear ganglion neurons in the starling Sturnus vulgaris. INSERM 68, 127-136 (1977).
5) Watanabe, T., Katsuki, Y.: Response patterns of single auditory neurons of the cat to species-specific vocalization. Jap.J.Physiol. 24, 135-155 (1974).

Encoding of Complex Sounds by Thalamic and Cortical Neurons

F.-C. HELLWEG, O. CREUTZFELDT and CHR. SCHREINER, Max-Planck-Institut für biophysikalische Chemie, Göttingen, W-Germany

In order to get an idea of the strategies used by a brain to process auditory signals we observed the discharges of single cortical and thalamic neurons recorded simultaneously in unanaesthetized guinea pigs. The question was how the complex structure of sounds was represented at the cortical and thalamic level.

We did not confine ourselves to ask how a sound is dissected into its spectral components and how these are represented by neuron discharges up through the auditory system. This would have resulted mainly in an investigation of tuning properties of individual neurons .

On the other hand we also did not try to find out, whether the presence or absence of an auditory signal could be represented as such by exclusively sound- or call-specific neuronal discriminators (Scheich et al., 1977; Leppelsack, 1974). This would - theoretically - require an infinite stimulus repertoire. An exclusive stimulation using species-specific vocalizations in the search for neuronal detectors is an unnecessary restriction. The organism usually has to handle and discriminate between a much larger number of sound signals and decide on their relevance.

We therefore used for auditory stimulation in this study - in addition to the classical AM - FM - click - signals - only sixteen complex sounds, including guinea pig vocalizations, cries of exotic birds and synthetized sounds at different intensities.

Results are derived from the responses of more than two hundred single neurons and over seventy thalamo-cortical neuron pairs, which yielded over four thousand plotted peri-stimulus-time-

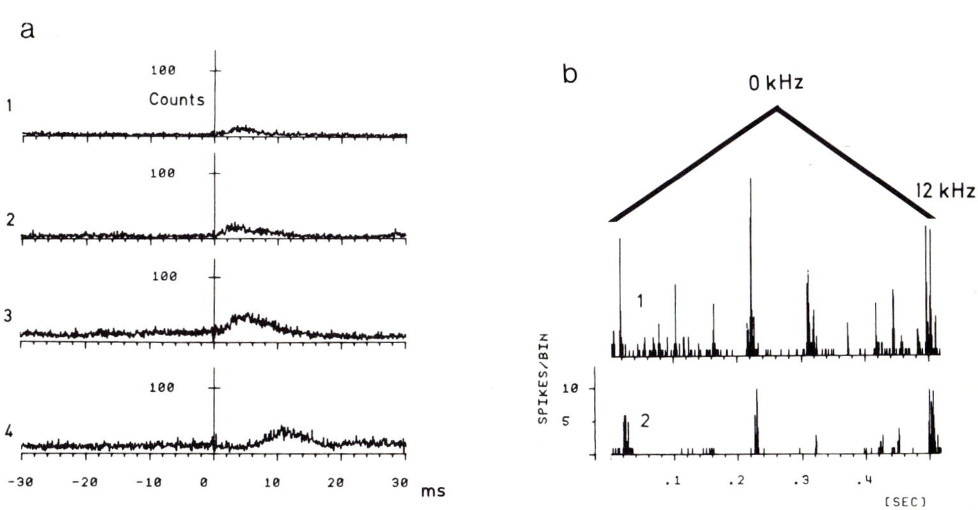

Fig. 1. A. Cross-correlation of four different thalamo-cortical unit pairs with different degrees of correlation of their spontaneous activity. Abscissa: Time of a cortical neuronal discharge relative to the thalamic neuronal discharges, which appear always at zero. Ordinate: Number of cortical discharges at different times preceding and following the thalamic discharges.
B: Response of a thalamo-cortical neuron pair to a frequency sweep from 12 to zero kHz and back. The main discharge peak corresponding to the CF appears at 1.8 kHz (0.22 and 0.32 sec, respectively), but the additional discharge peaks in the thalamic neuron (1) are less expressed in the cortical neuron (2). The discharge peaks at the beginning and the end of the PSTH are due to the on-set and the off-set of the frequency sweep at 12 kHz

histograms. The details of the methods, recording and test procedures are standard and will be described in detail in the main publication (Creutzfeldt et al., in press, 1979).

In short, once a thalamic cell had been isolated and its characteristic frequency been determined, a second electrode was lowered into the corresponding isofrequency stripe of the guinea pigs main large cochleotopic cortical field (Hellweg et al., 1978). If cell pairs were recorded simultaneously, a crosscorrelogram of both spike trains during spontaneous activity was performed. In nine out of seventy pairs we found a positive peak in the correlogram a few milliseconds after zero in the positive time axis. This indicated a synaptic connection between those cells (fig. 1A). Such a positive correlation was only seen between cells having the same best frequency (fig. 1B). This indicates a rather restricted thalamo-cortical convergence of excitatory inputs, at least as far as physiological coupling or functional synaptic linkage is concerned. This is somewhat in contrast with the broad divergent thalamo-cortical projection as demonstrated with radioactive and enzymatic tracer methods (Merzenich, this volume). The anatomical connections revealed with these methods, however, do not necessarily reflect a correspondingly strong functional synaptic linkage. Perhaps one should also take into account the possibility of trophic connections that have little relevance with respect to information transmission.

The difference between cortical and thalamic cell response patterns may be summarized as follows: thalamic cells generally show a higher spontaneous discharge rate and richer responses to stimuli than the cells of the main cochleotopic cortical field. The responses to individual modulations during stimulation with repetitive tone bursts or click-trains follow up to much higher repetition rates in thalamic cells (up to 120/sec at a one to one ratio) than in cortical cells (usually less than 30/sec). Therefore, also during more complex stimuli as for instance natural calls, repetitive contents of the stimulus that may still be represented by thalamic cells are not reflected in cortical cell discharge patterns (see fig. 2A and B; compare the histograms of the cortical versus the thalamic cell, which are synaptically linked in this case). Therefore, the detailed time structure of the sounds is not represented any more by the cortical responses, although still present in the thalamic neuronal response.

With respect to response specifity we found, that most cells of the large cochleotopic part of the guinea pig auditory cortex "responded" to more than one of the sixteen calls used. In two guinea pig cells no signal except for a certain call of the exotic mynah bird elicited a response (the guinea pig had not been exposed to mynah birds prior to the experiment). Such apparent response-specifities of cells, even if they respond exclusively to a few or even one species-specific call indicate merely, that such a call contains features to which the cell is responsive and which are not contained in the other calls tested.

Another phenomenon could be observed when the sound pressure level of the stimulating calls was varied. Many cortical as well as thalamic cells showed, at different intensities of the signal, qualitative differences in their response patterns.

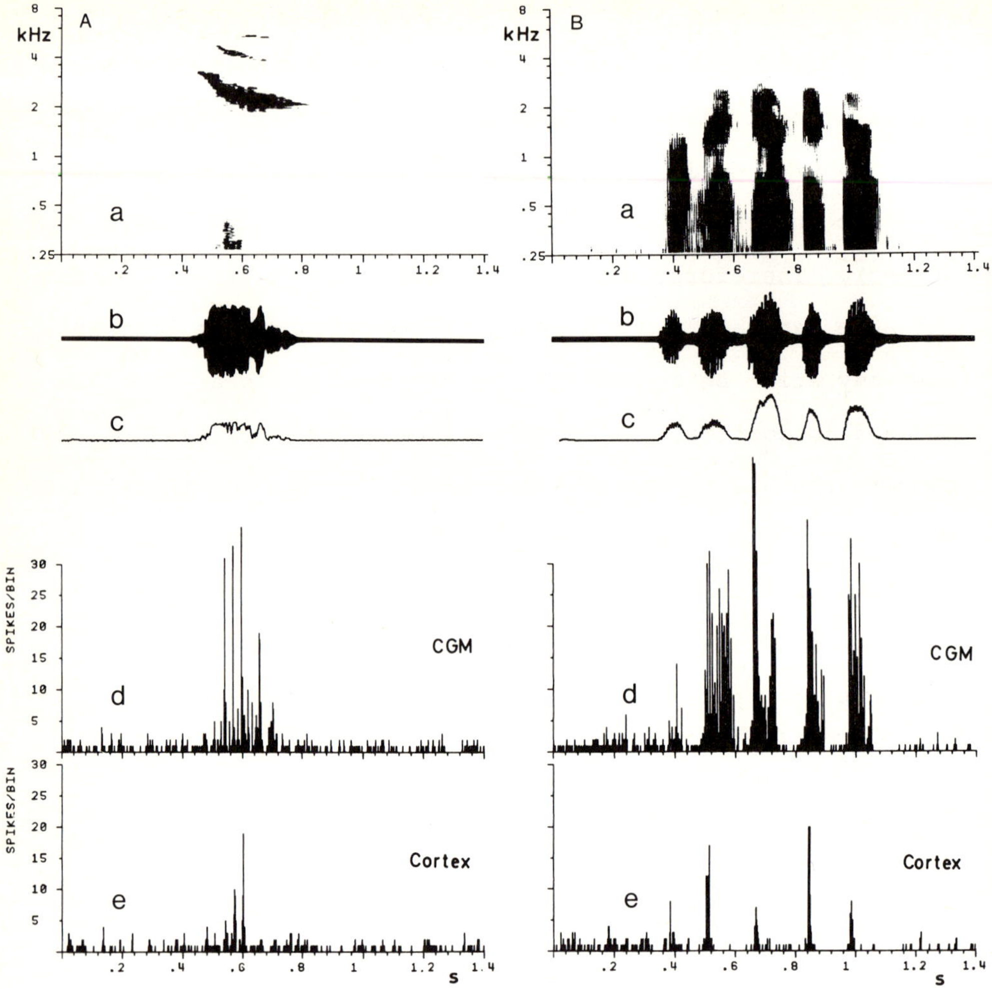

Fig. 2. Responses of a thalamo-cortical neuron pair to different natural sounds. The CGM and cortical neuron were synaptically connected as demonstrated by cross-correlation. In each record the various features of sounds are represented by the sonagram (a), the sound signal oscillograph (b) and the envelope (c). PSTH's are summed from 20 stimuli, bin width 2 msec, time in sec.
A: Whistle of a mynah bird. B: Repetitive rattling call of a mynah bird. For further details see text

Since conceptually a meaningful feature should be independant of intensity, this finding also does not support the suggestion, that single cells categorize in an all or none fashion complex parts of a meaningful stimulus.

References:

1) Creutzfeldt, O.; Hellweg, F.-C. and Schreiner, C.: Encoding of complex sounds in the thalamus and cortex of unanaesthetized guinea pigs. Exp. Brain Res., in press (1979).

2) Hellweg, F.C.; Koch, R. and Vollrath, M.: Representation of the cochlea in the Neocortex of guinea pigs. Exp. Brain Res. 29, 467-474 (1977).

3) Leppelsack, H.J.: Funktionelle Eigenschaften der Hörbahn im Feld L des Neostriatum Caudale des Staren (Sturnus vulgaris, Aves). J.Comp.Physiol. 88, 271-320 (1974).

4) Merzenich, M.M.: article see this volume.

5) Scheich, H.; Langner, G. and Koch, R.: Coding of narrow band and wide band vocalizations in the auditory midbrain nucleus of the guinea fowl (numida meleagris). J.Comp.Physiol. 117, 245-265 (1977).

This work was partly supported by the Deutsche Forschungsgemeinschaft, SFB 33, "Nervensystem und Information".

Time Segmentation in Central Analysis of Complex Signals

R. KOCH* and H. M. PIPER, Abt. Neurobiologie, Max-Planck-Institut f. biophys. Chemie, Göttingen. *Tierärztliche Hochschule Hannover, Med. Phys., Bischofsholer Damm 15, D-3000 Hannover, W-Germany

An auditory signal can be described as a function of frequency, intensity, and phase over time. While much experimental work is concerned with the representation of frequency, intensity and phase by neuronal activity in the brain, the temporal coding of a stimulus has somewhat been neglected. Two ranges of time representation may be discriminated: long-time and short-time analysis. The long-time analysis is concerned with a time range up to several seconds (words or sentences), while the short-time analysis works for sequences of some 100 msec up to a second (substructures of words like vowels or consonants). We are interested in mechanisms of short-time analysis of complex stimuli by the auditory system. We therefore asked first, which neuronal response parameter may code the time information of a stimulus?

In extracellular single unit records the responses of neurons of the colliculus inferior (CI) and the corpus geniculatum mediale (CGM) of unanaesthetized guinea pigs were analysed. We measured the tuning, intensity- and modulation transfer-characteristics as well as the reaction to different unmodified and modified natural sounds. At the best frequency (CF) three response types could be distinguished in accordance with other authors: tonic, phasic and mixed responses. The responses of most phasic neurons were extremely precise in temporal relation to certain signal parameters. This high temporal precision suggests that function of such responses may be the time marking of acoustical events. In addition these neurons carry information about frequency, intensity, modulation, direction and other parameters.

The responses of a neuron to tone pips of different frequencies and to different modified natural signals at 4 intensities are shown in the figure. For each stimulus the threshold intensity was determined independently and intensity values are given relative to the threshold for one stimulus condition. The spectral response width for pure tones depends on tone intensity, and at low sound pressure levels only a small frequency range evokes a response. At higher intensities the response area increases (fig. a). In all cases the response is strongly phasic.

In fig. b,c responses to amplitude modulated signals with different carrier frequencies are shown. It can be seen, that only the fast rising asymmetric triangular waveform elicits a response within the same frequency range and with the same intensity dependance of the spectral width of the spectral response region as seen with unmodulated tones. Figure d shows the response of the neuron to different bandpass ranges of a natural signal whose spectral composition is shown in fig. g. The signal was sent through a bandpass filter of 12 dB/oct. The center-frequencies of the bandpassfilter are the same as the tone frequencies used in fig. b and c. It is evident,

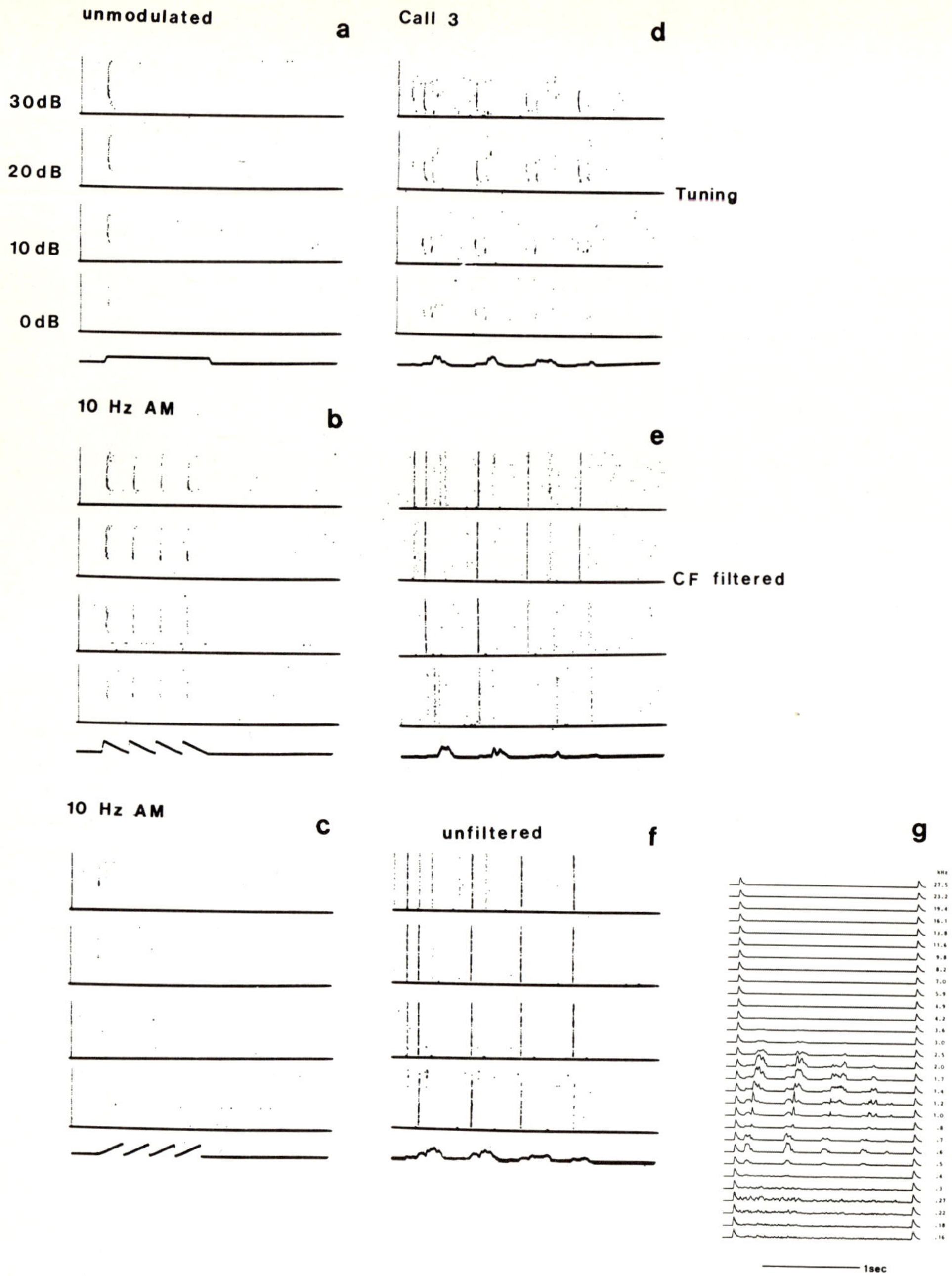

Fig. 1. Data of the inferior colliculus unit 22-5-78; CF = 2.5 kHz. The results are shown as dot-displays.
Each stimulus is presented at four different intensities as indicated on the left. The threshold condition corresponds to 0 dB. Below the diagrams the envelopes of the stimuli are shown. In figures a - d the carrier frequency of the

that the spectral sensitivity range and the intensity characteristics of the neuron are the same for natural signals as for synthetic stimuli. The small shift to lower frequencies can be due to the slope of the filter, which is not adapted to the slopes of the tuning curve of the neuron, and to the high intensity of low frequencies in the spectrogramm of the signal. These low frequencies were below the bestfrequency of the neuron (CF 2.5 kHz).

In part f of the figure the whole signal, and in part e the center-frequency band is used as stimulus. There is no significant difference in the time pattern of the response in all three presentation types of the natural sound. This behaviour is typical for the phasic responding neurons.

These results indicate, that already at the level of the inferior colliculus and the medial geniculate body neurons may exclusively respond to fast changes of the envelope of spectral signal components that fall into the tuning-range of this neuron. Different neurons may represent different parameters

---

Cont. Fig. 1.
stimuli is varied along the ordinate, which is divided into 30 frequency steps, thus scanning the range from 0.16 to 37.5 kHz in a logarithmis scale. The duration of the signals (abszissa) is 1 sec for synthetic stimuli and 2 sec for natural stimuli.
a. Tuning with tone bursts.
b and c. Tuning with amplitude modulated tone bursts, modulated by an asymmetric triangle.
d. Tuning with a natural sound of a guinea pig. The sound is sent through a bandpass filter (12 dB/octave) with center frequencies and envelopes of the output signals as shown in part g.
e. Thirty representations of a filtered natural call at four intensities. The center frequency of the filter is at 2.5kHz, which corresponds to the CF of the neuron.
f: Thirty representations of a unfiltered natural call

of the envelope like risetime, repetition rate and precision in time. Different complex stimuli may thus lead to different response patterns of time marks and comparable signals to comparable time patterns. Such a mechanism may make auditory signal analysis to some extent independent of carrier frequency as long as the temporal pattern is preserved.

References:

1) Funkenstein, H.H. and Winter, P.: Responses to a certain stimuli of units in the auditory cortex of awake squirrel monkeys. Exp. Brain Res. 29, 467-474 (1973).
2) Koch, R.: Akustische Signalverarbeitung in der zentralen Hörbahn. Diss. Göttingen (1975).
3) Piper, H.-M.: Akustische Signalübertragungseigenschaften im Colliculus inferior und Corpus geniculatum des Meerschweinchens. Diss. Göttingen (1979).
4) Winter, P. and Funkenstein, H.H.: The effect of species specific vocalizations on the discharge of auditory cortical cells in the awake squirrel monkey (saimiri sciureus). Exp. Brain Res. 18, 489-504 (1973).

This work was partly supported by the Deutsche Forschungsgemeinschaft, SFB 33, "Nervensystem und Information".

Temporal Suppression and Speech Processing

CHRISTOPH SCHREINER, Max-Planck-Institute for Biophysical Chemistry, D-3400 Göttingen-Nikolausberg, Am Faßberg, W-Germany

In order to get some insight in the processing of speech sounds in the auditory system, it is necessary to compare the response of auditory neurons to simple sounds (like sinusoidal stimuli) with the response of the neuron to complex or speech-like sounds. The classification of single neuron responses by simple sounds included for example tuning-properties, dynamic range, side-band inhibition, and the modulation-transfer characteristic (for review s. Keidel and Neff, 1975). In spite of such a detailed description of the neuronal response, it is difficult to predict out of this knowledge the response to speech-like signals. That means, that either not all properties of the unit can be obtained by using simple sounds, or that further properties of the unit response have to be investigated with simple sounds. One of these properties could be the temporal succession of parts of the signal.

It is well known, that the time segmentation of stimuli is an important aspect of signal processing and perception. An example is the influence of a gap between a consonant and the following vowel on the perception of the syllable (Liberman et al., 1967; Marcus, 1978). In neurophysiology it could be shown by several authors, that the response of a neuron to speech segments is - in addition to other parameters - a function of the neurons preceding activity and the context in which the information is embedded (Rupert et al., 1977; Watanabe et al., 1978). This suggests, that temporal effects seem to be very important for the representation of speech signals, especially at the upper auditory levels. In these regions the poststimulatory inhibition is strongly marked. As a consequence we may find a response reduction to a test stimulus if this is preceded by another stimulus, so-called temporal suppression.

To get more information about the behavior of the temporal suppression of simple sounds, alternating signals were used (Schreiner, 1979a). A masker and a test tone of 100 ms were presented alternately 5 times per second for about 1 minute. This corresponds to a certain degree with the temporal structure of syllables. Responses of single neurons in the mediale geniculate body (MGB) of the unanaesthetized guinea pig to each of the two signals were recorded.

In fig. 1 some results are displayed in diagrams. The upper left one shows the firing-rate connected with the test tone at the CF of the unit as a function of the level of the test tone. Parameter is the level of the preceding noise maker. An increase of the masker level yields a shift of the rate-intensity function to higher levels of the test tone. That means, that the temporal suppression causes a threshold shift for poststimulatory signals. The dynamic range of the response remains uninfluenced in this case of alternating stimuli.

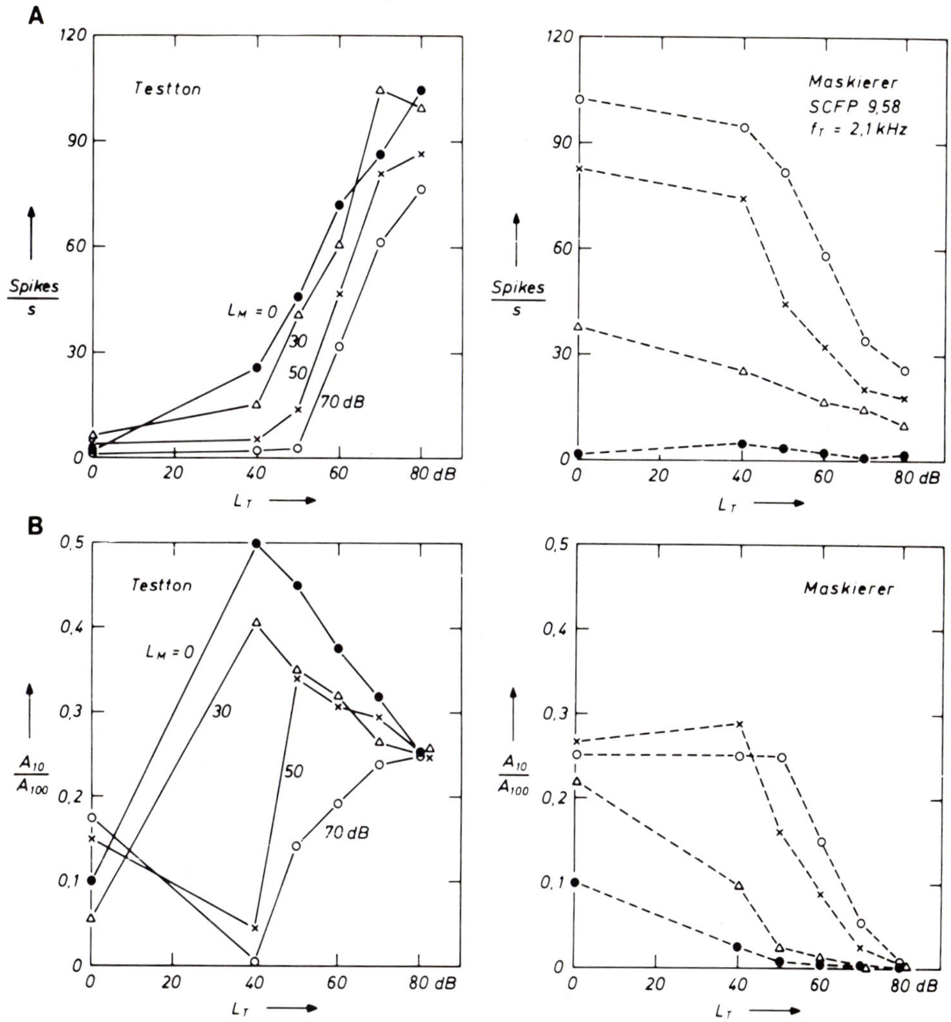

Fig. 1. A) Response of a thalamic neuron (MGB, CF = 2.1 kHz) to a test tone of 2.1 kHz (solid lines) and a masker noise (dashed lines) as a function of the level of the test tone. Parameter is the level of the noise. Test- and masker-stimuli of 100 msec duration were alternately presented. Binwidth: 100 msec.
b) Ratio of the phasic component (first 10 msec) to the complete activity (100 msec) of the response. Test tone: solid lines; masker: dashed lines

In the lower part of the diagram the ratio of the phasic part to the whole response is plotted as a function of the testtone level. By this way differences of the temporal influence on the phasic and tonic part of the response can be illustrated. The rapid change of the plotted ratio (as well as of the absolute amplitude of the phasic response) for a masker of 50 dB indicates, that a small change of test-tone level yields a rebound of the phasic part of the test-tone response within a small dynamic range, whereas the recovery of the tonic response stretches over a wider range. This rapid change of the on-set response within a small region of a parameter looks like a threshold transition, separating two regions of different responsiveness. The sudden increase of the test-tone response goes parallel with a sudden decrease of the masker response (dashed curves in fig. 1).

In the next step we want to compare the results of suppression between non-simultaneously presented signals with the suppression between simultaneously presented stimuli. For this purpose an iso-intensity tuning of the neurons was done. The full line in fig. 2 shows the response to test tones at various frequencies (90 dB SPL). The best frequency of the unit is about 10 kHz. The dash-dotted line represents the result for presenting a fixed 10 kHz-tone simultaneously with the variable test tone. We notice a clear two-tone inhibition in the frequency region of 1 to 7 kHz and, in addition, around 13 kHz. The response of the fixed 10 kHz-tone is reduced in the lower inhibition area down to the spontaneous activity of the unit.

The dashed line in fig. 2 shows the response of the fixed 10 kHz-tone plotted versus the frequency of a preceding variable test tone. In other words, the fixed and the variable tone are presented non-simultaneously. We can observe a reduction

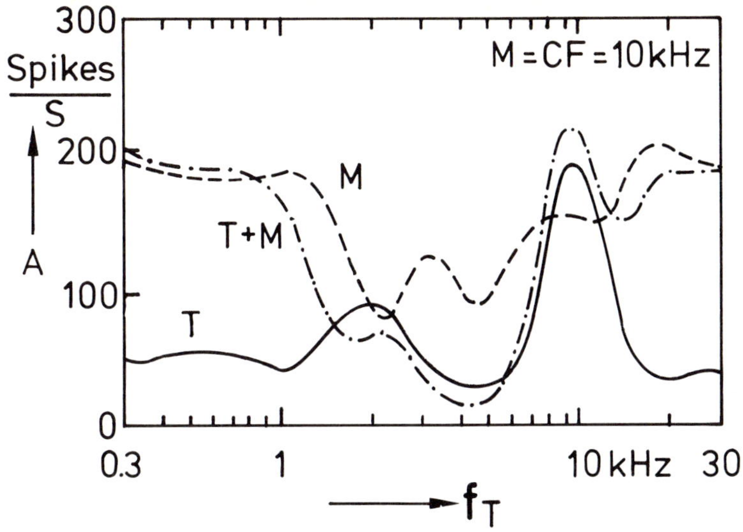

Fig. 2. Two-tone inhibition of simultaneously presented test tone (T) and masker (M) (dash-dotted line) and alternately presented test tone and masker (dashed line) as function of the frequency of the test tone (90 dB SPL). The masker was a fixed tone of 10 kHz (CF) and 90 dB SPL. The solid line is the result of an iso-intensity tuning of the test tone (90 dB SPL). MGB; CF = 10 kHz; binwidth: 100 msec

of the response of the fixed tone, too. The frequency region of the suppression is narrower than the inhibitory area of the simultaneously presented signals. However, the resemblance between both suppression regions is evident. The non-simultaneous suppression of the response is less strong than in case of the simultaneous suppression. In addition a suppression takes place at the best frequency itself, in contrast to simultaneous presentation. Psychoacoustical measurements of non-simultaneous loudness reduction yield similar suppression areas (Schreiner, 1979b).

To distinguish, whether there is a difference in the temporal suppression evoked by a preceding excitatory or inhibitory response, the following measurement was performed on inferior-

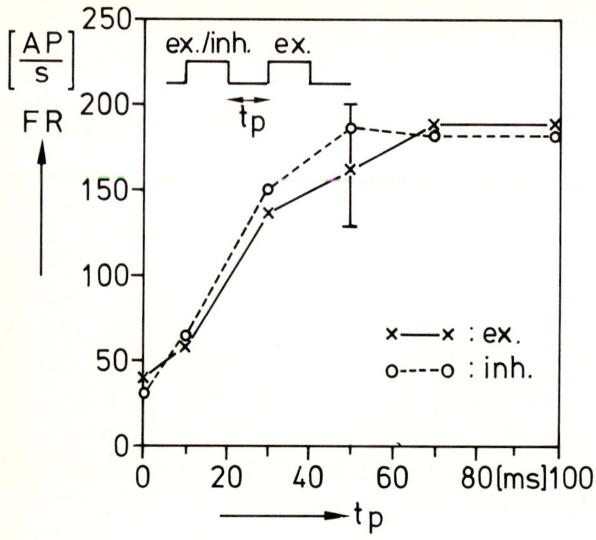

Fig. 3. Poststimulatory inhibition of the on-set response of 6 inferior-colliculus neurons as a function of the time gap between the conditioning stimulus and the following excitatory (CF) test stimulus. Solid line: excitatory conditioning signal. Dashed line: inhibitory conditioning signal. Binwidth: 10 msec

colliculus (CI) neurons (fig. 3): The phasic response of an excitatory stimulus was obtained as a function of the time gap between the end of a preceding signal and the beginning of the excitatory stimulus. The curves show, that the recovery of the phasic response of the second stimulus is nearly the same for an excitatory and an inhibitory signal serving as conditioning (first) stimulus. The time course of the recovery is similar to phoneme boundaries, e.g. between "slit" and "split" in dependence on the silent-interval duration between "s" and "l" (Marcus, 1978).

The similarity of the simultaneous and the non-simultaneous suppression and of the recovery of the onset after inhibitory and excitatory conditioning suggest, that the temporal suppression seen in CI and MGB seems to be an inhibitory process and not an effect of peripheral adaptation or even of mechanical/ cochlear origin. Furthermore, the temporal suppression seems not to be a side-band inhibition, but a process which is spread over the whole response area of the neuron. The time constant of the temporal suppression corresponds to the inhibition in CI and MGB, measured with clicks by Aitkin and Dunlop (1969).

In connection with the processing of speech in upper levels of the auditory system, the temporal-suppression effect indicates, that the succession of spectral components has a strong influence on the internal representation of a signal by neuronal responses. This corresponds to the influence of context on the perception of vowels and consonants known from psychophysical investigations.

References:

1) Aitkin, L.M. and Dunlop, C.W.: Inhibition in the medial geniculate body of the cat. Exp. Brain Res. 7, 68-83 (1969).
2) Keidel, W.D. and Neff, W.D. (eds.): Handbook of Sensory Physiology, V/2 Auditory System, Springer-Verlag (1975).
3) Liberman, A.; Cooper, F.; Shankweiler, D. and Studdert-Kennedy, M.: Perception of the speech code. Psychol. Review 74, 431-461 (1967).
4) Marcus, S.M.: Distinguishing "slit" and "split" - an invariant timing cue in speech perception. Perception & Psychophysics 23, 58-60 (1978).
5) Rupert, A.L.; Caspary, D.M. and Moushegian, G.: Response characteristics of the cochlear nucleus neurons to vowel sounds. Ann.Otol. 86, 37-48 (1977).
6) Schreiner, Chr.: Darstellung alternierender akustischer Signale in der zentralen Hörbahn von Meerschweinchen. Med. Dissertation, Göttingen (1979).
7) Schreiner, Chr.: Nichtsimultane Lautheitsdrosselung und ihr Einfluß auf die Pulsationsschwelle. Acustica 42, 158-165, (1979).
8) Watanabe, T. and Sakai, H.: Responses of the cat's collicular neuron to human speech. J.Acoust.Soc.Am. 64, 333-337 (1978).

This work was partly supported by the Deutsche Forschungsgemeinschaft, SFB 33, "Nervensystem und Information".

Feature Detection by Single Units in Squirrel Monkey Auditory Cortex

J. D. NEWMAN and D. SYMMES, Laboratory of Developmental Neurobiology, National Institute of Child Health and Human Development, National Institutes of Health, Bethesda, Md. 20205, USA

Studies of the responses of central auditory neurons to species-specific vocalizations and other natural sounds inevitably converge on the issue of what acoustic dimensions within these sounds trigger neural activation. This issue is central to hypotheses of the representation of natural sounds by single neurons, particularly with respect to whether vocalizations are represented as individual entities, as structural or functional classes, or as smaller units consisting of limited numbers of acoustic features. Hypothetical "call detectors" have been postulated whose activation depends on the occurrence in the same vocalization of several acoustic dimensions or features, which together uniquely specify that particular call. Two kinds of detectors may be postulated. Detectors activated by calls rich in harmonic or formant structure would be sensitive to a particular contemporaneous combination of spectral peaks. In these cases, <u>spectral facilitation</u> plays a significant role. On the other hand, detectors of vocalizations characterized by a sequence of FM elements (typical of contact calls in the squirrel monkey) would require for activation <u>temporal facilitation</u> by the summative effect of several features occurring sequentially. This latter supposition has not been adequately tested experimentally. One possible outcome of such testing would be to demonstrate that temporal facilitation is required for activation. An alternative outcome, however, would be to demonstrate that a restricted segment within a vocalization by itself triggers a response equivalent to the response evoked by the entire call. This alternative implies a process of feature detection, whereby acoustic features residing at discrete loci whithin the structural framework of the vocalization are not additive in their effectiveness in driving a neuron. We have directly tested the role of temporal facilitation in cortical neurons by comparing the rate of response during an active segment of an intact vocalization with rate of response to the same segment presented as an isolated vocal fragment. The results of this testing clearly characterize the neurons studied by us as "feature detectors" rather than "call detectors".

Methods:

Extracellular discharges of single cortical units were obtained from unanesthetized monkeys using methods outlined in detail elsewhere (1). Our previous studies indicated that stable, temporally discrete responses are more often recorded from cells lying in primary auditory cortex (PAC) than from cells lying more ventral on the lateral surface of the superior temporal gyrus. Since this response characteristic is an asset in identifying active segments of a test vocalization, we have limited our penetrations to cortex of the upper 2 mm below the lateral fissure. We have utilized as test stimuli natural or spontaneously occurring vocalizations of the squirrel monkey chosen from the major vocal classes of that species (2). Nine tokens from our library of tape-recorded vocalizations were presented via a pair of Sennheiser HD 414 ear phones coupled to each ear by a latex form. The frequency response of the system at the entry to the external meatus was linear ± 5 dB over 600-19000 Hz. Our goal was to select from the 9 tokens one that was optimally effective in driving the unit under study. This goal was facilitated by first determining the best frequency (BF), threshold intensity of the BF, and optimal aural presentation configuration (binaural, contra-, or ipsilateral) utilizing pure tone stimuli. This helped us to choose the intensity and aural pattern for testing with vocal tokens. It also provided data for comparisons of the responses of the same unit to artificial and vocal stimuli, an aspect of our studies not covered here.

In more than half of the units, testing near threshold intensity resulted in only one or two vocalizations driving the unit, allowing us to select the token most consistently producing a response. This token was then tested by itself over a range of 60-80 dB SPL to determine the intensity producing the strongest and most consistent response. This intensity was used thereafter to compare the unit's response to the intact call vs. isolated fragments. Fragments were isolated through the use of a programmable gate (5 ms rise-fall time) by which we deleted all but a restricted part of the vocalization. The average rate of the unit to the fragment producing the strongest response was computed over 10 - 20 presentations, and compared with the average rate of the unit computed in like manner for the corresponding temporal segment within the intact, undeleted call. Data for these two rate comparisons were collected within a few minutes of each other to control for a drift in the unit's overall responsiveness.

Results:

We have made rate comparisons in 17 units. In no case was the response rate to the intact vocalization stronger than to the isolated fragment. In 7 units, the rate to the fragment and to the intact call was nearly the same (the rates being within - or +25% of each other). In the rest of the units, the driven rate to the frament was up to 3 times greater than to the intact call. These results are summarized in Fig. 1.

Conclusions:

As stated in the introductory comments, the property of feature detection is manifest in a single neuron if the neuron responds

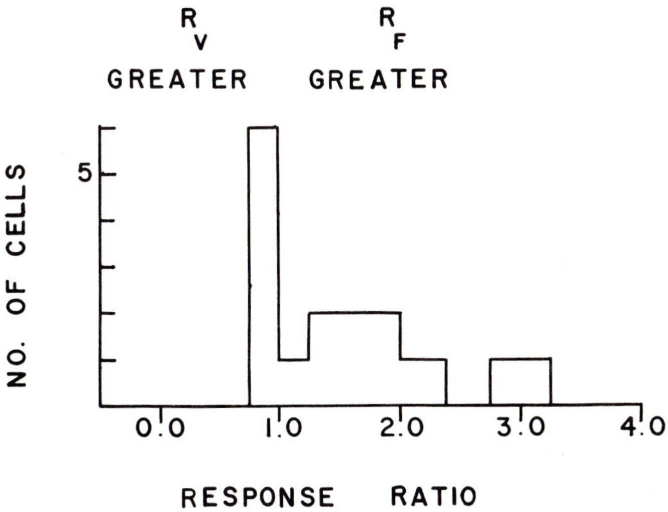

Fig. 1. Ratio of response evoked by isolated vocal fragment (R_F) to response evoked by same fragment imbedded in intact cell (R_V) as measured in 17 PAC neurons. A ratio of 1.0 implies equal response rates in the two conditions, and a ratio of zero implies that the response disappeared when the fragment was isolated. Seven of the 9 vocalizations in our test series are represented at least once

as strongly to an isolated fragment as it does to the fragment embedded within the rest of the vocalization. Our results clearly demonstrate that PAC neurons are properly labelled "feature detectors" by this criterion. We may conclude from these findings that temporal facilitation does not play a significant role in influencing the response vigor of PAC units to vocalizations. On the other hand, the fact that in a majority of our units the optimal fragment actually produced a stronger response suggests that temporal inhibition is present. This means that an antecedent part of a vocalization, even though not triggering a response by itself, may depress the driven rate of a unit to a later part of the call. We have found further evidence for temporal inhibition by the fact that, in a few units, testing with isolated fragments revealed additional responses not evident in testing with the intact call. The functional significance of temporal inhibition requires further clarification. We suggest, however, that it may play a role in sharpening the response to an effective fragment, as well as increasing the relative importance of acoustic features within that fragment by suppressing responses to weaker, less optimal features residing in other segments of the same vocalization. This would have the effect of increasing the differences between similar features or vocal elements, thereby improving discrimination between them. Since we have found that natural variants of a particular call type differ in one or more structural detail according to the vocalizer (Isolation Peep; Chuck) or context (Chuck; Twitter), neural circuitry capable of detecting these differences is likely to exist. The results presented here suggest that PAC neurons are part of that circuity.

References:

1) Newman, J.D., Wollberg, Z.: Multiple coding of species-specific vocalizations in squirrel monkey auditory cortex. Brain Res. 54, 287-304 (1973).

2) Ploog, D., Hupfer, K., Juergens, U., Newman, J.D.: Neuroethological studies of vocalization in squirrel monkeys with special reference to genetic differences of calling in two subspecies. In: M.A.B. Brazier (ed.) Growth and Development of the Brain, Raven Press (New York), 231-254 (1975).

Processing of Self-produced Vocalizations by Single Neurons in the Auditory Cortex of the Squirrel Monkey (Saimiri Sciureus)

P. MÜLLER-PREUSS, Max-Planck-Institut für Psychiatrie, München, FRG

Two systems in the brain have been shown by anatomical and physiological studies to deal with acoustic communication; motor structures which produce vocalizations and sensory structures which process auditory information. The first system is anatomically not well defined, however it is suggested that the area around the genu of the corpus callosum in the limbic cortex and the central grey matter in the midbrain play an important role in phonation[1]. The other system, which processes auditory information, is the anatomically well-defined auditory pathway. In general the purpose of this work has been to study the relationships between these two systems. Two questions arising from this complex of problems are: 1) Does the auditory system process self-produced vocalizations differently from vocalizations coming from the environment? 2) Does the auditory system receive neuronal information from structures which are involved in phonation before vocalizations are emitted by the larynx? In a partial attempt to answer these questions the activity of single cells in the auditory cortex of the squirrel monkey was extracellularly recorded during phonation. Because it is difficult to evoke vocalization from these monkeys in a controlled behavioral situation, vocal activity was mainly elicited through electrical stimulation of the central grey. In a few cases it was possible to record the activity of cells during spontaneously emitted calls. The stimulation and recording sites are schematically shown in fig. 1.

Only those stimulation points were used, which elicited vocalizations 100-800 ms after the end of the electrical stimulation. Stimulus duration was 1-1.5 sec, the pulse lenght 1 ms, the intensity up to 400 micro-Amps and the frequency 30 Hz. The stimulation of individual electrodes consistently evoked the same call, differing only slightly in amplitude. The auditory pathway was at first stimulated during phonation with these self-produced vocalizations. Then as a comparable

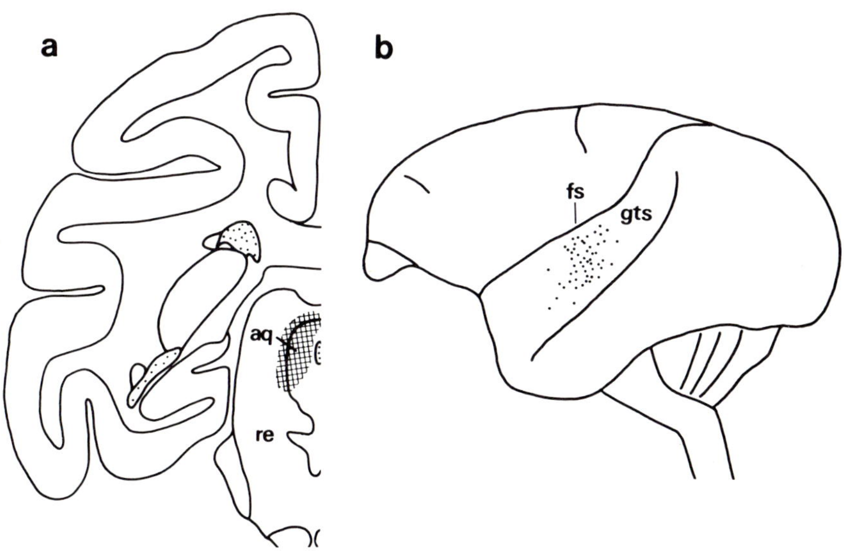

Fig. 1. (a): Site of brain stimulation shown by cross-hatching.
(b): Site of recording, shown by black dots.

aq: central grey matter
fs: fissura sylvii
gts: superior temporal gyrus
re: reticular formation

acoustic stimulus without effects of phonation, these self-produced vocalizations were recorded on an endless-loop tape, later played back to the monkeys. The auditory input during play-back of the self-produced vocalizations was similar to the original input during phonation, even given changes caused by bone conduction[2], and is therefore appropriate for comparison of the neural responses. The played-back calls were presented at different sound-intensities in the range of 40-80 dB SPL to characterize the intensity/response-relationships of the cells. Finally to test in general the acoustic reactivity of the neurons, various species-specific vocalizations and artificial sounds such as white noise were used. With 185 cells it was possible to observe the activity shortly before and during phonation evoked by electrical brain-stimulation. In about 10 neurons activity was recorded during spontaneously emitted vocalizations. Taking these latter data into account is a little bit problematic, because only one or two spontaneous calls can be compared with longer series of electrically evoked or loudspeaker transmitted calls. No cells were observed in which a significant change in spontaneous activity occurred before the beginning of the vocalizations. In the case of the electrically evoked vocalizations the observation-time was at least from the end of the electrical stimulation to the beginning of the call on average 400 ms. One hundred five cells have been studied with the full acoustic test-programm, the most important part of which was the play-back of the electrically evoked vocalizations. Less than 50 % of the tested cells displayed no significant difference in response pattern throughout the duration of a self-produced call in comparison to play-back and other vocalizations. More than 50 % of the tested neurons in the auditory cortex showed a significant difference in the response to self-produced compared with loudspeaker transmitted vocalizations. In these cells responses are either much weaker or totally absent during own vocal activity. Two examples of this type of cells are shown in fig. 2. Both cells respond to loudspeaker transmitted calls with a sustained excitation, but as can be seen in the upper

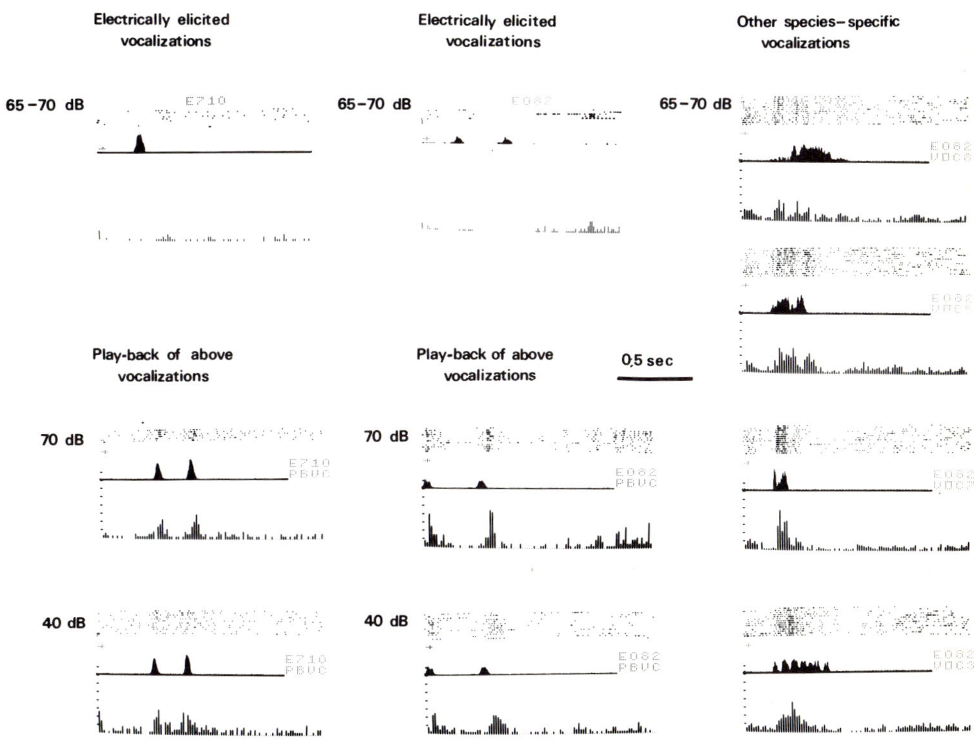

Fig. 2. Two examples of cells which differentiate between self-produced and loudspeaker transmitted calls. In each section the upper traces are raster diagrams in which each dot represents one actionpotential. The middle trace in each section shows the time course of the call and the lower trace a PST-Histogram (Binwidth 15 ms)

left and middle part of the figure do not react to the self-produced call. A qualitatively similar reaction is shown by those neurons which were tested during spontaneous calls. In these cells a comparison of the reactivity was only possible with other species-specific calls, not for play-back calls. In two cases the cells respond to all presented acoustic stimuli, but not to the self-produced vocalization. To investigate the possible influence of electrical stimulation on the acoustic reactivity of the neurons, some cells were stimulated almost simultaneously with loudspeaker transmitted and self-produced vocalizations. Shortly after the end of the electrical stimulation and before phonation a previously recorded call was presented. These cells responded to the loudspeaker transmitted calls, even when preceeded by electrical stimulation, but not always to the self-produced vocalizations. Together with the results from the reaction to spontaneously self-produced calls, this is evidence that the observed inhibitory effects on the acoustic reactivity during phonation is not caused directly by the electrical stimulation.

As there were no cells which showed a significant change in spontaneous activity before the beginning of a call, either during electrical elicitation or spontaneous phonation, it may be concluded that the auditory cortex does not receive at this time information about the activity of structures involved in phonation. This would indicate that at the cortical level the auditory system does not receive information from the motor structures during the time of neuronal preparation for vocalization in the sense of a corollary discharge[3]. The fact that more than 50 % of the investigated cells differed in their response to self-produced versus loudspeaker transmitted calls seems an indication that the auditory cortex receives different information depending upon the source of the call. It is suggested that this inhibition during self-vocalization is caused by the activated vocalization structures and might be the result of corollary discharges from motor structures to subcortical parts of the auditory system. In bats neural attenuation during phonation has been demonstrated at the level of the lateral lemniscus[4]. The biological value of a processing mechanism which differentiates in this way or such an inhibitory influence during an animal's own activity is obvious: One part of the auditory cortex would receive full information about phonation, information which might be important for learning or modulating vocalizations. One part would not be occupied and perhaps not blocked during phonation which might be important for the processing of essential signals coming from the environment during this time.

References:

1) Békésy G.v.: The structure of the middle ear and the hearing of one's own voice by bone conduction. J.Acoust.Soc.Am. 21, 217-232 (1949).
2) Evarts, E.V.: Feedback and corollary discharge: A merging of the concepts. Neurosc.Res.Symp.Summ. 6, 86-112 (1972).
3) Jürgens, U.: Reinforcing concomitans of electrically elicited vocalizations. Exp.Brain Res. 26, 203-214 (1976).
4) Suga, N., Shimozawa, T.: Site of neural attenuation of responses to self-vocalized sounds in echolocating bats. Science 183, 1211-1213 (1974).

Encoding Processes of Speech Sounds in the Auditory System

FINKENZELLER, P.[1], THUMFART, W.[2], FELLNER, E.[1]
[1] Institut für Physiologie und Biokybernetik, Universität Erlangen-Nürnberg, Universitätsstr. 17, D-8520 Erlangen
[2] Universitäts-Hals-Nasen-Ohren-Klinik, Waldstr. 1, D-8520 Erlangen, FRG

Auditory prosthesis represent an ideal possibility of checking neurophysiological results and of combining individual findings in hearing research to form an integrated whole. Progress in microsurgery and microelectronics requires from the neurophysiologist the information as to how many independent stimulation channels need to be provided, and how speech needs to be processed for transmission by these channels in order to restore hearing ability by a given amount.

Starting with the coding and decoding mechanisms of the inner ear with respect to intensity, frequency, and periodicity of sound, it would seem possible to predict the performance of an auditory prosthesis. Hereby, it does not matter if such a prosthesis is based on electrical, vibrotactile, or optical stimulation, or on effective use of residual hearing.

As an example, a method of frequency transposition for matching speech frequencies to the frequency range of neural excitation, developed during the last six years at Erlangen, is described. In contrast to attempts to perform the frequency transposition by the use of segmented rotating tape heads (Oeken, 1966) or by frequency warping (Ohnsorge and Boerger, 1977), which are optimal for the conservation of the spectral distribution, we isolated segments of the speech signal of 5 to 20 ms duration and expanded them in time at the cost of redundant segments (Kusch, 1971). In the meantime we have succeeded in constructing a device which permits the selection of a transposition ratio between 1:1 and 1:3.75 in 12 steps. The expanded segments are connected with inaudible transitions. This method conserves phase relations and envelope of the signal which, in the context of periodicity hearing, would seem to be very important for speech recognition (Keidel, 1974; Finkenzeller und Keidel, 1976).

On the basis of hearing tests and learning time, the advantages of this on-line transposition device are demonstrated for low frequency hearing and vibrotactile stimulation. Confusion matrices show that some transposed sounds cannot be recognized as expected. The attempt to explain this phenomenon is of particular neurophysiological interest since, after retransformation of the transposed speech signals, without further processing, they again become intelligible and discriminable.

To derive objective criteria for the perception of complex sounds, we averaged auditory evoked potentials of several seconds duration based on the dc-recorded vertex-EEG in man. The properties of these potentials were determined by systematically varying the stimulus with respect to intensity, frequency, and time resolution and by investigating the interaction of stimuli of different modalities (Keidel, 1976). It was established that every perceived acoustic event gave rise to an evoked potential provided that a minimum interval of 80 ms between events was observed. This held true right down to the subjective threshold level and makes this technique of interest also for the application of words as stimulus (Finkenzeller, 1979).

When, for example, the two digit numeral "achtundsiebzig" (78) of the Freiburger word test is presented, the resulting evoked potential largely corresponds to the envelope curve of the sound pressure. This can be shown by means of an appropriately modulated sinusoidal signal which produces similar results. Close to the threshold the potential latencies increase steeply, mirroring the mean loss of discrimination of the word list.

In order further to investigate the basis of prosthetic stimulation of the ear, we implanted electrodes, using the transoccipital approach, in the cochlear nerve of the cat near the porus acusticus internus. On one hand these electrodes permitted registration of the activity of adjacent nerve fibers following acoustic stimulation, while on the other they could be used to apply an appropriate current for electrostimulation. In particular with respect to the clinical application, objective criteria are necessary to check the selectivity of the different stimulus channels and to prove the adequacy of the electrical stimulation.

In a first series of experiments, enamelled electrodes of 100 μm diameter were securely implanted over a five month experimental period. During this time the threshold for electrical stimulation remained constant at 150 μA. But a systematic change of the shape of evoked responses from addiionally implanted cortical electrodes indicated an unwanted spread of current at higher intensities - which would appear to confirm that pitch perception is intensity dependent. To avoid this effect we then implanted a set of 4 teflon-isolated steel electrodes, electrolytically sharpened to 5µm, with a distance between them of 200 µm. With electrodes of this size single unit activity can sometimes be recorded. In any case the compound action potential obtained originates only from a number of fibers in a nerve fascicle.

These potentials were investigated carefully under various stimulation conditions. One result, which may be of particular importance for an understanding of the information processing in higher parts of the auditory pathway, namely the emphasizing of sound transients, is demonstrated here.

If we apply a tone burst of 25 ms duration, tonic and phasic parts can be isolated from the compound AP by the usual phase reversal of the stimulus with an appropriate addition (phase independent response), or subtraction (phase dependent response) of the raw signal obtained.

The phasic part behaves like the frequency following response with a clear amplitude maximum at 1 kHz, extending approximately from 200 Hz to 4 kHz (Fig. 1). After an initial P_1-N_1-P_2-complex, the classical AP, the tonic part lasts for some 15 ms with little frequency dependence. This is shown in Fig. 2 for different intensities and it is worth noting that at lower intensities the periodicity of the response develops with a delay of one or two periods.

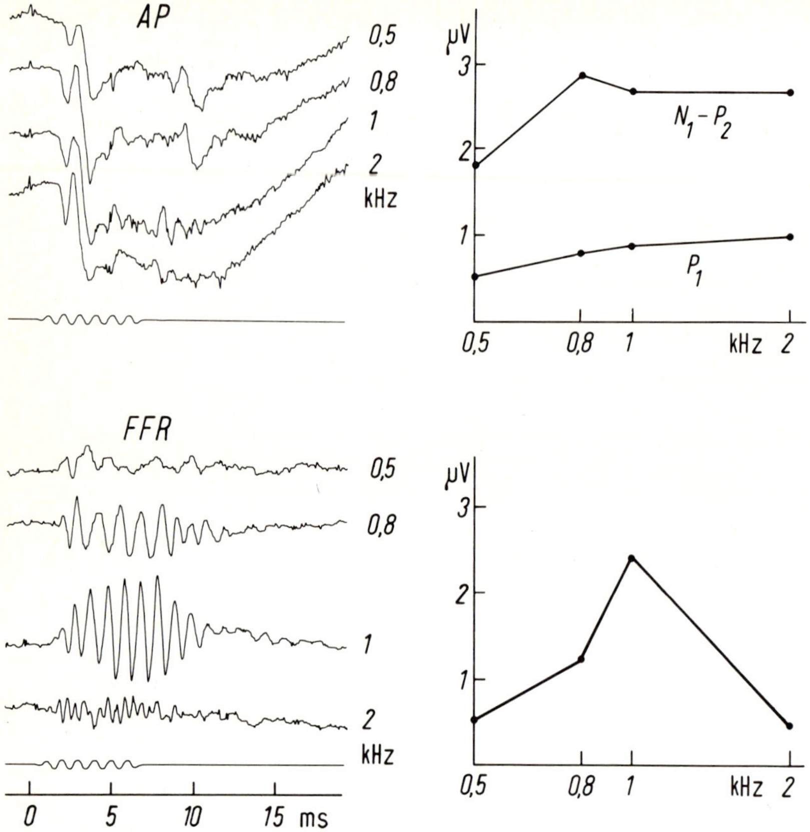

Fig. 1. Potentials from long-term implanted electrodes in the cochlear nerve of the cat.
Above: Mass potentials recorded with phase reversal of tone burst stimulus for the frequencies indicated.
Below: Same experiment, but the two potentials elicited by tones of reversed phase subtracted from each other in order to isolate phase dependent part (frequency following response).
Right: Amplitude-frequency characteristics of the evoked potential (above) and the frequency following response

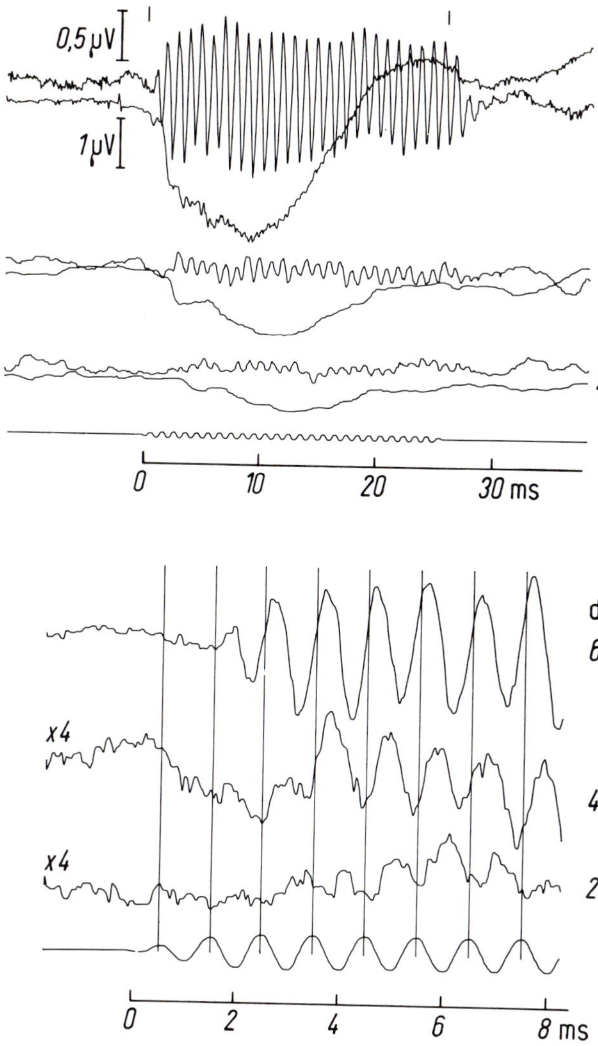

Fig. 2. Isolated tonic APs and frequency following responses recorded for 3 intensities of a 25 ms tone burst as indicated. Below, onsets of frequency following responses shown with expanded time scale

The question arises as to whether for the decoding of complex sounds the degree of synchronized activity in single groups of nerve fibers or neurons is evaluated, possibly by coincidence and anticoincidence networks, to realize the simultaneously required high intensity- and frequency selectivity.

References:

1) Finkenzeller, P.: Auditory evoked potentials - late cortical responses. In: H.A. Beagley (ed.), Technological Basis of Auditory Investigation, Oxford University Press (1979).
2) Finkenzeller, P.; Keidel, W.D.: The intelligibility of frequency transposed speech. Int. Congress of Audiology, Florence, p. 172 (A) (1979).
3) Keidel, W.D.: The cochlear model in skin stimulation. In: F.A. Geldard (ed.): Conference on vibrotactile communication. Psychonomic Society, Austin/Texas (1974).
4) Keidel, W.D.: The physiological background of the electric response audiometry. In: W.D. Keidel, W.D. Neff (eds.): Handbook of Sensory Physiology, Vol. V/3, 106-231, Springer-Verlag, Berlin, Heidelberg, New York (1976).
5) Kusch, H.: Ein neues Verfahren zur Verbesserung der Sprache in Heliumatmosphäre. Acustica 25, 42-46 (1971).
6) Oeken, F.-W.: Frequenztransposition zur Hörverbesserung? Hals-, Nasen- und Ohrenheilkunde 17, 88 (1966).
7) Ohnsorge, H.; Boerger, G.: Aufbereitung von Sprachsignalen zur Kommunikation mit Schwersthörigen. Abschlußbericht zum Projekt (1977).

Verb and Noun Meaning of Homophone Words Activate Different Cortical Generators: A Topographical Study of Evoked Potential Fields

W. S. BROWN and D. LEHMANN, Dept. of Neurology, Univ. Hospitals,
8091 Zürich, Switzerland

Certain aspects of language have been hypothesized to be processed in different cortical areas or by different neural elements.

In addition to the classical differentiation between expressive and receptive aphasia, preferential impairment of noun or verb word finding was reported by Kleist (1934, p.801), and Brown (1972, p.26 and 29). Recent research (Brown et al., 1973, 1976; Marsh and Brown, 1977) has shown that different contextual meanings of homophone words evoke different EEG response waveforms. Discriminant analysis of this data showed maximal differences between responses at different electrode sites for individual response epochs (Brown et al., 1976).

The present paper investigates the scalp topography of EEG responses evoked by the noun or verb meanings of homophones in sentence context. The main features of EEG scalp-fields are simple (Lehmann, 1971, 1977; Lehmann et al., 1977b; Ragot et al., 1976) and can be described at a moment in time by the location of the maximal and minimal field values (Lehmann, 1971, 1977). If neural populations for the processing of nouns and verbs differ, different locations of maximal and minimal evoked field values are expected.

The choice of the reference does not influence the configuration of scalp-field distribution, and thus does not affect the location of the maximal and minimal values, or the voltage differences between any recording points at a given moment in time; however, the waveshapes (in time) recorded from any single electrode are influenced by the choice of the reference (Lehmann, 1971, 1977).

One stimulus paradigm was English and the other Swiss-German: "a pretty rose" and "the boatman rows"; and "e schöni chlini Flüüge" (a pretty little fly) and "en Vogel chunnt z'flüüge" (a bird comes flying). The test sentences were tape-recorded, and the stimulus word, with an associated trigger pulse, was spliced into the two sentences from each paradigm.

To rule out any effects of the acoustic differences in the words preceding the stimulus word, a blurred, speech-like tone sequence was produced by amplitude modulating a 500 Hz tone with a rectified and low-pass filtered original test sentence. The resulting sound sequence was not understandable; upon suggestion of wordings ("e schöni chlini Flüüge" or "en Vogel chunnt z'flüüge") either wording was judged to be equally likely. Thus, depending on the instructions to the subject (S), the identical blurred stimulus could elicit a noun or verb interpretation.

The 21 Ss were all right-handed, healthy females (age 18-35). The English sentences were presented to seven native English speaking Ss, and the Swiss German sentences, as well as the blurred sentences, to native Swiss-German speaking Ss (seven in either group).

Electrodes were attached in a transverse 2 x 4 array (15 x 20 cm) around the vertex (Fig. 1A). Data were recorded in 13 channels against the right ear (6 dB down at 0.3 and 70 Hz, 256 s/sec A/D rate).

The Ss were seated in a sound-attenuated chamber and instructed to listen with eyes closed to the sentences, particularly attending to the meaning of the test word in the specific sentence context. Sentences were presented by loundspeaker (1.5 m behind the S, 70 dB at Ss' ears) over a low-level continuous background random noise. Each recording run consisted of 30 sentence presentations (4.8 sec cycle time) followed by a 2.5 min. pause. Data collection was started after the first presentation in each run.

For each S, evoked potentials in all channels were averaged (N=30) during seven runs with each of the two stimulus words. Average evoked potentials showed wave-shapes typical of auditory responses (a negative peak at 110-120 msec and a positive peak at 180-200 msec) as described by G. Goff et al. (1977) and Pieton et al. (1974). Each of the resulting 14 sets of 12 averaged evoked potentials was transformed into maps of scalp-field distributions (in Fig. 1A) for 40 analysis times, in intervals of 15.6 msec, between 33 and 642 msec after stimulus onset. In each map, the location of the electrode with the maximal and minimal potential value was determined.

For each S, condition, and analysis time, the median location of the maximal and minimal values was computed over the 7 runs. Since we wanted to examine the topographical differences between noun and verb-evoked scalp fields, the verb-evoked extreme value

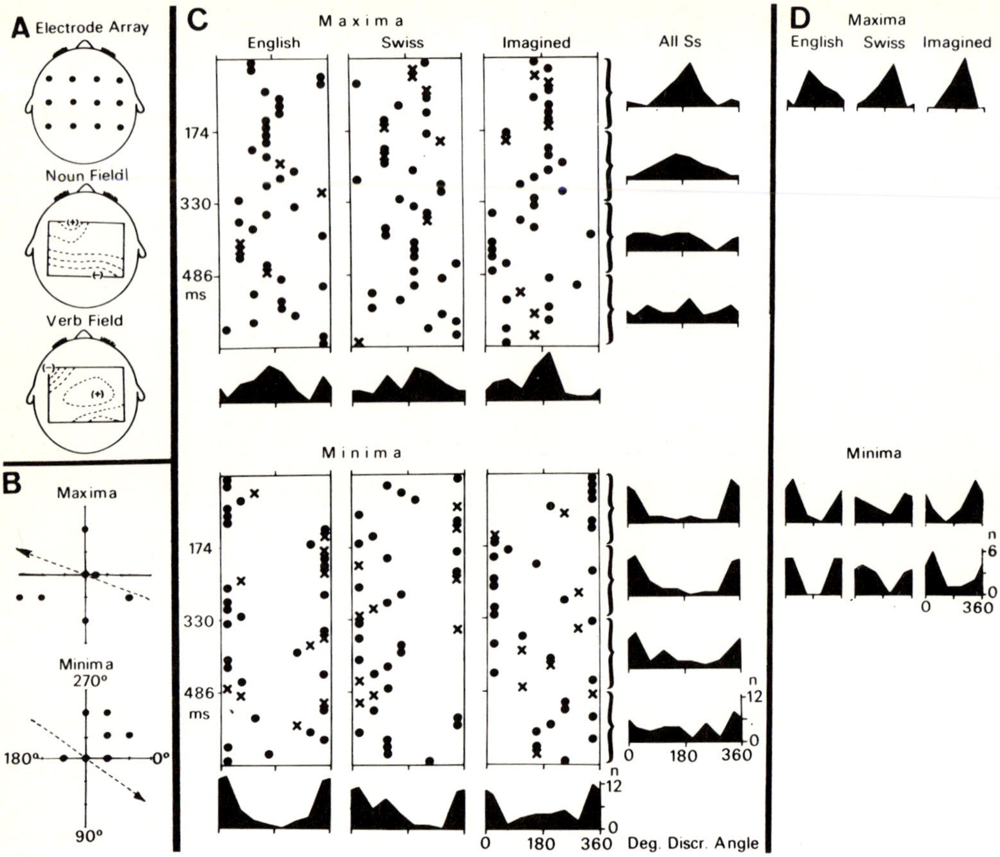

Fig 1. A. Electrode array and sample average scalp-field distributions in one S. Field lines linearly interpolated between electrode positions. +=maximal and -=minimal field values. B. Relative positions of maximal and minimal values of verb fields (dots) of 7 Ss, plotted in spatial reference to noun field extreme values (at origin of co-ordinate system) at one analysis time. Scale marker: 5 cm. Dashed line shows the discriminant angle (p=.249 for maxima; p=.046 for minima). C. Discriminant angles (horizontal) between the relative scalp locations of verb- and noun-evoked maximal and minimal field values, for English, Swiss-German and Imagined sentences, as a function of time (vertical) after word onset (crosses=p .06, dots=N.S.). Sums over all 40 analysis times shown at bottom. Sums over epochs of 10 analysis times over all Ss shown at right. D. Discriminant angles summed over 10 analysis times for each S group. Significance values see text. (from Brown and Lehmann, in preparation)

locations were plotted as relative positions in a co-ordinate system where the comparable noun location was at the origin. For each analysis time, the median locations for each of the 7 Ss from one experiment were entered into separate plots for maxima and minima (example Fig. 1B).

The difference between the relative locations of the extreme field values for nouns and verbs were then evaluated in a spatial discriminant analysis. A vector was rotated through the origin of the co-ordinate system to determine the line wich divided the plot into two halves, so that the highest sum of signed ranked distances, and the highest sum of signed distances of the plotted verb locations from the vector was obtained (Fig. 1B). Significances of the discriminations were determined by onetailed Wilcoxon tests.

For each group, the discriminant vector angles of all analysis times were entered into graphs (Fig. 1C). The three subject groups showed similar results. The sums of all entries during the entire analysis period (histograms at the bottom of each graph of Fig. 1C) indicate a predominant angle of about 180 degrees for maximal field values, and approximately 0 (or 360) degrees for minimal values. Chi-square tests for non-randomness for maxima/minima yielded $p<.02/<.001$ (English); $<.10/<.001$ (Swiss-German); $<.001/<.01$ (Imagined). - If we examine changes over time by summing over only 10 analysis times across the 3 groups (Fig. 1C, "All Ss") and test for randomness of the distribution, we find that the locations of the maxima are clearly separate in the noun and verb conditions in an anterior-posterior direction (angles between 135 and 225 degrees) during the first 174 msec after stimulus onset, and the locations of the minima are separate in the opposite direction (angles between 315 and 45 degrees) during the first 330 msec, whereafter the clear preference of the discriminant angles begins to fade (Chi-square (two-tailed) for non-randomness for maxima: $<.001$ between 33 and 174 msec, and N.S. for the last three epochs; for minima, $p<.001$ for the first two epochs up to 330 msec, p .02 for the third, and N.S. for the last). The shape of the distribution for each of the three experimental groups is similar for epochs where significant distributions occur across all Ss (Fig. 1D; Chi-square (two-tailed) for non-randomness for maxima: English, $<.15$; Swiss-German, $<.05$; imagined, $<.001$. For minima (first and second epochs): English, $<.05$ and $<.02$; Swiss-German, $>.2$ and $>.2$; and imagined, $<.06$ and $<.08$).

The literature to our knowledge does not report on vertical eye movements related to perceived word meaning. However, vertical eye movements were recorded from electrodes above and below the eye from 3 Ss in the English, 4 in the Swiss-German, and 4 in the imagined sentence paradigms. These data exhibited no significant differences between the two experimental conditions at analysis time, which excludes any role of eye movements in our results.

The results obtained demonstrate consistent differences of the locations of extreme scalp field values between the noun and the verb stimulus conditions. For the first 175 msec after stimulus onset, the maximal field value is more anteriorly located in the noun condition; and for the first 330 msec, the minimal field value is more posteriorly located in the noun condition than in the verb condition (example of fields see Fig. 2). Apparently, the neural elements whose activity constitutes the evoked response are not identical in the two stimulus conditions: a critical subpopulation is different for noun and verb. This may mean different locations, or different orientations of the active elements.

The distance between field peaks cannot be interpreted. Even a large distance may be caused by roughly identically located elements with different orientations. The mean distances between noun and verb locations for the first 10 analysis times for maxima/minima were 11mm/21mm (English), 12mm/16mm (Swiss-German), 18mm/16mm (imagined).

The topographical differences are constant over two languages, using different sentence meaning, and different stimulus-word meanings. They are also constant over at least two sets of

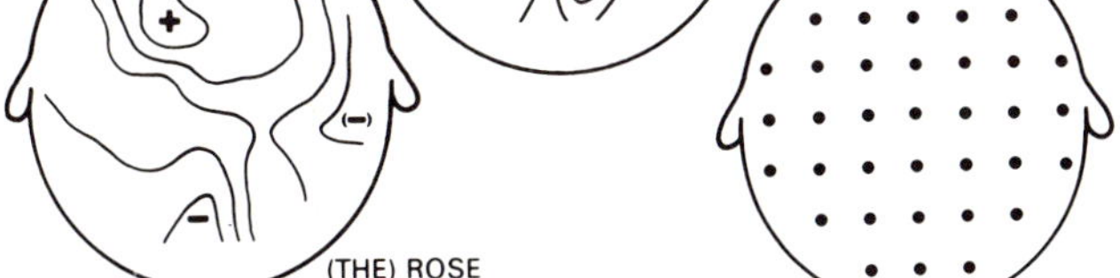

Fig. 2. Evoked, average scalp field distributions on the scalp, 72 msec after onset of "rose" and "rows", recorded simultaneously from 37 channels (electrode positions see schema). Equipotential field lines are computer-interpolated in 0.25 uV steps. Maximal values +, minimal values -, lesser extreme values (+) and (-); head seen from above, nose up. (from Brown and Lehmann, in preparation)

phonetic representations. The most obvious common difference of meaning between the two sentences in the three experiments is the verb-noun syntactic difference, but other connotative differences may also be implied by the particular nouns and verbs (i.e. passive/active, contemplative/strenuous).

It appears that it is not the decoding process of the physical stimulus which is manifested in the differences in scalp-field topography, since the blurred sound sequence with instructions to the S evoked results which were comparable to those from understandable sentences. Rather, it is the syntactic or connotative meaning which is reflected by the evoked potential topography. Thus, different internally generated word meanings are associated with evoked potential characteristics which are similar to those produced by the same meanings when conveyed by speech.

Other reports have shown that internal information, or mental classification of stimulus content, determined evoked waveforms independent of the nature of the physical stimulus (John et al., 1967; Herrington et al., 1968; Teyler et al., 1973; Johnston et al., 1974; Brown et al., 1976; Lehmann et al., 1977a; Chapman et al., 1977; John and Thatcher, 1977). Our topographical analysis is unlike waveform analysis used in other evoked potential studies of language meaning (Brown et al., 1976; Marsh and Brown, 1977; Chapman et al., 1977; Teyler et al., 1973). Therefore, direct comparison of the results is not possible.

Acknowledgements: The authors thank C. Mätzener for collaboration in data collection and analysis.
The study was supported in part by Swiss National Science Foundation, EMDO Foundation, Hartmann Müller Foundation, and Stiftung für Wiss. Forschung, Zürich.

References:

1) Brown, J.W.: Aphasia, apraxia and agnosia. Springfield, Ill.; Thomas (1972).
2) Brown, W.S.; Marsh, J.T.; Smith, J.C.: Contextual meaning effects on speech-evoked potentials. Behav.Biol. 9, 755-761 (1973).
3) Brown, W.S.; Marsh, J.T.; Smith, J.C.: Evoked potential wave-form differences produced by the perception of different meanings of an ambiguous phrase. Electroencephalogr.Clin. Neurophysiol. 41, 113-123 (1976).
4) Chapman, R.; Bragdon, M.; Chapman, J.; McCrary, J.: Semantic meaning of words and average evoked potentials. In: Desmedt, J. (ed.) Language and hemispheric specialization in man. Basel, Karger, 36-47 (1977).
5) Goff, G.D.; Matsumiya, Y.; Allison, T.; Goff, W.R.: The scalp topography of human somatosensory and auditory evoked potentials. Electroenceph.Clin.Neurophysiol. 42, 57-76 (1977).
6) John, E.R.; Thatcher, R.: Functional Neuroscience Vol. 1, Foundations of cognitive processes. Hillsdale, N.J., Erlbaum (1977).
7) Johnston, V.; Chesney, G.: Electrophysiological correlates of meaning. Science 186, 944-946 (1974).
8) Kleist, K.: Gehirnpathologie, vornehmlich aufgrund der Kriegserfahrungen. Leipzig, Johann Ambrosius Barth (1934).
9)Lehmann, D.: EEG Analyse und psychische Funktionen. Nervenarzt 42, 257-262 (1971).
10) Lehmann, D.: The EEG as scalp field distribution. In: EEG informatics. Rémond, A. (ed.) Amsterdam, Elsevier/North Holland (1977).
11) Lehmann, D., Koukkou, M., Dittrich, A.: Pattern evoked average EEG potentials and dichoptic visual percepts. Perception 6, 77-84 (1977a).
12) Lehmann, D.; Meles, H.P.; Mir, Z.: Average multichannel EEG potential fields evoked from upper and lower hemiretina: latency differences. Electroenceph.Clin.Neurophysiol. 43, 725-731 (1977b).
13) Marsh, J.T.; Brown, W.S.: Evoked potentials correlates of meaning in the perception of language. In: Language and hemishperic spezialisation in man. Desmedt, J.E. (ed.), Basel, Karger, 60-72 (1977).
14) Picton, T.W.; Hillyard, S.A.; Krausz, H.U.; Galambos, R.: Human auditory evoked potentials. Evaluation of components. Electroenceph.Clin.Neurophysiol. 36, 179-190 (1974).
15) Ragot, R., Cecchini, A.; Rémond, A.: Les possibilités de la saisie topographieque et du traitement cartographique des signaux EEG. Rev. Electroenceph.Neurophysiol.Clin. 6, 278-284 (1976).

16) Teyler, T.; Harrison, T.; Roemer, R.; Thompson, R.: Human scalp recorded evoked potential correlates of linguistic stimuli. Psychonom.Soc.Bull. 1, 333-334 (1973).

III) Brain Mechanisms of Speech Perception and Production

Anatomical and Functional Cerebral Organization of Phonation in Animals

U. JÜRGENS, Max-Planck-Institut für Psychiatrie, München, FRG

Vocal utterances can be innate, i.e. genetically preprogrammed, or learnt, i.e. imitated from a model by exercise. The cerebral mechanisms underlying the production of these two types are different. A transection of the brain at the rostral mesencephalic level in the dog neither abolishes its species-specific barking calls nor changes their quality (Onodi, 1902). The same holds for the cat; its species-specific meowing, purring and growling calls can still be obtained in animals with the whole forebrain and rostral midbrain removed (Bazett & Penfield, 1922). On the other hand, it is possible to disturb severely human speech, the songs of song-birds and the word imitations of parrots by relatively small lesions within the forebrain (Broca, 1861; Nottebohm et al., 1976; Kalischer 1905). The whole telencephalon, diencephalon and rostral midbrain thus is dispensable for the generation of species-specific calls, whereas these structures are clearly needed for the production of learnt vocal utterances.

The present report will deal only with those brain mechanisms responsible for the production of species-specific, i.e. innate, vocal utterances and leave out the discussion of those brain structures specifically related to human speech or birds' songs and vocal imitations. It should be kept in mind, however, that species-specific vocalizations not only occur in animals but also in man. Laughing, for instance, shrieking, moaning as well as the baby's babbling are all vocal utterances made also by the deaf-born (Eible-Eibesfeldt, 1967; Lenneberg, 1967) and thus do not need an external model from which they have to be learnt. Furthermore, a number of emotionally determined intonation patterns in speech - as used during shouting, lamenting, caressing or jubilating - are very similar across cultures and thus also point to a genetically determined basis (Kramer, 1964).

Our own approach to the question of which brain structures are involved in the control of species-specific vocalizations started with a systematic exploration of the brain of the squirrel monkey with electrical stimulation (Jürgens et al., 1967; Jürgens & Ploog, 1970). Fig. 1 gives a schematic summary of the results. All brain areas yielding vocalization when electrically stimulated are shown in black; the call types elicitable from the different areas are indicated by the sonagrams below each brain diagram. It can be seen that the vocalization-eliciting substrate is not a small discrete area but an extensive system reaching from the forebrain down into the medulla. Furthermore, this system is not a continuous one but is made up of islands of vocalization-eliciting areas separated by unresponsive areas. From the fact that the vocalization-eliciting areas are so widely scattered, it may be concluded that they probably do not all represent specific

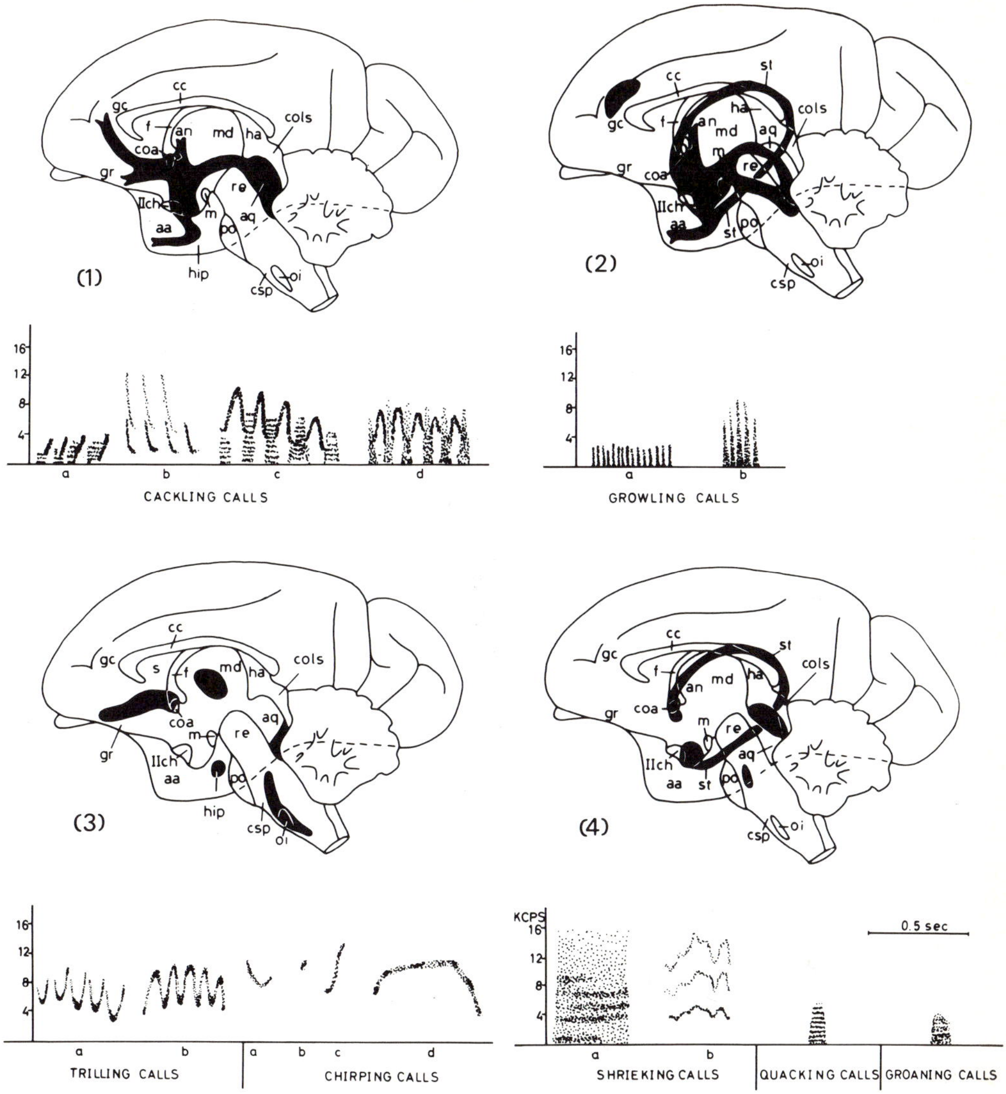

Fig. 1. For explanation see text

vocalization areas, that is areas which control directly the phonatory motor-coordinating mechanisms.

Fig. 1 also shows that there is some correlation between the brain structure stimulated and the call type elicited, with some brain structures yielding only one or a few call types functionally related to each other. This fact together with the wide distribution of vocalization-eliciting areas and their close relationship to the limbic system suggests that at least some of the electrically elicitable vocalizations probably do not represent pure motor responses but rather should be interpreted as vocal expressions of stimulation-induced motivational changes.

In order to test this hypothesis, we have made a self-stimulation study in which the aversive and pleasurable effects accompanying electrically elicited vocalizations were investigated (Jürgens, 1976a). The results of this study are summarized schematically in Fig. 2. The black areas in the diagram represent vocalization-eliciting areas which showed a strict

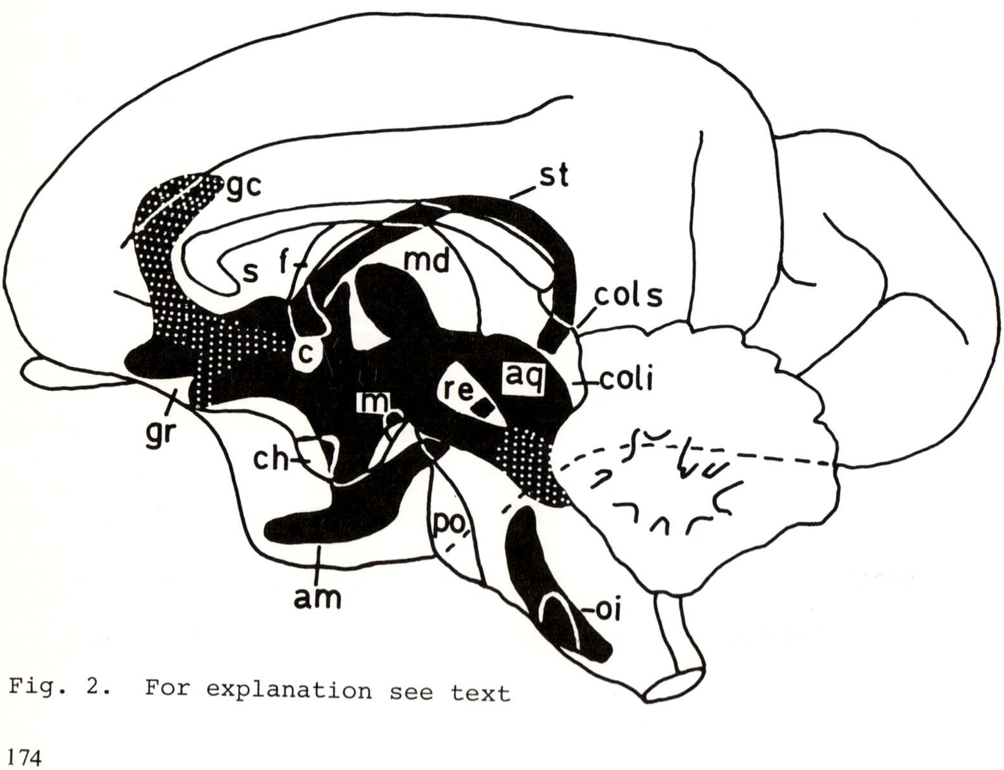

Fig. 2. For explanation see text

correlation between elicited call type and accompanying motivational effects as measured by the self-stimulation procedure. The stippled areas represent vocalization areas in which there was no correlation, which means that one and the same call type dependent upon the electrode site was accompanied by either positive self-stimulation (approach to the vocalization-inducing stimulation) or negative self-stimulation (escape from vocalization-inducing stimulation) or neither of them. The only two areas showing such a lack of correlation between elicited call type and accompanying motivational effect are the anterior limbic cortex with the dorsally adjacent supplementary motor area and the caudal periaqueductal grey with the laterally adjacent tegmentum. These two areas thus take an outstanding position within the vocalization-eliciting system; more specifically stated, vocalizations elicitable from these areas probably do not represent vocal expressions of stimulation-induced motivational changes but are triggered directly.

This suggestion is further corroborated by the results of an anatomical study, in which we studied the projections from the cortical larynx area (Jürgens, 1976b). This area lies in the inferior precentral cortex and yields isolated movements of the vocal folds when electrically stimulated. It thus seems to have a quite direct relationship to the phonatory apparatus, and it can be assumed that a vocalization-eliciting area directly connected with it also is related quite directly to phonation. The study showed that the only vocalization-eliciting areas receiving direct afferents from the cortical larynx area are the cortex around the anterior cingulate sulcus and the tegmentum bordering the caudal periaqueductal grey. With other words, direct connections exist only with those areas showing a lack of correlation between call type and motivational effect according to the self-stimulation study.

In order to further specify the role of the cingular and periaqueductal vocalization areas, we tested the effects of lesions within these areas (Jürgens & Pratt, 1979; Jürgens & Pratt, in press). It was found that destruction of the periaqueductal vocalization area abolishes all spontaneous as well as electrically elicitable species-specific calls. This points to a very fundamental role in vocalization production. On the other hand, it must be assumed that the periaqueductal region does not participate in the motor-coordination of vocalization itself as the calls elicitable from this region sound natural and do not show a stimulus-dependent artificial character. The periaqueductal region thus seems to take an intermediate position between those areas mediating vocalization inducing motivations and those areas responsible for the motor-coordination of vocalization. According to this interpretation, this region would couple specific motivations to the corresponding vocal expressions; or, with other words, the diverse external and internal stimuli which normally induce an animal to vocalize must activate the periaqueductal region in order to generate a call.

As regards the cingular vocalization area, we neither found an effect of its destruction on spontaneous nor on electrically elicitable calls. There are, however, two observations, made by Sutton and co-workers (Sutton et al., 1974, 1978) which shed some light on the possible role of this area for vocalization. They trained rhesus monkeys to vocalize for food reward. After the animals had mastered this vocal operant conditioning task, they underwent bilateral ablation of the cingular vocalization area. After these lesions, the animals were unable to do this task anymore. The other observation concerns a single-unit recording study (Sutton et al., 1978) in which the authors found a number of cells within the cingular vocalization area which consistently fired 200 - 800 msec <u>before</u> the conditioned vocalization occured. These observations point to a possible role of the anterior cingular cortex in the voluntary initiation of vocalization.

In a recent study, we have tried to outline the pathway along which the cingular vocalization area transmits its vocalization-initiating activity down to the motor-coordinating mechanisms in the lower brain stem (Jürgens & Pratt, 1979). In this study, vocalization-eliciting electrodes were implanted in the anterior cingulate cortex and lesions were placed throughout the projection system of this area as outlined in a prior anatomical study (Müller-Preuß & Jürgens, 1976). The lesion sites effective in abolishing cingularly elicited vocalizations are indicated in Fig. 3. It can be seen that the route by which the cingular vocalization area triggers vocalization follows the internal capsule down to the caudal diencephalon, then sweeps dorsalward to a periventricular position and runs through the periaqueductal grey throughout its length. At the level of the caudal midbrain the pathway leaves the periaqueductal grey laterally and descends through the lateral pons

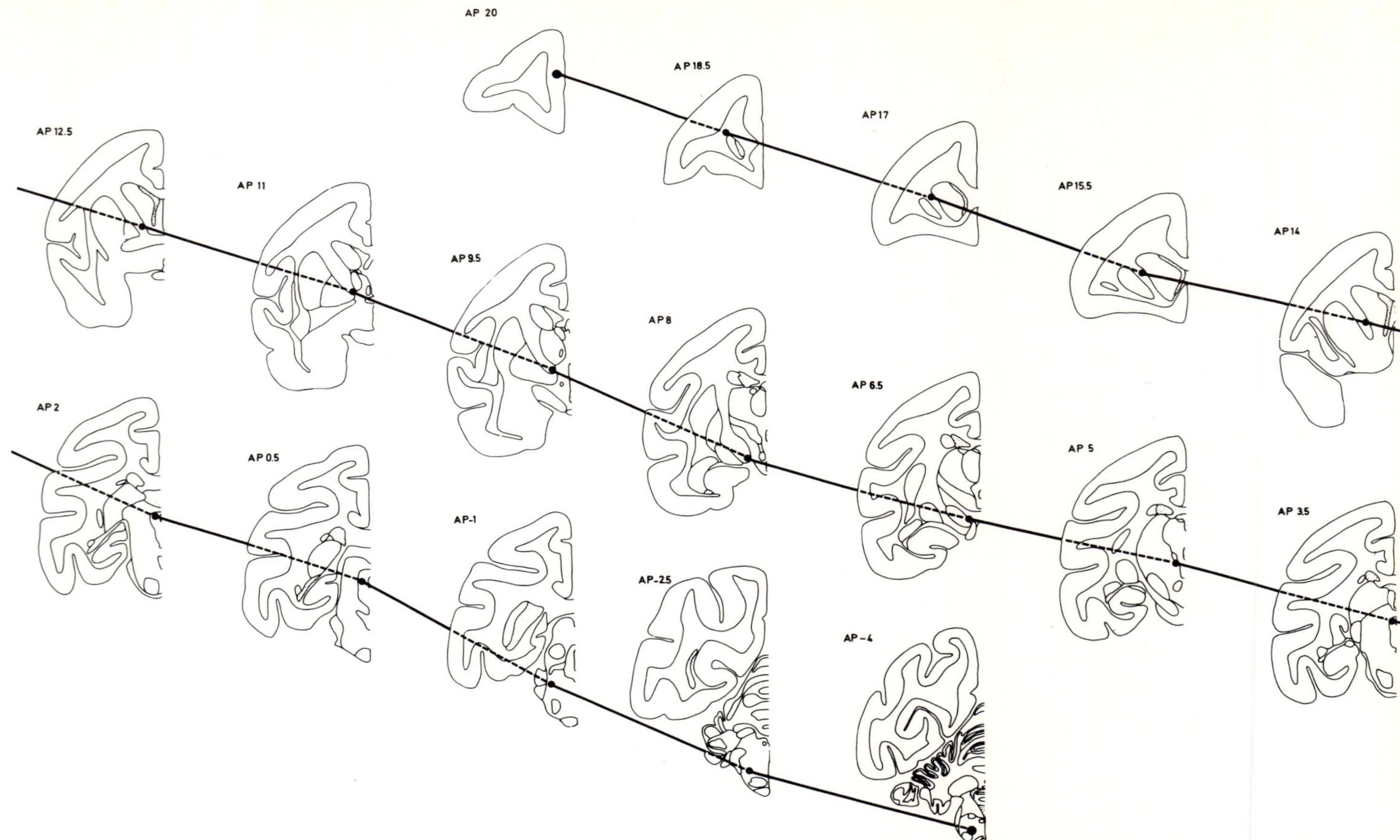

Fig. 3. For explanation see text

and medulla until it reaches the nucl. ambiguus, that is the site of the laryngeal motoneurones. As there is a direct anatomical connection between the anterior cingulate cortex and the periaqueductal region (Müller-Preuß & Jürgens, 1976) and between the latter and the nucl. ambiguus (Jürgens & Pratt, in press), but no projection from the cingulate cortex directly to the nucl. ambiguus, it follows that there exists a well-delineated anatomical pathway related to vocalization which runs from the anterior cingulate cortex down to the laryngeal motoneurones with at least one synapse in the periaqueductal region.

That the motor-coordination of vocalization, that is the integration of vocal fold tensioning, respiratory movements and articulation, is most probably done caudal to the periaqueductal region is suggested by two observations (Jürgens, in press): 1. Only lesions below the level of the midbrain change the acoustic structure of vocalizations. 2. Electrically elicitable vocalization with a stimulus-dependent artificial character are only found caudal to the midbrain. In which way the pontine, medullary and spinal motoneurones involved in phonation are coordinated in their activity to finally accomplish the generation of a species-specific call is, however, still unknown.

At the end, it should be mentioned that electrically elicitable vocalizations have been obtained not only in various mammals but also in birds, reptiles and amphibians (for review see Jürgens & Ploog, 1976). In those non-mammalian animals which have been explored more thoroughly, it has been found, similarly to mammals, that the vocalization-eliciting substrate is not a single discrete area but a widely scattered one. As we do not know what the homologue of the anterior cingulate cortex is in birds, reptiles and amphibians, a comparison at that level of the vocalization system is not possible. We do know, however, the homologue of the caudal periaqueductal grey and laterally adjacent tegmentum. A comparison between the four vertebrate classes capable of phonation reveals that vocalization can be obtained from this area in all of them. (e.g. Hunsperger, 1956; Brown, 1965; Kennedy, 1975; Schmidt, 1966). In addition, it has been reported that even in fish swim bladder-produced sounds can be elicited by stimulation of this area (Demski & Gerald, 1974). These observations point to a phylogenetically very old role of this area in phonation and furthermore, because of the different sound-producing apparatus and innervation in fish, birds and mammals, support the above-mentioned hypothesis that this area rather serves to trigger than to integrate phonation. That this integration, as we suggested already for mammals, is carried out also in birds and amphibians below the level of the midbrain is indicated, firstly, by the finding that in the frog only lesions caudal but not rostral to the midbrain-pons transition change the acoustic structure of the calls (Schmidt, 1976) and, secondly, that in birds neurones which fire synchronously with the calls also are found only caudal to the midbrain (Phillips & Youngren, 1976).

References:

1) Bazett, H.D.; Penfield, W.G.: A study of the Sherrington decerebrate animal in the chronic as well as the acute condition. Brain 45, 185-265 (1922).
2) Broca, P. (1861) cited by Ajuriaguerra, J. de, Hécaen, H.: Le Cortex Cérébral. Masson, Paris (1964).
3) Brown, J.L.: Vocalization evoked from the optic lobe of a song-bird. Science 149, 1002-1003 (1965).
4) Demski, L.S.; Gerald, J.W.: Sound production and other behavioural effects of midbrain stimulation in free-swimming toadfish, Opsanus beta. Brain Behav. Evol. 9, 41-59 (1974).
5) Eibl-Eibesfeldt, I.: Grundriß der vergleichenden Verhaltensforschung. Piper, München (1967).
6) Hunsperger, R.W.: Affektreaktionen auf elektrische Reizung im Hirnstamm der Katze. Helv.physiol.pharmacol.Acta 14, 70-92 (1956).
7) Jürgens, U.: Reinforcing concomitants of electrically-elicited vocalization. Exp. Brain Res. 26, 203-214 (1976a).
8) Jürgens, U.: Projections from the cortical larynx area in the squirrel monkey. Exp. Brain Res. 25, 401-411 (1976b).
9) Jürgens, U.: Neural control of vocalization in non-human primates. In: Steklis, H.D., Raleigh, M.J. (eds.): Neurobiology of Social Communication in Primates: An Evolutionary Perspective. Academic Press, New York (in press).
10) Jürgens, U.; Maurus, M.; Plogg, D.; Winter, P.: Vocalization in the squirrel monkey (Saimiri sciureus) elicited by brain stimulation. Exp. Brain Res. 4, 114-117 (1967).
11) Jürgens, U.; Ploog, D.: Cerebral representation of vocalization in the squirrel monkey. Exp. Brain Res. 10, 532-554 (1970).
12) Jürgens, U.; Ploog, D.: Zur Evolution der Stimme. Arch. Psychiat. Nervenkr. 222, 117-137 (1976).
13) Jürgens, U.; Pratt, R.: The cingular vocalization pathway in the squirrel monkey. Exp. Brain Res. 34, 499-510 (1979).
14) Jürgens, U.; Pratt, R.: Role of the periaqueductal grey in vocal expression of emotion. Brain Res. (in press).
15) Kalischer, O.: Das Großhirn der Papageien in anatomischer und physiologischer Beziehung. Abhandlgn.Kgl.Preuss.Akad.Wiss. 4, 1-105 (1905).
16) Kennedy, M.C.: Vocalization elicited in a lizard by electrical stimulation of the midbrain. Brain Res. 91, 321-325 (1975).
17) Kramer, E.: Elimination of verbal cues in judgement of emotion from voice. J.abnorm.soc.Psychol. 68, 390-396 (1964).
18) Lenneberg, E.H.: Biological Foundations of Language. Wiley, New York (1967).
19) Müller-Preuß, P.; Jürgens, U.: Projections from the 'cingular' vocalization area in the squirrel monkey. Brain Res. 103, 29-43 (1976).
20) Nottebom, F.; Stokes, T.M.; Leonard, C.M.: Central control of song in the canary, Serinus canarius. J. Comp. Neurol. 165, 457-486 (1976).
21) Onodi, A.: Die Anatomie und Physiologie der Kehlkopfnerven. Coblentz, Berlin (1902).

22) Phillips, R.E.; Youngren, O.M.: Pattern generator for repetitive avian vocalization: preliminary localization and functional characterization. Brain Behav.Evol. 13, 165-178 (1976).
23) Schmidt, R.S.: Central mechanisms of frog calling. Behaviour 26, 251-285 (1966).
24) Schmidt, R.S.: Neural correlates of frog calling. J. comp. Physiol. 108, 99-103 (1976).
25) Sutton, D.; Larson, C.; Lindemann, R.C.: Neocortical and limbic lesion effects on primate phonation. Brain Res. 71, 61-75 (1974).
26) Sutton, D.; Samson, H.H.; Larson, C.R.: Brain mechanisms in learned phonation of Macaca mulatta. In: Chiver, D.J.; Herbert, J. (eds.): Recent Advances in Primatology I. Academic Press, New York (1978).

Basal Ganglia Participation in Aphasia

KORNHUBER, H. H.; BRUNNER, R. J.; WALLESCH, C. W., Abteilung Neurologie, Universität Ulm, D-7900 Ulm, W-Germany

In a series of papers (Kornhuber, 1974; Kornhuber, 1977) we have pointed out the participation of the basal ganglia in language and speech production and their role in the pathogenesis of global aphasia.

A study in up to now 24 patients with large infarcts in the territory of the medial cerebral artery in the speech dominant hemisphere was conducted. The site and extent of lesion was confirmed by computerised axial tomography. The infarcts were well demarkated. A test of expressive language functions which was developed by our group (Brunner and Wallesch, in preperation) was used.

The following preliminary results were obtained (see table 1):
1. In the majority of patients with infarcts leading to a more than transient aphasia there was basal ganglia involvement, mostly of the nc. lenticularis, in addition to a lesion of cortex and white matter. We have the impression that this is true for the majority of aphasic patients studied so far, who usually have suffered a cerebrovascular accident. In the recently published study of Naeser and Hayward (1978) the same anatomical situation can be demonstrated. The obvious

Table 1. Types of aphasia occuring in anatomically different vascular infarct lesions in the speech-domirant hemisphere and occurence of repetitive verbal behaviour.
*Indicates patients with the full syndrome of global asphasia, including sterotyped verbal behaviour. The other patients diagnosed as global only suffered from a marked impairment in all linguistic capabilities.
"Highly repetitive verbal behavior" indicates at least 25% of speech output.

	cortical lesion						
	prerolandic		retrorolandic		pre-as well as retrorolandic		none
basal ganglia involvement	-	+	-	+	-	+	+
no. of patients	1	4	4	4	2	4	5
type of aphasia	1 Broca	2 global, partially recovered; 1 Broca; 1 nominal, well re-covered	2 global, partially recovered; 1 Broca, partially recovered; 1 nominal, well re-covered	2 global*; 2 Broca, both ini-tially global, well re-covered	2nominál, well re-covered	3 global*; 1 Wernicke	2 nominal, well recovered; 1 initially Broca, fully recovered 1 inititally nominal, fully recovered 1 none
repetitive ver-bal behaviour	none	none	none	2 global aphasics with high-ly repe-titive ver-bal be-haviour none to slight in the 2 Broca	none	3 global aphasics with high-ly repe-titive ver-bal behaviour 1 Wernicke with marked repetitive features in jargon	none

reason for this is the territory of supply of the medial cerebral artery. This piece of data has been overlooked in most of the aphasiological research up to now, and it casts doubt on the view of aphasia as an exclusively cortical and/or connective syndrome.

Especially the role of Broca's area and the adjacent cortical regions as the sole origin of Broca's aphasia, a point of view still held by Geschwind (1973) and Kerschensteiner et al. (1978) appears to be no longer tenable. Even with rigid diagnostic criteria there are a number of Broca's aphasias with other than left frontal cortical lesions. One of our patients showed Broca's aphasia for more than 6 weeks after a lesion confined to the left nc. lenticularis. Quite consistent with these findings are the data obtained by Mohr et al. (1978) who also found Broca's aphasia in patients with no cortical lesion at all but substantial damage to the left basal ganglia.

2. In all patients in whom the constituent characteristics of global aphasia as outlined by Stachowiak et al. (1977, reduction of speech production, repetitive verbal behaviour, severe impairment of all linguistic capabilities) were present there was massive basal ganglia involvement in combination with a posterior cortical lesion (5 patients, indicated by asterixes in table 1). In 4 of 5 patients the cortical lesion included Wernicke's area, in the fifth the lesion was situated more posteriorly. In those patients who had an anterior cortical lesion with or without basal ganglia pathology or a posterior lesion without basal ganglia lesion there were aphasic language disturbances in most cases but not the following types of re-

petitive verbal behaviour: verbal sterotypes, echolalia, perseveration, recurring utterances.

Repetitive verbal behaviour in our view is an indicator of basal ganglia involvement in the pathogenetic process of aphasia (Kornhuber, 1977).

3. We conclude from our limited data that the aphasic syndrome is more severe and has less tendency to improve if there is basal ganglia involvement. The same holds true for hemiplegia and some types of apraxia.

Aphasic language disturbance resulting from basal ganglia lesions alone seem to improve rapidly. The repetitive verbal and behavioural phenomena in those cases are under further investigation in a longitudinal study.

Discussion:

There is a body of evidence concerning the participation of the basal ganglia in language production. Language disturbances following sterotaxic surgery in the treatment of movement disorders are well-known side-effects (Darley et al., 1975 e.g.).

Quite interesting for the discussion of our data are Dr. Ojemann's findings (later this workshop) who could demonstrate in his stimulation experiments in patients a marked tendency to perseverate verbally during stimulation of nc. ventrolateralis thalami (VL) but never during cortical stimulation. Anatomical data suggest, that VL with its strong pallidal afferents acts as a regulator of input from the basal ganglia to the cortex. Perseverative behaviour, as we found in the

speech fo aphasics with basal ganglia involvement in addition to a cortical lesion is a well known feature of basal ganglia pathology (Kirkby, 1975; Kornhuber, 1974, 1977).
Perseveration was previously held to be a nonspecific symptom of forebrain lesions, and there is probably some truth in this opinion, especially in states of blurred consciousness and in the later stages of bilateral cortical atrophy. However, there is some doubt whether perseveration is due to cortical dysfunction (as stated by Helmick and Berg, 1976) even in these cases. Certainly it is not an exclusively cortical phenomenon. Furthermore, it seems unlikely from our data so far that it is just due to a mass effect of hemispheric damage. This point, however, is under further investigation.

Conclusions:

There is evidence for a participation of the basal ganglia in speech and language. A basal ganglia lesion is considered to be a necessary factor in the pathogenesis of the complete syndrome of global aphasia.

References:

1) Brunner, R.J.; Wallesch, C.W.: Assessment of expressive language functions. In preparation.
2) Darley, F.L.; Brown, J.R.; Swenson, W.M.: Language changes after neurosurgery for parkinson. Brain Lang. 2,1, 65-69 (1975).
3) Geschwind, N.: The Brain and Language. In: G.A. Miller (ed.): Communication, Language, and Meaning. New York (1973).
4) Helmick, J.W.; Berg, C.B.: Perseveration in brain injured adults. J.Comm.Dis. 9, 143-156 (1976).
5) Kerschensteiner, M.; Poeck, K.; Huber, W.; Stachowiak, H.J.; Weniger, D.: Die Broca-Aphasie. J.Neurol. 217, 223-242 (1978).
6) Kirkby, R.J.: Caudate nucleus lesions and perseverative behaviour. Physiology and Behaviour 4, 451-454 (1975).
7) Kornhuber, H.H.: Cerebral cortex, cerebellum and basal ganglia: An introduction to their motor functions. In: F.O. Schmitt; F.G. Worden (eds.): The Neurosciences: Third Study Program. Cambridge, Mass. and London (1974).

8) Kornhuber, H.H.: A reconsideration of the cortical and subcortical mechanisms involved in speech and languge. In: J.E. Desmedt (ed.): Language and Hemispheric Specialisation in Man: Cerebral ERP's. Prog.Clin.Neurophysiol. 3, Basel (1977).
9) Mohr, J.P.; Pessin, M.S.; Finkelstein, S.; Funkenstein, H.H.; Duncan, G.W.; Davis, K.R.: Broca aphasia: Pathologic and clinical. Neurology (Minneap) 28, 311-324 (1978).
10) Naeser, M.A.; Hayward, M.D.: Lesion localization in aphasia with cranial computed tomography and the Boston Diagnostic Aphasia Exam. Neurology (Minneap) 28, 545-551 (1978).
11) Stachowiak, F.J.; Huber, W.; Kerschensteiner, M.; Poeck, K.; Weniger, D.: Die globale Aphasie. J.Neurol. 214, 75-87 (1977).

Participation of Mesial Cortex in Speech: Evidence from Cerebral Potentials Preceding Speech Production in Man

GRÖZINGER, B.; KORNHUBER, H. H. and KRIEBEL, J., Department of Neurology and Neurophysiology, University of Ulm, Oberer Eselsberg, D-7900 Ulm, West Germany

Foerster (1936) and Penfield (1938) first described the role of the "supplementary motor cortex" (SMA) in motor functions in man. There is increasing evidence for the participation of the SMA in speech production. This is supported by electrical stimulation studies (Brickner, 1940; Penfield and Rasmussen, 1949), analysis of the effects of brain lesions (Bancaud et al., 1967; Környey, 1975; Rubens, 1975; Laplan et al., 1977; Caplan et al., 1978) and speech related measurements of regional cerebral bloodflow (Lassen et al., 1978). These data were obtained from post-mortem pathological observations, electrical stimulation and/or invasive diagnostic procedures. Our data, on the other hand, were gathered from healthy subjects using scalp EEG recordings and event related averaging (Grözinger et al., 1972, 1975, 1977).

Results:

Figure 1 shows the results of two experiments with two subjects. In both experiments the subjects repeated the word "PUPPE" (in English, "doll"). In upper traces a more pronounced Bereitschaftspotential (BP) (readiness-potential) is recorded over the vertex than over bilateral frontal electrode positions. The BP is superimposed on a respiration correlated

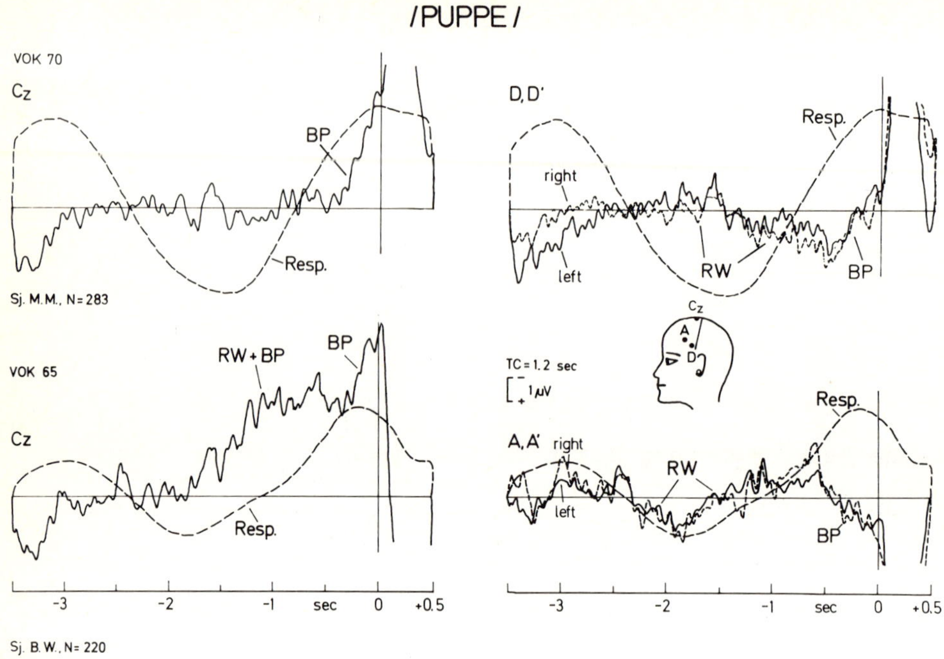

Fig. 1. Averaged brain potentials preceding repetitive speaking of /PUPPE/ from two experiments. Recordings from vertex (C_Z) and bilateral frontal positions as indicated. Time of analysis is 4 sec, vertical lines indicate activity onset via mouth myogram. Dashed lines mark averaged respiration (thermocouple in the nose). The experiment in the upper part of the diagram shows a Bereitschaftspotential (BP), onset about 500 msec prior to speech onset. The experiments in the lower part show a superposition of respiratory waves (RW) and BP. The BP of the bifrontal sites are of positive polarity. Altogether the vertex has the greatest RW and BP. Reference electrode = linked ears

cerebral potential (R-wave), especially notable in the experiment shown in the lower trace. The BP over the vertex is negative while the BP over the frontal electrodes is positiv. Since it can be assumed that negativity indicates the electrode is close to brain areas exhibiting greater activity, prominence of the vertex responses is of particular note.

Figure 2 summarizes amplitudes of the BP prior to speech (10

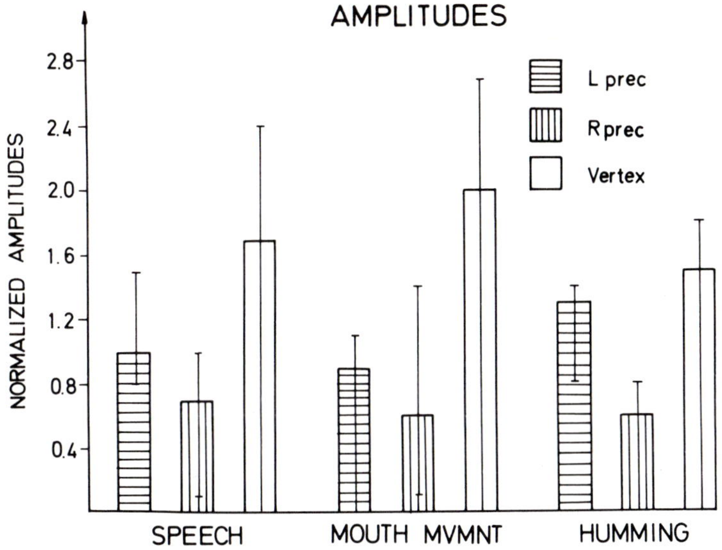

Fig. 2. Medians and 95% confidence intervalls of normalized amplitudes (smallest value was set zero) of the BP preceding speech (10 subjects), mouth movement (11 subjects) and humming (14 subjects). Under all conditions the vertex amplitudes are highest, especially in activities involving articulatory movements. Monopolar recordings vs. linked ears

subjects), mouth movement (11 subjects) and humming (14 subjects). The data were normalized. Under all three conditions, the vertex potentials are highest in amplitude. However, the vertex BP does not depend on speech exclusively; it is highest preceding a complex motor task (articulatory movement of the mouth and face).

Discussion:

Our EEG recordings emphasize the importance of the SMA in speech production and facial movements and are in agreement with the findings reported by other methods. As regards function, the SMA may have some role in the translation of motivation into action, for it is juxtaposed to and connected with the limbic cortex (Jürgens et al., 1977).

References:

1) Bancaud, J.; Talairach, J. and Bonis, A.: Physiopathogenie des epilepsies-sursaut. (A propos d'une epilepsie de l'aire motorice supplementaire). Rev.Neurol. (Paris) 117, 441-453 (1967).
2) Brickner, R.M.: A human cortical area producing repetive phenomena when stimulated. J.Neurophysiol. 3, 128-130 (1940).
3) Caplan, L.R. and Zervas, N.T.: Speech arrest in a dextral with a right mesial frontal astrocytoma. Arch.Neurol. 35, 252-253 (1978).
4) Foerster, O.: Motor cortex in man in the light of Hughlings Jackson's doctrines. Brain 59, 135-159 (1936).
5) Grözinger, B.; Kornhuber, H.H. and Kriebel, J.: Methodological problems in the investigation of cerebral potentials preceding speech: determining the onset and suppressing artefacts caused by speech. Neurophysiol. 13, 263-270 (1975).
6) Grözinger, B.; Kornhuber, H.H. and Kriebel, J.: Human cerebral potentials preceding speech production, phonation, and movements of the mouth and tongue, with reference to respiratory and extracerebral potentials. In: Desmedt: Language and hemispheric spezialisation in man: Cerebral event-related potentials. Karger, Basel, 87-103 (1977).
7) Grözinger, B.; Kornhuber, H.H.; Kriebel, J. and Murata, K.: Menschliche Hirnpotentiale vor dem Sprechen. Pflügers Arch. ges.Physiol. 332, Suppl., R100, 200 (1972).
8) Jürgens, U. and Müller-Preuss, P.: Convergent projections of different limbic vocalization areas in the Squirrel Monkey. Exp. Brain Res. 29, 75-83 (1977).
9) Környey, E.: Aphasie transcorticale et écholalie; le probleme de l'initiative de la parole. Rev.Neurol. (Paris) 131, 347-363 (1975).
10) Laplane, D.; Talairach, J.; Meininger, V.; Bancaud, J. and Orgogozo, J.M.: Clinical consequences of corticectomies involving the supplementary motor area. J.Neurol.Sci. 34, 301-314 (1977).
11) Lassen, N.A.; Ingvar, D.H. and Skinhøj, E.: Brain function and blood flow. Scientif.Amer. 10, 50-59 (1978).
12) Penfield, W.: The cerebral cortex in man: I. The Cerebral Cortex and Consciousness. Arch. Neurol. & Psychiat. 40, 417-442 (1938).
13) Penfield, W. and Rasmussen, T.: Vocalization and arrest of speech. Arch. Neurol. & Psychiat. 61, 21-27 (1949).
14) Rubens, A.B.: Aphasia with infarction in the territory of the anterior cerebral artery. Cortex 11, 239-250 (1975).

Electrical Stimulation Mapping of Language Cortex

HARRY A. WHITAKER, Dept. of Psychology, The University of Rochester, New York 14627, USA

Introduction:

Just over half a century ago, Wilder Penfield began a remarkable series of neurosurgical procedures for the relief of medically intractable focal epilepsy, inspired by his six-month period of study in Breslau with Otfrid Foerster. From the standpoint of brain research, an important aspect of the epilepsy operation is the functional mapping of the cerebral cortex by electrical stimulation in the awake patient. Since the 1930's, stimulation mapping has provided a number of insights into speech and language representation in the brain, most notably in the work of Penfield and his colleagues, and more recently, in the work of George Ojemann, John Van Buren and their colleagues. The former studies, summarized in Penfield & Jasper (1954) and Penfield & Roberts (1959) and recently up-dated by Rasmussen & Milner (1975), resulted in the now-classic map of the speech areas: a frontal region comparable to Broca's area, a larger posterior region including posterior temporal and inferior parietal cortex and a smaller region in the mesial frontal lobe. The data of Penfield's stimulation studies are both dysarthric and aphasic responses: arrest of speech, slowing, distortion, misnaming, substitution and repetition. The evidence seemed to indicate that this map accurately reflected the speech and language system of the dominant, usually left, hemisphere in the majority of persons; as noted by Rasmussen & Milner (1975) the exceptional individual with bilateral speech and language presentation was found in 15-18% of the left-handed or ambidextrous population. Our recent work has considerably extended and somewhat modified these observations.

Penfield's procedures and data:

It is not generally appreciated that the aphasic errors reported in Penfield & Roberts (1959) were infrequently elicited from patients. A total of 132 aphasic errors were reported for 110 patients studied; of these 51 were inability to name with a retained ability to speak, 27 were perseverative errors and 19 were paraphasic misnaming errors. On the average, 1.2 aphasic errors were elicited for each patient in the study. As noted in Penfield & Jasper (1954), typically only positive responses to electrical stimulation were recorded. Exceptionally, a location at which stimulation failed to produce a response would be noted if it would influence the extent of the surgical resection. Overall, approximately half of the stimulation of the cortex by Penfield produced no response in a patient. Penfield & Roberts (1959) did note, however, that "if exact placement is achieved by a fixed electrode, remarkably constant results are obtained from the motor area and from Broca's area" (p.134). With respect to the content of the elicited data, in spite of the fact that a substantial number of Penfield's patients were bilingual, there were only a few unsystematic observations made on the effect of stimulation on two or more languages. For example, in Penfield & Jasper (1954) Case L.G., responses to stimulation were noted in both French and English without any special notice taken of the different locations; French was disturbed in a mid-parietal and a mid-first temporal locus and English was disturbed at a posterior third temporal, two posterior second temporal and a mid-posterior first temporal locus. No indication is given whether the two languages were sampled at the same sites or not. In response to a direct question, Rasmussen & Milner (1975) noted "we have had trilingual patients and the speech interference and the dysphasia did not seem to follow any specific pattern"(p.255).

Electrical stimulation parameters:

Over the years Penfield and colleagues used a number of different stimulation parameters, including sine waves, saw-toothed waves and square waves, delivered through monopolar and bipolar electrodes. Evidently, these were all monophasic (unidirectional) waves. Fedio & Van Buren (1974) used symmetric, biphasic waves delivered through a monopolar electrode.
Ojemann & Whitaker (1978) used symmetric, biphasic waves delivered through a bipolar electrode. At the current levels used in these studies, typically under 5 milliamps peak, there is no evidence that the different types of stimulation produce any differences in responses, as noted by Rasmussen & Milner (1975). Stimulating in epileptic cortex in which the likelihood of getting after-discharges is greater, may have an effect on the type of response; otherwise, current studies of naming find the same kinds of speech and language effects as noted

by Penfield and colleagues. Ojemann's most recent work, this volume, shows that electrical stimulation can also affect sequential oral movements and phonemic discrimination. This seems to imply that the acquisition of new data is limited by the questions asked of the patient, not by any intrinsic shortcoming of electrical stimulation of the cortex per se. As noted above, Penfield & Roberts (1959) believed that stimulating the site in the cortex would produce a constant result, with the proviso that repetitive stimulation at brief intervals was known to cause instability, facilitation or displacement of responses (ref. to Penfield & Jasper, 1954: 240-241). This opinion seems to be born out in the studies of Brindley & Lewin (1968) and Dobelle & Mladejovsky (1974) using implanted eletrodes in calcarine cortex as a visual prosthesis for the blind. The phosphenes so produced turn out to be remarkably stable over time, even though the phosphene map produced by identical electrodes is quite different in different patients. The weight of the evidence at present indicates that, with a suitable interval elapsing, stimulation of the same site will produce the same effect when repeated.

Current studies:

The current research by Ojemann, Van Buren and colleagues, has considered subcortical speech and language mechanisms (reviewed in Ojemann, 1978) and cortical speech and language mechanisms, to be reviewed in this paper. In the fall of 1976 we asked ourselves two questions (1) is the cortical map for language for an individual as extensive as the pooled-subjects map of Penfield & Roberts (1959) and (2) is there any evidence that different parts of the individual's cortical language map may be differentially or unequally committed? We chose to investigate these questions with a picture-naming paradigm for two important reasons: first, naming data would be easiest to relate to the pioneering work of Penfield and his colleagues, and second, a century of aphasia studies in brain lesioned subjects has convincingly shown that naming per se is not easily localized in the cortex. If any language function were likely to be affected by electrical stimulation over the whole extent of language cortex, it would be naming. As described in Whitaker & Ojemann (1977) we proceeded to map language cortex in a manner analogous to Penfield's, with three important exceptions: we placed sterile numbered tickets over the whole cortical exposure in a gridwork pattern prior to stimulation mapping, using the tickets as reference points for multiple samplings at each labelled site, and, we systematically exposed the picture stimuli using a slide projector for a period of 5 seconds each (on a timer), employing 80 stimulus slides in a carousel tray that continually cycled, and, we controlled for speech arrest data by using a written test phrase placed above each picture to be named in the test. These written phrases randomly were: "This is a", "That is a", "Here is a", and the like. We noted speech arrests, when the patient neither read the test phrase nor named the pictured object, we noted all aphasic responses, typically omission of the name of the object with retained ability to read the test phrase, we noted all trials in which stimulation failed to produce any speech, language or other effects, and we counted the number of errors in naming which occured on trials during which no electrical stimulation was applied (this is the non-stimulation control trial error rate, see Table 1). On all subjects we had the results of neuropsychological testing and the results of intracarotid sodium amytal testing. Further details of our procedure are given in Whitaker & Ojemann (1977) and Ojemann & Whitaker (1978a, 1978b).

Graded localization:

Our first finding has been given the name "graded localization", by which we intend to convey the principle that, under the same conditions of stimulation and testing, some sites in the cortical language system exhibit a greater or lesser involvement in the naming function. Electrical stimulation may produce a naming error on every trial at one site, on a majority of

---

Summary Data on 10 Left Hemisphere Operated Patients

(1) All patients were left hemisphere dominant for language as measured by the intracarotid sodium amytal test (Wada Test)

(2) Two of the 10 patients were left handed, the rest were right handed

(3) Nine patients had seizure onset before 6 years of age; the remaining patient's seizures onset was at 21 years of age.

(4) Mean age at operation = 27 years old; range = 17-35 years

(5) Mean Full Scale I.Q. = 94.3; range = 77-110

(6) Mean Verbal I.Q. = 97.7; range = 69-115

(7) Mean stimulating current used for mapping = 7.1 milliamps; range = 5-10 ma

(8) Mean number of sites sampled on lateral cortex = 12.8; range = 5-28

(9) Mean number of stimulation trials per site = 2.8; range = 1.8-4.8

(10) Mean control-trials error rate = 4.6%; range = 0-15%

---

trials at the next site, and never on any trials at a third site, all sites being in relatively close proximity to each other. This phenomenon has pertained in every patient studied since we began multiple stimulations at the same site, clearly off-setting the possible criticism that in any one patient we may only have sampled each site on an average of 2 or 3 times (see Table 1). The potential significance of this finding was discussed in Ojemann (1979); resection near a 100% naming site was followed by a marked postoperative aphasia, but removal of partial naming sites has not been followed by such sequelae. Although we cannot rule out the possibility that graded localization is an idiosyncratic brain response to electrical stimulation, we can rule out the possibility that it is an idiosyncratic subject variable, since it appears in every subject tested. As noted in most of our previous studies, the cortical language map produced by electrical stimulation appears unique to each patient, another piece of evidence favorable to the hypothesis of significant individual differences in cortical organization (see Fig. 1).

The extent of language cortex:

Whitaker & Ojemann (1977), Ojemann & Whitaker (1978a) and Van Buren, Fedio & Frederick (1978) have all addressed the question of how much (exposed) cortex may exhibit language functions using the stimulation mapping technique. Perhaps the most noteworthy discovery in this regard, in view of the historical precedent of Pierre Marie, is that the Insula may be language cortex. Ojemann & Whitaker (1978a) mapped two sites in an Insula exposed by a temporal lobectomy, and found one site,

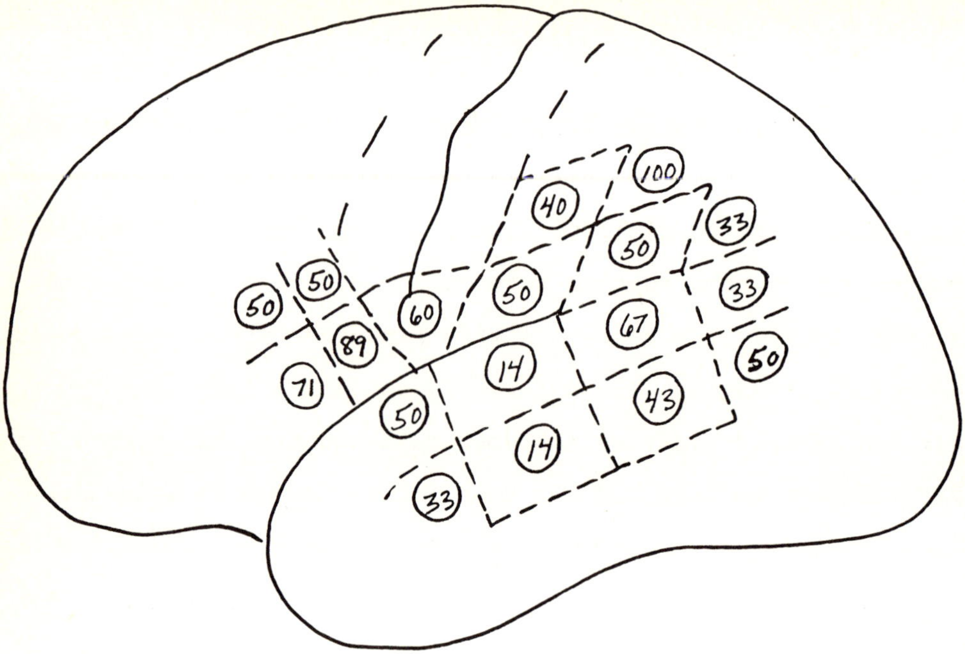

Fig. 1. Inter-individual Variability in Language Functions: Numbers represent percent (%) naming errors elicited with electrical stimulation from 2-9 patients sampled at that site. Data is from the 10 patients summarized in Table 1

directly below Rolandic cortex, to be 100% involved in naming functions. Stimulation at this site did not produce the sensory or motor responses of pre- and post-Rolandic cortex. Although this does not attest to whether or not Insula is routinely part of the language system, it does prove that it may be employed in the language system to the same extent as the supra-Sylvian cortex. In our studies we routinely obtained naming errors from a wide expanse of lateral cortex, ranging from high, second frontal gyrus, to posterior-superior parietal zone to anterior temporal lobe. In view of the fact that our patients have, for the most part, suffered from seizures from early in life, and in view of the fact that early brain lesions are more likely to cause a shift in cortical representation of functions (Rasmussen & Milner, 1975), it seems probable that to some (unknown) degree our data does not reflect the true state of affairs in the normal brain. What we have shown, however, is that a wide expanse of lateral cortex, including the Insula, may be recruited into the language function. Further, Van Buren, Fedio & Frederick (1978) have produced naming impairments from stimulation of sites all the way back close to the parietal mid-line and the occipital pole. If we make the plausible assumption that within the language area, there is language representation in the sulci as well as on the exposed gyri, then one is forced to conclude that the language system may occupy up to 50% of the lateral cortex in a hemisphere. As already noted, the actual map over this expanse of cortex for any individual, seems to be quite variable. In order to compare this data with that of Penfield, we pooled naming errors across subjects at (arbitrarily chosen) sites, in those instances in which we had a sufficient number of patients sampled at those sites. The results are pictured in Figure 1, showing the variability of language representation at 18 sites within the left hemisphere; the dotted lines are the arbitrary divisions into these 18 sites. Ten patients contributed the data for this variability map; summary characteristics of these patients are in Table 1. It is immediately apparent that a number of the sites shown in Figure 1 are outside of the classical language map of Penfield. It is also immediately apparent that the sites which are more committed to language (naming) functions, lie above the Sylvian fissure, within cortex supplied by the upper division of the middle cerebral artery.

Bilingual representation:

Ojemann & Whitaker (1978b) presented data on two bilingual subjects which were part of this series; one was a native speaker of Dutch and secondarily fluent in English, the other was a native speaker of English with near-native fluency (from very early childhood) in Spanish. Stimulation mapping of each language at the same sites but at different times, resulted in a pattern which we called partial overlapping representation. There were sites at which both languages were equally represented (100%, or partial, or not at all); there were sites at which one language was represented and not the other; and there were sites at which one language was represented differentially more, or less, than the other. Ojemann has had occasion to test one more bilingual subject, in this case the two languages were English and Greek. The same basic phenomenon of partial overlapping was again observed. As we noted in Ojemann & Whitaker (1978b), one implication of this finding is that the often-reported mystery of differential impairment and differential recovery in bilingual aphasia, may have a simple anatomic basis: the two or more languages may or may not occupy the same pieces of brain. As an aside, the naming errors and the phenomenon of graded localization were the same in these bilingual patients as in the other patients.

Other observations:

As in the patients reported on by Penfield & Roberts (1959), we did not observe naming changes from stimulation in the non-dominant hemisphere. The lack of naming errors when stimulating the right hemisphere of a left hemisphere language dominant individual, not only implies that lateralization for language can be relatively clear-cut, but it also implies that the effects of the elctrical stimulation are being confined to the hemisphere of operation and are not being transmitted across the corpus callosum.

We have observed rather remarkable degrees of displacement and re-organization of the basic functional sites in a hemisphere. In one case, sensory responses were evoked from pre-Rolandic sites and motor responses from post-Rolandic sites in the same patient. In another instance, evoked motor responses like those obtained from Rolandic cortex, were obtained in a band running in an anteropostero direction across the mid-Parietal lobe, back at least to a point above what should have been angular gyrus.

In two instances stimulation in post-Rolandic (sensory) cortex, in the general vicinity of the arm/hand area, produced an easily noticed change in speech intonation contours. Pitch was lowered, syllable durations were changed but there was no dysarthric manifestation. These effects are reminiscent of the dysprosody evidence of Monrad-Krohn, Pick, Critchley and others. In one of our patients at the site in question, stimulation seemed also to affect the production of vowels such that the vowel targets were incorrect. The limited samples of this type do not really permit further speculation.

Electrical stimulation of the brain during epilepsy procedures has proved to be a remarkable tool for the analysis of cortical language representation. Just sampling picture naming alone has produced a number of results that will modify our concept-ions of language representation in the brain. The current group of studies being conducted by Ojemann and colleagues, is extending speech and language studies into tests of sequential oro-facial movements, phonemic (speech) perception and syntactic functions in sentence reading. What can be accomplished in the future with this clinical/research tool is likely to be limited only by the inventiveness of the experiments in which it is employed.

References:

1) Brindley, G.S. and W.S. Lewin: The sensations produced by electrical stimulation of the visual cortex. Journal of Physiology 196, 479-493 (1968).
2) Dobelle, W.H. and M.G. Mladejovsky: Phosphenes produced by electrical stimulation of a prosthesis for the blind. Journal of Physiology 243, 553-576 (1974).
3) Fedio, P. and J.M. Van Buren: Memory deficits during electrical stimulation of the speech cortex in conscious man. Brain & Language, 1, 29-42 (1974).
4) Ojemann, G.: Subcortical language mechanisms. in H. Whitaker & H.A. Whitaker (eds.) Studies in Neurolinguistics, I, New York, 103-138, Academic Press (1976).
5) Ojemann, G.: Organization of short term verbal memory in language areas of human cortex: evidence from electrial stimulation. Brain & Language, 5, 331-340 (1978).
6) Ojemann, G.: Individual variability in cortical localization of language. Journal of Neurosurgery, 50, 164-169 (1979).
7) Ojemann, G. and H.A. Whitaker: Language localization and variability. Brain & Language, 6, 239-260 (1978a).
8) Ojemann, G. and H.A. Whitaker: The bilingual brain. Archives of Neurology, 35, 409-412 (1978b).
9) Penfield, W. and H. Jasper: Epilepsy and the Functional Anatomy of the Human Brain, Boston, Little, Brown (1954).
10) Penfield, W. and L. Roberts: Speech and Brain Mechanisms. Princeton, Princeton University Press (1959).
11) Rasmussen, T. and B. Milner: Clinical and surgical studies of the cerebral speech areas in man. in K. Zülch O. Creutzfeldt & G.C. Galbraith (eds.) Cerebral Localization. New York, Springer-Verlag, 238-257 (1975).
12) Van Buren, J.M, P. Fedio and G.C. Frederick: Mechanism and localization of speech in the parietotemporal cortex. Neurosurgery, 2, 233-239 (1978).
13) Whitaker, H.A. and G. Ojemann: Graded localization of naming from electrical stimulation mapping of left cerebral cortex. Nature 270, 50-51 (1977).

Human Language Cortex: Identification of Common Sites for Sequencing Motor Activity and Speech Discrimination

G. OJEMANN, C. MATEER, Department of Neurological Surgery, University of Washington, Seattle, Washington, USA

The production and understanding of speech seem to share a common cerebral organization. Evidence of this common substrate comes from two sources. First is evidence from the study of patients with cortical lesions that produce language deficits. Patients with expressive aphasias also show at least minor receptive deficits on careful testing (DeRenzi and Vignolo 1962). Most aphasic patients, including those with predominantly receptive defects, show abnormalities in sequential control of oral movements (Mateer and Kimura, 1977). Second, is evidence from the study of the factors that influence perception of speech sounds, where the perception of a phoneme appears to be more closely correlated with its articulation than its acoustics (Liberman et al., 1967). This evidence forms the basis for the motor theory of speech perception.

Using the electrical stimulation mapping technique during craniotomy under local anesthesia for resection of epileptic foci, we have investigated the effects of stimulation of multiple cortical sites on several measures of language: naming and reading, a test of short-term verbal memory, another of repetitive and sequential oral facial movements and one of phonemic discrimination. This study then, was designed to determine the role of different areas of language cortex in motor movement, phonemic understanding, and short-term verbal memory. Mapping data with these tests have been obtained from four patients undergoing craniotomy for resection of epileptic foci in the left hemisphere, previously shown to be language dominant by intracarotid sodium amytal testing. Naming, reading and short-term memory were tested with a visually presented task from 52 sites in periSylvian cortex of these 4 patients, with no fewer than 10 nor more than 15 sites from each patient. At least 3 samples of each type of language behavior were obtained at each site, using stimulation mapping through bipolar electrodes 5 mm apart, with 4-8 second trains of 60 Hz 2 1/2 msec biphasic square wave pulses from a constant current stimulation at the largest currents that did not evoke after-discharges: a mean of 5.75 milliamps between peaks of the biphasic pulses (Range: 3-8 milliamps). At 25 of these sites (5-10 per patient), stimulation effects were also measured during mimicry of single and sequential oral movements, and during a presentation period only of a taped live voice series of imbedded stop consonants. The 4 patients were 2 male and 2 female, with a mean verbal IQ of 95 (Range: 90-98), and mean age of 21.5 (Range: 17-32). The tests used in this study, the techniques for using them during stimulation, and the scoring methods have been described in detail elsewhere (Ojemann and Mateer, 1979). Statistical significance of changes in performance during stimulation at each site on each test condition were evaluated with the binomial single sample test and only changes at a significance level of .05 or less are included.

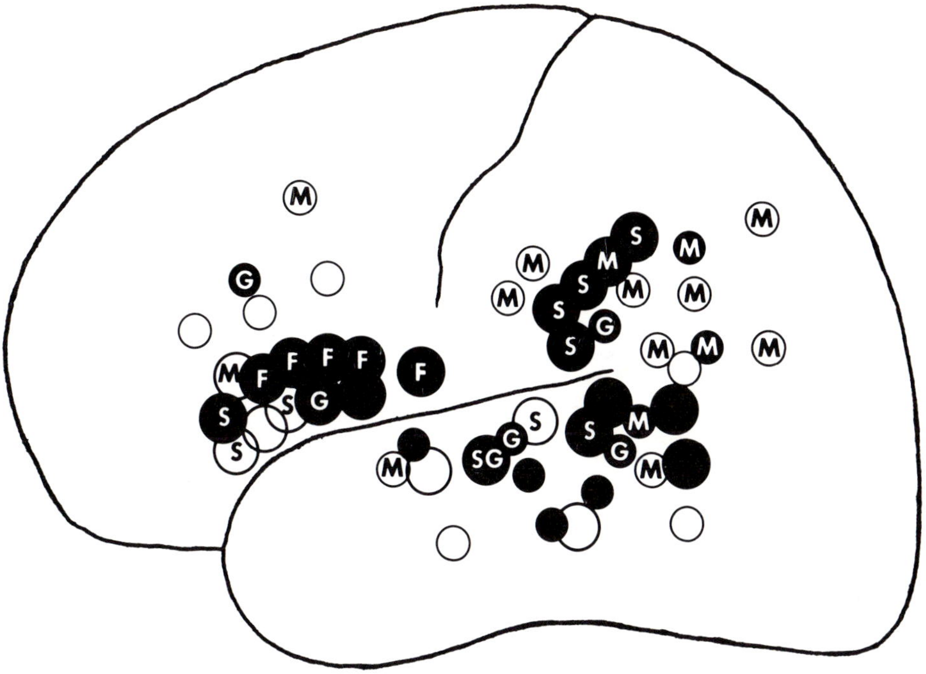

Location of different system in language cortex of the four patients described in this paper. Large cicles indicate sites where naming, reading, short-term verbal memory, repetitive and sequential oral movements and phonemic discrimination were measured. Small circles: sites where only naming, reading and short-term memory were measured. Filled circles: naming and/or reading errors at that site. Letters identify several systems in language cortex as defined in the text: F = final motor pathway; S = system common to sequencing movement and phonemic discrimination; M = short-term verbal memory; G = system for syntax. (SG = one site showing both sequential movement - phonemic discrimination and syntax changes)

The illustration shows the sites stimulated. The pattern of statistically significant changes evoked in one or more of these tests identified several different systems in language cortex:

1. A series of 5 sites (at least one in each patient) in motor cortex and immediate premotor cortex in which stimulation interrupted all types of oral movements and evoked an arrest of language, regardless of how measured. This seems to represent a final motor pathway for speech ("F" on illustration). Two of

the 4 of these sites tested demonstrated disturbed phonemic discrimination.

2. Ten sites (at least 2 in each patient) in periSylvian cortex of frontal, superior temporal and parietal lobe where sequential but not repetitive oral movements were disturbed ("S" on illustration). Nine of these 10 sites also showed disruption of phonemic discrimination. Outside of these two motor systems, no other sites showed disturbed phonemic discrimination. Eight showed either naming or reading changes as well, but none showed short-term memory changes. These sites identify an area of periSylvian cortex in dominant hemisphere that is common to sequencing motor movements and discrimination of phonemes. The presence of this common cortex would explain the close association between motor speech production and language understanding. The relatively crucial nature of this cortex for language function is suggested by the inclusion of part of it in almost every cortical lesion that gives rise to a persisting language disorder.

3. Another system in language cortex is identified by the 15 sites, 2 or more in each patient, where short-term verbal memory was altered ("M" on illustration). At 9 sites in parietal or temporal, but not frontal lobe, the memory errors followed stimulation during input or storage phases of the memory task and not output. At the remaining frontal and parietal sites, most errors occurred with output stimulation. In general, the memory system is wholly separate from the sequential motor system, and generally separate from other aspects of the language system since naming or reading was altered at only 4 of

these memory sites. These findings are similar to that reported earlier for a series of 6 other patients (Ojemann, 1978). This short-term memory system surrounds the motor discrimination system frontally, parietally and temporally.

4. Naming or reading changes only were evoked at 13 sites that are not part of one of these other systems. Generally, naming and reading were altered by stimulation at separate sites. These isolated sites of reading errors tended to be of a particular type, where most mistakes were in verb tenses, or omission of prepositions or conjunctions, errors in the grammar of sentences. By contrast, when reading errors overlapped one of the other systems, the errors were most often the production of jargon. The grammatic errors were evoked from sites that seem to lie between the sequential motor-speech discrimination and memory systems scattered in frontal, temporal parietal lobe of 3 patients ("G" on illustration). They identify specific cortical sites concerned with syntax.

Similar mapping was carried out in the right nondominant hemisphere in one patient. No sequential motor, phonemic discrimination, short-term verbal memory, naming or reading errors were identified at any of the eight sampled sites outside of motor cortex. All types of oral-facial movements could be altered from motor cortex; then phonemic discrimination was intact. These studies indicate the presence of a dominant hemisphere periSylvian area of cortex that is a common system for sequencing motor movements and decoding speech sounds, a system that would seem to provide the central link between auditory input and speech production. Surrounding it is a cortical system for short-term verbal memory, with storage aspects particularly in parietal and temporal lobes, and retrieval in frontal lobe. We suggest that language develops in the interaction of these two systems, with such specialized aspects of language as syntax allocated to cortex between them. Indeed, there are other sites lying between these systems that show only evoked changes in naming or partial arrests of reading, behavioral changes that indicate sites with a role in language that our present tests do not further identify.

The relative relationships between these systems have been quite constant in the series of patients studied to date, but the exact cortical regions involved in each system have shown considerable individual variability. This has been quantitated for areas showing evoked changes in naming (Ojemann, 1979). Whether this degree of variability is a characteristic of normal human brain, or related to the early brain damage that gives rise to the seizures and indications for operation in our patient population is unknown.

Based on our model, then, the phylogenetic developments leading to language should be characterized by the development of lateralized systems for sequential motor control and for short-term memory. The latter has been identified in monkey (Dewson, 1977). This would also suggest that language arises, at least in part, in brain areas that originally had predominantly motor function. This suggestion has previously been advanced by Kimura (1976), based on motor changes in aphasic patients. And it is also supported by the evidence that subcortical language mechanisms also involve motor portions of the brain, for example the effects evoked from left ventrolateral thalamus (Ojemann, 1977). The development of language seems to have incorporated brain mechanisms originally developed for motor learning.

Acknowledgements: This research was supported by NIH Grant No. NS 04053, awarded by the National Institute of Neurological and Communicative Disorders and Stroke, PHS/DHEW, and NINCDS Fellowship 1 F32 NS 05847-01. Dr. Ojemann is an Affiliate of the Child Development and Mental Retardation Center, University of Washington, Seattle, Washington, USA. Dr. Mateer's correspondence may be addressed to the Department of Speech Pathology, University of Toronto, Ontario, Canada. Two of the cases were under the care of Dr. A.A. Ward,Jr. Dr. C. Dodrill provided IQ and Amytal data.

References:

1) De Renzi, E. and Vignolo, L.: The token test: a sensitive test to detect reception disturbances in aphasics. Brain 85, 665-678 (1962).
2) Dewson, J.: Preliminary evidence of hemispheric asymmetry of auditory function in monkeys. In: Harnard, S., Doty, R., Goldstein, L., Saynes, J. and Krauthamer, G. (eds.) Lateralization in the Nervous System. New York, Academic Press, 63-74 (1977).
3) Kimura, D.: The neural basis of language qua gesture. Studies in Neurolinguistics 2, 145-156 (1976).
4) Liberman, A., Cooper, F., Shankweiler, D., Studdert-Kennedy, M.: Perception of the speech code. Psychol.Review, 74, 431-461 (1967).
5) Mateer, C. and Kimura, D.: Impairment of non-verbal oral movements in aphasia. Brain and Language 5, 331-340 (1978).
6) Ojemann, G.: Organization of short-term memory in language areas of human cortex: Evidence from electrical stimulation. Brain and Language 5, 331-340 (1978).
7) Ojemann, G. and Mateer, C.: Cortical and subcortical organization of human communication: Evidence from stimulation studies. In: Steklis, H. and Raleigh, M. (eds.) Neurobiology of Social Communication in Primates. New York, Academic Press, in press (1979).
8) Ojemann, G.: Individual variability in cortical localization of language. J.Neurosurg. 50, 164-169 (1979).
9) Ojemann, G.: Asymmetric function of the thalamus in man. Annals New York Academy of Sciences 299, 380-396 (1977).

Studies on Language Comprehension in Hemispherectomy, Split Brain and Aphasic Patients. A Possible Contribution to the Knowledge of the Psychological Mechanisms of Speech Comprehension.

KLAUS POECK, Abteilung Neurologie der Rheinisch-Westfälischen Technischen Hochschule Aachen, 5100 Aachen, Goethestr. 27-29, W-Germany

Neuropsychological and in particular neurolinguistic studies can make only very limited contribution to the knowledge of the physiological mechanisms of speech comprehension. The main reason for this negative statement is that the processes we call "understanding of spoken language" have more psychological than physiological implications which will be discussed in the third part of this paper. I am going to give a "state of the art" review on investigations into the language understanding capacity of the left (language dominant) and right (non-dominant, so-called minor) hemisphere in man. I am going to speak on language processing in the right hemisphere after left (dominant) hemispherectomy, then I am going to report old and new findings on the capacity of the right, non-dominant hemisphere in split brain patients to understand verbal material, and, finally, I shall consider the results of investigations into language comprehension of aphasic patients.

Evidence from hemispherectomy cases

With respect to our particular problem, the processing of language understanding within the brain, the hemispherectomy evidence is scanty and controversial. Hemispherectomy has been performed mainly in the fifties and sixties as a treatment for intractable epilepsy in patients with infantile hemiplegia. These patients had either sustained the injury before acquiring speech or during the process of speech acquisition. Unfortunately, most of these patients have been studied only by clinical observation and by the Wechsler Intelligence Scale, and the reports on their faculty of speech are based on comparison of the verbal and the performance scale of the Wechsler Test. This, however, is a rather crude method of assessing linguistic performances. The only conclusions that can be drawn from the reports of Basser (1962) and other authors, are the following: Even when the injury had damaged the left hemisphere and even if the left hemisphere was removed, language performance either remained unaffected or returned to the preoperative level, sometimes even beyond the preoperative level, and as a rule language understanding was better preserved than expressive language. This holds true irrespective of stock-handedness in the respective families.

Recently Gott (1973) has reported the case of a 12-year-old girl who underwent left hemispherectomy for a cerebral malignancy. This case is particularly illustrative because the malignant tumor had certainly not started to develop prior to age 11. Yet even at this age the right hemisphere was able to take on receptive language functions to a remarkable degree. The girl was able to follow commands, to give proper Yes or No answers to declarative statements, and her verbal intelligence measured by the Peabody Picture Vocabulary Test, where the response is given by pointing to a multiple choice set of pictures, was 70. The age beyond which speech functions cannot be satisfactorily acquired by the opposite hemisphere seems variable and has not been sharply determined.

Experience with unilateral brain lesions and with hemispherectomy permit the following statements: Lesions to either side of the brain during the first few years of language development disrupt speech with almost equal probability. The deficits are temporary and are largely expressive rather than receptive (Lenneberg, 1967). After dominant hemispherectomy the opposite half of the brain is endowed to take on full or at east satisfactory control of language, and understanding is always better than expressive speech - just as it is the case in the development of language, in healthy adults learning a foreign language or in adult patients with aphasia, at least in the great majority of cases.

Removal of the language dominant hemisphere in adults is rarely performed, and the reason is mostly because of a malignant glioma. The hemispherectomy is followed by a complete or almost complete loss of all language functions. Over a period of several weeks or months varying degrees of recovery are observed, but only language comprehension approximates normal levels one year post operatively. The observation period in these cases is necessarily short, because the malignant tumor tends to recurr after approximately one year.

The first case was described by Smith and Burklund (1966) and in more detail by Smith (1969). Receptive language functions in this patient, and also in patients reported in the following years, were initially less impaired than expressive speech. In general the patients show improving language comprehension, they understand oral messages whereas their speech output is limited to single utterances, to swearing and some degree of singing.

In hemispherectomy patients it has been demonstrated that the right hemisphere is capable of processing language in the oral receptive modality to a fairly satisfactory degree after dominant hemispherectomy in adults (Smith, 1972). It is known that removal of one hemisphere is followed quite often by an improvement in the number of epileptic seizures and also in social behaviour. These observations have led to the conclusion that the lesioned hemisphere has a disturbing or inhibitory influence on the (relatively) intact half of the brain. Unfortunately nobody has so far examined patients with dominant hemispherectomy and patients with global aphasia who harbour a large lesion destroying virtually all of the speech area with exactly the same methods. Only a comparison of these groups of patients would permit an answer to the question whether the damaged dominant hemisphere exerts an inhibitory influence on the language capacity of the opposite side, as some authors have speculated. Were this the case, then the logical consequence would be to perform a split brain operation in patients with long standing and stable severe global aphasia, in order to relieve the intact right hemisphere from the inhibitory influcence of the damaged left. This idea is not as bizarre as it might appear. This point will be illustrated when we consider the language functions in split brain patients.

Split brain evidence

In the split brain operations in humans surgical separation of the hemispheres is produced by complete transection of the corpus callosum plus the anterior and hippocampal commissures and with separation of the massa intermedia of the thalamus.

Split brain patients have virtually no expressive language preserved within the right hemisphere. Sperry and Gazzaniga (1967), and Gazzaniga (for review, 1974) have demonstrated that the isolated right (non-dominant) hemisphere has some comprehension of simple nouns, it was, however, unable to process verbs and short sentences. Gazzaniga and Hillyard (1971) have examined, with negative results, the abilities of the right hemisphere to process more complicated syntactic structures.

The findings and conclusions of Gazzaniga have recently been challenged by Zaidel (1978) who was able to demonstrate that the receptive ability of the non-dominant hemisphere far exceeded the range described by Gazzaniga and collaborators. Zaidel has examined, in commissurotomy patients, the linguistic processing of auditory stimuli in the right hemisphere following the experimental paradigm used by Gazzaniga. In short, the tasks require the subject to respond with the left hand (right hemisphere) to a visual stimulus flashed to the left visual half-field (right hemisphere). The task is to select, among a choice of various objects the one fitting best the name of the word flashed to the left half-field tachistoscopally.

Zaidel was able to demonstrate that the right hemisphere could analyze a spoken input into its phonetic components. At the semantic level Zaidel found the right hemisphere inferior to the left, but the difference was relatively small. The disconnected and isolated right hemisphere seemed to have access to a substantial auditory vocabulary. A very important finding is that the performance of both hemispheres showed the same dependancy on word frequency which is also exhibited by normal and aphasic adults and normal children. This finding is very remarkable because word frequency is taken to reflect the effects of linguistic experience.

With Carrol's test for auditory language comprehension Zaidel found that the right hemisphere could make various syntactical discriminations and attained a mental age equal to or above that of five years.

Evidence from patients with aphasia

In aphasiology, research has been focussed on comprehension for at least a decade in almost all centers. The outcome of the many sophisticated studies, however, has been quite disappointing. Up to a period around 1970 language understanding had been treated in the aphasiological literature as if it were a onedimensional function. Whereas expressive language was considered as a complex of various functions which could be impaired differentially in aphasia, depending on the locus of brain lesion, most authors had given their judgement on language understanding in a very crude way as intact, slightly impaired, severely impaired and so on. Some of the many studies on language understanding published after 1970 gave the insight that language understanding is equally complex as language expression and that under this heading are subsumed a great variety of quite different performances. Surprisingly enough it did not emerge from the studies that the well defined aphasiological syndromes, for instance Broca's amnesic, Wernicke's and global aphasia which are easily differentiated on the basis of language production had an equally defined receptive aspect. Most differences between the aphasiological subgroups that were found were only quantitative in nature, and quite often patients with Broca's aphasia performed as well as patients with right hemispheric lesion without aphasia. These negative findings were not attributable to poor methods of examination.

At the phonemic level, Luria (1970) had asserted that a phoneme discrimination impairment is operative in the comprehension deficit of patients with Wernicke's aphasia. This view was not supported by experiments of Basso et al. (1977) and Blumstein et al. (1977). However, it was found (Blumstein et al., 1977) that those patients who had severe problems in producing phonemes in proper form and order were also particularly impaired in phoneme discrimination. So it appeared as if the examinations had demonstrated a supramodal organisation which worked in a similar way in production and reception.

Tests of word comprehension have not been very revealing. Some years ago we reported (Poeck et al., 1973) that three examinations, which are standard in clinical aphasiology, i.e. understanding of object names, of colour names, and of simple commands did not discriminate between brain damaged patients with and without aphasia. Also a test with correct and incorrect statements did not yield conclusive results. Tasks, which are derived from intelligence tests, evidently do not assess the specific aphasic nature of the language understanding deficit in aphasic patients.

At the level of sentences, where syntactical analysis comes into play, Parisi and Pizzamiglio (1970) as well as Shewan and Canter (1971) have established that the expressive impairment and the impairment in comprehension for sentences in aphasic patients varied independently. The knowledge of an aphasic's expressive language deficit was not a good predictive indicator of his receptive abilities. They concluded that input and output problems may be largely independent in aphasia and not necessarily part of a common central integrative problem. The language deficits evident in the verbal output of aphasic patients differed both qualitatively and quantitatively. By contrast, receptive deficits for sentences seemed to differ only along a quantitative dimension.

In the normal communicative situation, however, language comprehension requires not only the understanding of phonemes, words and sentences but also the processing of discourse or text. In order to reconstruct the content of a text the semantically most relevant constituents and their relations must be stored and remembered. Language comprehension at this level requires lexical and grammatical knowledge as well as pragmatic strategies and memory. This means that the understanding of lexical and grammatical units must be supplemented by processes of inference, deduction and problem solving. These processes are related to verbal as well as situational aspects of a given discourse. For the hearer to understand the information conveyed, he has to reconstruct both verbal and situational aspects.

In order to study language comprehension at the textual level, we have developed a text comprehension test (Stachowiak et al., 1977) which was given to aphasics of different subtypes, to brain damaged patients without aphasia and to normal controls. The paradigm was, as usual, the identification of a target sentence in a story read to the patient by pointing to the appropriate drawing in a multiple choice set of pictures. Much to our surprise, our aphasic patients were not selectively impaired in this text comprehension task. We also did not find any qualitative differences between the performance of the major aphasic subgroups. Obviously, the greater redundancy of texts as compared to single words and isolated sentences makes up for an eventual deficit of the aphasic patients at the word and sentence level. If a particular word or sentence structure within a text is not understood, there are nevertheless enough cues in the context from which the missing part can be inferred.

These largely negative findings leave the question open, what the aphasic nature of the comprehension deficit in aphasic patients might be.

With regards to the organisation of language understanding in the human brain the studies reviewed so far lead to five conclusions:

1. The well delineated expressive syndromes of aphasia have no qualitative counterpart in language comprehension.

2. Comprehension is apparently much less lateralized to the

language dominant hemisphere, usually the left, than language production.

3. Within the language dominant hemisphere language understanding has a much less focal organisation than other aspects of language, such as, for instance, word finding or the ability to produce syntactic constructions.

4. It appears likely that different aspects of language understanding such as linguistic analysis in a restricted sense of the word and the analysis of features like intonation contours are processed simultaneously in both hemispheres, the right hemisphere contributing essential elements to the process of language understanding.

5. It appears that even in aphasic patients general pragmatic strategies of language understanding remain intact or not too profoundly disturbed, which might compensate the impairment at more specific levels such as analysis of the meaning of words or sentences.

The vast literature on language understanding deficits in aphasic patients has contributed very little to the problem why aphasic patients are impaired in the natural use of language in communicative situations.

There is, however, a group of data considered to be specific for the aphasic deficit in the comprehension of spoken language. Many authors have considered the Token Test by De Renzi and Vignolo (1962) to assess a specifically aphasic impairment in language understanding. The test was introduced with the hope that it would be a sensitive test to detect receptive disturbance in aphasics. In this test, the patient is presented with 10 or 20 tokens which differ in colour (5 colours), in form (circles and squares) and size (large and small ones). Instructions are rigorously standardized and require the patient to perform single operations with these tokens such as picking up a blue circle and pointing to the large white rectangle and so on. The test consists of five parts where the commands are of increasing complexity. The Token Test has been subject of very extensive studies mainly centered on its psychometric aspects. It was clearly established that the test is very valuable for the purpose of selecting aphasic subjects out of a population of brain damaged patients. It turned out very early (Orgass and Poeck, 1966) that aphasic patients of all subtypes fell below the range of brain damaged non-aphasic controls, even patients with Broca's aphasia or amnesic aphasia with apparently little or no sizeable understanding deficit.

On the face of it, the test requires three chains of performances: the acoustic and semantic/syntactic analysis of the spoken command, the processing of the command in that hypothetical analyzer which Whitaker (1971) has termed the Central Language System and the ability to direct a pointing response in the correct way. Disturbance of brain function at any one of these levels could lead to identical results, i.e. failure to carry out the action correctly. We have recently done a study (Hartje and Poeck, 1978; Poeck and Hartje, in press) where we compared two versions of the Token Test, one in which the instructions were given via the acoustic input (vocal instructions as usual) and one where the input was visual (written instructions). In this study, we found no significant difference, neither in the performance of the total group of aphasics nor in the performance of the aphasic subgroups in the two modes of presentation (vocal vs. visual). Obviously, the test is sensitive not only for oral comprehension, but taps a supramodal deficit in aphasic patients.

On the other hand acoustic factors of course do play a role in performance in this test: We have carried out another study (Poeck and Pietron, unpublished results) with aphasic patients, where the commands of the Token Test were given in two versions, both on magnetic tapes, one spoken in a normal way and one with stretched speech, where the single signals were stretched by the factor 1.25 without altering the frequency. It was found that in the stretched version the number of errors was significantly smaller than in the normal version. Unfortunately we could not perform a control experiment on the possible influence of stretched speech in right brain damaged patients, because these make so few errors that no significant improvement could have been expected.

I have reported these two studies because they illustrate how challenging the task is to detect brain mechanisms by aphasiological methods. Two patients may fail in the Token Test, quantitatively, to the same degree, but the reason might be deficient temporal processing of language signals in one case and a supramodal integrative deficit in the other.

Concluding remarks

What are the conclusions suggested by a review on language comprehension in the three conditions: hemispherectomy, split brain and circumscribed aphasia producing lesion.

The ability of the disconnected right hemisphere to produce appropriate speech is, if present at all, remarkably lower than the ability to comprehend spoken words and sentences. These findings speak against motor theories of speech perception at least in so far as motor aspects of speech are not necessary to account for speech perception on the phonetic and lexical levels. Evidently speech is much more lateralized than auditory language comprehension, and the onogenesis of cerebral specialization for the two functions has a quite different natural history. Until the age of about 4 to 5 years the two hemispheres develop substantially parallel competence for language skills. At that point the competence for some components such as speech declines in the right hemisphere in order to permit left hemisphere specialization for fine motor programming and better control of the speech apparatus. Other components such as the auditory or reading lexicon continue to develop in the right hemisphere even though at a reduced rate relative to the left. It is not clear whether the relatively rich lexical semantics of the right hemisphere is used in cooperation with left hemisphere language processing or whether they only serve the non-verbal cognitive needs of the right. It could be that normal language perception involves the simultaneous analysis of the linguistic input in both hemispheres with the analysis of the phonetic and semantic components of language conducted primarily in the left hemisphere and the analysis of intonational components of the speech signal conducted primarily in the right hemisphere.

Comparison of right hemisphere performance with language development in children shows striking and gross discrepancies. Right hemisphere auditory comprehension cannot be characterized uniformly as the receptive competence of a child at a given age. There is no normal stage in the development of language comprehension such that the child may possess both a vocabulary of a 12-year-old and the apparent syntax of a 6 or 4-year-old. Obviously lateralization of language to the left does not occur at the same age or to the same degree for all components of the comprehension system.

Also, the comprehension performance of the right hemisphere does not permit analogies with any one aphasic subtype. There is some similarity, for instance the dependancy on word frequency, a feature which holds for the vocabularies of children as well and which apparently reflects a universal linguistic pattern. In general, however, there are consistent differences between aphasic patients behaviour and performances of the right hemisphere. There are also large individual differences in the normal dextrous right hemisphere language competence, and its ability to take over language functions cannot be predicted. By the same token, any consideration of right hemisphere contribution in a healthy individual must necessarily remain speculative.

References:

1) Basser, L.S.: Hemiplegia of early onset and the faculty of speech with special reference to the effects of hemispherectomy. Brain 85, 427-460 (1962).

2) Basso, A.; G. Casati and L.A. Vignolo: Phonemic identification defect in aphasia. Cortex 13, 85-95 (1977).
3) Blumstein, S.; E. Baker and H. Goodglass: Phonological factors in auditory comprehension in aphasia. Neuropsychologia 15, 19-30 (1977).
4) De Renzi, E. and L.A. Vignolo: The Token Test: a sensitive test to detect receptive disturbance in aphasia. Brain 85, 665-678 (1962).
5) Gazzaniga, M.: Cerebral dominance viewed as a decision system. In: Dimond, S. and J. Graham Beaumont (eds.), Hemisphere Function in the Human Brain. London: Elk Science, 367-382 (1974).
6) Gazzaniga, M.S. and S.A. Hillyard: Language and speech capacity of the right hemisphere. Neuropsychologia 9, 273-280 (1971).
7) Gott, P.S.: Cognitive abilities following right and left hemispherectomy. Cortex 9, 266-274 (1973).
8) Hartje, W. and K. Poeck: Token-Test-Leistung aphasischer Patienten bei vokaler und visueller Testanweisung. Nervenarzt 49, 654-657 (1978).
9) Lenneberg, E.H.: Biological foundations of language. New York: Wiley (1967).
10) Luria, A.R.: Traumatic aphasia. The Hague: Mouton, pp. 155, 127 (1970).
11) Orgass, B. and K. Poeck: Clinical validation of a new test for aphasia: an experimental study on the Token Test. Cortex 2, 222-243 (1966).
12) Parisi, D. and L. Pizzamiglio: Syntactic comprehension in aphasia. Cortex 6, 204-215 (1970).
13) Poeck, K. and W. Hartje: Performance of aphasic patients in visual versus auditory presentation of the Token Test (in press).
14) Poeck, K., W. Hartje, M. Kerschensteiner and B. Orgass: Sprachverständnisstörungen bei aphasischen und nicht aphasischen Hirnkranken. Dtsch.med.Wschr. 98, 139-147 (1973).
15) Shewan, C.M. and G. Canter: Effects of vocabulary, syntax and sentence length on auditory comprehension. Cortex 7, 209-226 (1971).
16) Smith, A.: Nondominant hemispherectomy. Neurology 19, 442-445 (1969).
17) Smith, A. and C.W. Burklund: Dominant hemispherectomy: preliminary report on neuropsychological sequelae. Science 153, 1280-1282 (1966).
18) Smith, A.: Dominant and nondominant hemispherectomy. In: Smith, W.L. (ed.), Drugs, Development and Cerebral Function. Springfield: Thomas, 37-68 (1972).
19) Sperry, R.W. and M.S. Gazzaniga: Language following surgical disconnection of the hemispheres. In: Millikan, C.H. and F.L. Darley (eds.): Brain Mechanisms Underlying Speech and Language. New York and London: Grune and Stratton, 108-115 (1967).
20) Stachowiak, F.-J.; W. Huber, K. Poeck and M. Kerschensteiner: Text comprehension in aphasia. Brain and Language 4, 177-195 (1977).
21) Whitaker, H.A.: On the representation of language in the human brain. Edmonton/Champaign Linguistic Research Inc.,(1971).

22) Zaidel, E.: Auditory Language Comprehension in the Right Hemisphere Following Cerebral Commissurotomy and Hemispherectomy: A Comparison with Child Language and Aphasia. In: Zurif, E. and A. Caramazza (eds.): The Acquisition and Breakdown of Language, Parallels and Divergencies. Baltimore: Johns Hopkins University Press, 229-277 (1978).

Timing in Speech Production: Aspects of (German) Hesitation Vowels

E. BRÜSER and D. TODT, Verhaltensforschung, Lehr- und Forschungsbereich der FU Berlin, FB 23 - WE 4, Haderslebenerstr. 9, 1000 Berlin 41, FRG

As part of the DFG project "Wortfindungs- und Wortformulierungsstörungen beim Menschen" (supported by the SFB 70 (Teilprojekt: TODT) we have studied the temporal and sequential ordering of vocal units (of a special category) normally occuring in spontaneous speech, but, while characterized as nonverbal vocalisations, are often excluded from linguistic investigations. (Todt, 1976; Wolfgramm, 1976; Brüser, 1977); Todt & Brüser, 1979). In the German language these units sound like [ɛ] ("äh"), or [ɛm] ("ähm"); in American they are more like an [ɤ], [ə] ("ah"). As their features resemble those of a vowel, and as they occur predominantly when a speaker hesitates, we call them "hesitation vowels" (HVs). Synonymous terms are "hesitation phenomena", "filled pauses" (in contrast to "silent pauses"), "äh-units", or just "äh" (lit. Maclay & Osgood, 1959; Hawkins, 1971; Cook & Smith & Lalljee, 1974; MCK Mercer, 1976; Conrad & Schönle, 1979). Hesitation phenomena in speech have been investigated by several research groups; in particular Goldman-Eisler and her team published a considerable number of contributions (lit.: Goldman-Eisler, 1972, 1968). Hesitation vowels are utterances which - within limits - are not pathological. On the other hand they may be regarded as deviations of language norms: Their occurrence is not systematically described by any grammar, however, they can be detected easily in recorded speech. Assuming that the HVs are not voluntarily produced they can be analysed as indicators of involuntary processes especially of hesitations during the processing of speech.

Methods:

The methodological procedure chosen for this investigation was tested in pilot studies. The speakers in our experiments were 14 female biology students, aging from 22 to 28 years. They had been instructed to first read aloud a text of 611 words and then to speak about it for at least 25 min. The persons were free to refer to the "story" repeatedly, to improvise on it and to add to it. The behaviour of the speakers was recorded on magnetic tape, and in addition, audio-visually. The spoken material was analysed by sonagramms, oscillogramms and type written transcripts. All non-verbal vocalisations within the speech samples were also registered and 2 co-workers independently punctuated according to the German grammar.

Results:

1. Is there more than one type of HV? Which temporal features characterize 'them'?

As regards the temporal parameters of the HV we analysed its duration (length) as well as the duration of the pauses (silent intervals) preceding and following it. We found that the duration of HVs covered a wide range (30-840 msec.) "Normal" vowels comparable to the HVs in question, are obviously shorter and less variable than the latter. In most subjects the classed duration of HVs formed a bimodal frequency distribution, thereby indicating 2 HV types: "Short" $\leq$300 msec., and "long" ones >300 msec. (fig. 1,B). "Short" hesitation vowels correspond in length to "long" German vowels, which within words show an average duration of 250 msec. (Rietveld, 1975). "Long" hesitation vowels (400 to 650 msec.) were equivalent to "short" German words. The frequency distributions of silent intervals preceding (fig. 1,A) respectively following (fig. 1,C) the HVs (classed according to length) obviously differed. Further analysis showed that the values of silent intervals preceding short HVs were distributed similarly to those values preceding long HVs. On the other hand, short HVs were predominantly followed by short silent intervals, whereas long HVs were followed more often by long silent intervals (fig. 1, lower part). Based on these differences, we included the pauses preceding the HV in our analysis. To test whether the length of the intervals preceding HVs were related to special combinations of the hesitation vowel and the following interval, we formed for a clearer distinction 3 classes of the following intervals:

1. Short intervals: < 320 msec.
2. Medium intervals: 320 - 360 msec.
3. Long intervals: > 920 msec.

The distribution of the preceding intervals was analyed according to the following 4 combinations of HV with following intervals:

1. short hesitation vowel → short following interval
2. short hesitation vowel → long following interval

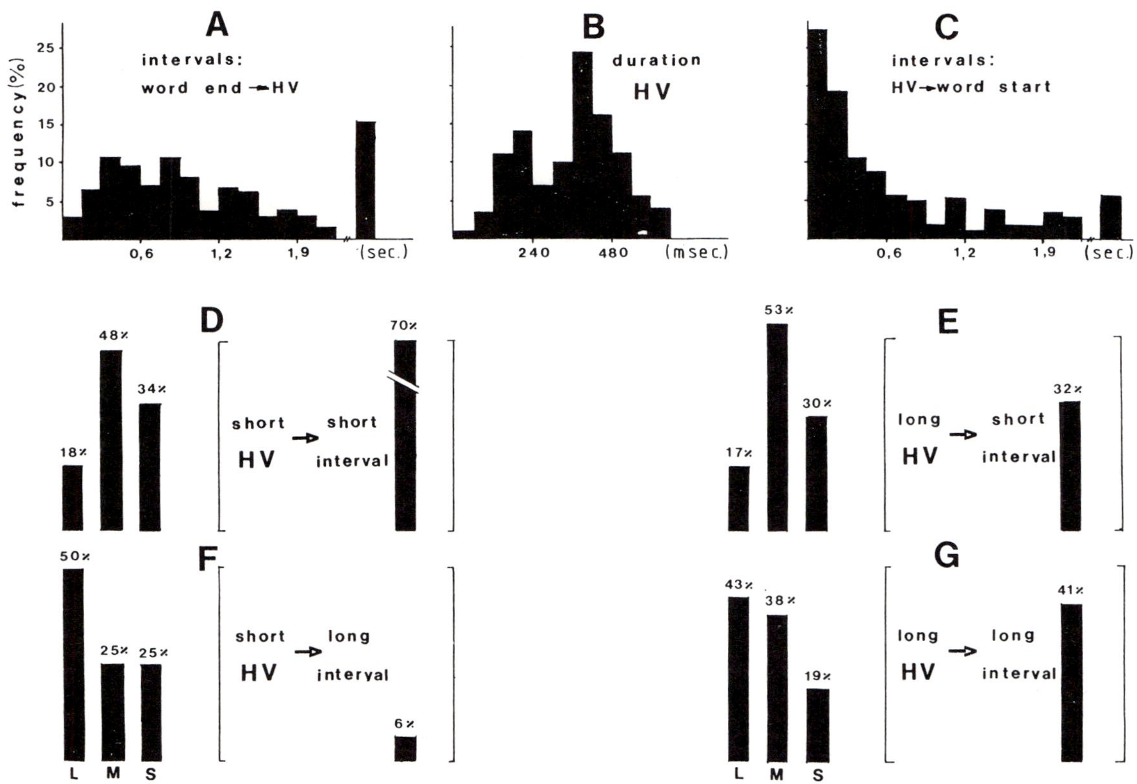

Fig. 1. Upper part: 3 frequency distributions of time classes for durations of hesitation vowels (HVs) in (B), intervals preceding (A), and following (C) HVs. NOte diversal shapes. Based on the bimodal distribution of HV durations we distinguished "short" and "long" HV types. Lower part: As shown in the figure short HVs are mostly followed by short silent intervals (E) and seldom by long ones (D). Long HVs are more often followed by long (F) than by short intervals depends on the length of the following interval and obviously not on the duration of the HV

3. long hesitation vowel → short following interval

4. long hesitation vowel → long following interval.

As shown in Fig. 1 (D,E,F,G) the length of intervals preceding the HV were correlated to specific combination of HV and the following interval.

2. Are the hesitation vowels preferentially uttered at specific locations in the text and avoided at others?
Former studies had shown, that hesitation vowels occurred predominantly (about 95%) between but seldom within words. Based on the occurrence for all interword positions of the text, according to the formula $\gamma = \frac{e-o}{e}$ (γ = variable showing preference strength; o= observed value; e= expected value). Expected values were calculated under assumption of random occurrence of HVs. As shown in Fig. 2 the distribution of HVs was not random. They occurred more frequent than random at interword positions at clause (respectively sentence) boundaries. At the beginning of a clause (Fig. 2: +p1 +p2 +p3) HVs were still more frequent than random. At clause end (Fig. 2: -p1 -p2 -p3) they were avoided.
It is evident that words at the beginning of a clause are normally "function" words (in the sense of Maclay & Osgood, 1959) and according to German frequency dictionaries are of high usage, (in more than 95% the word at +p1 in Fig. 2 was one of the hundred most frequent German words). Words at clause end, however, are normally content words and comparatively rare. - The question whether the HV occurrence depends on the quality of the conjunction and its logical implications, is still under study.

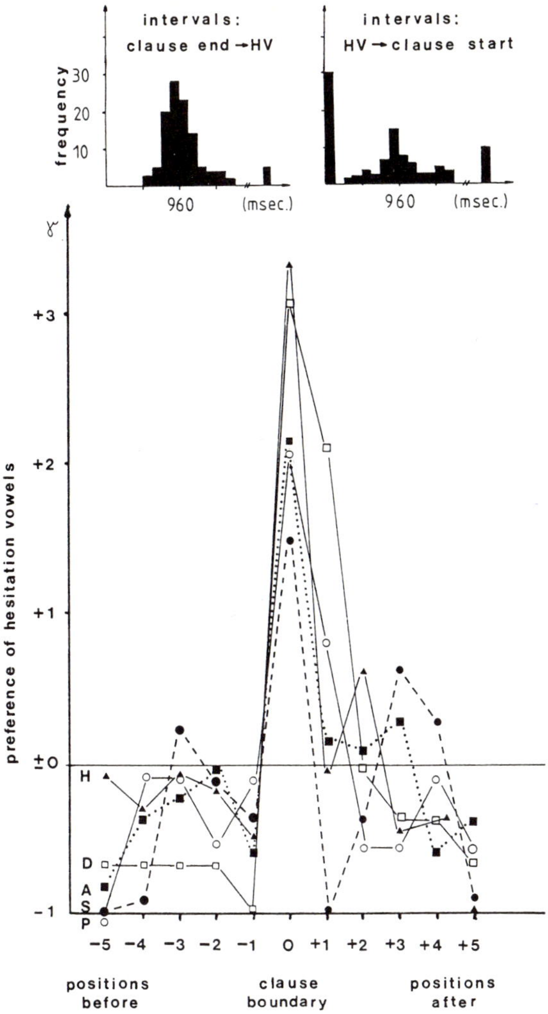

Fig. 2. Upper part: Interval distribution at clause boundaries on the left and multimodal interval distribution on the right (see text). Lower part: Representation of preference strength of HVs at clause (respectively sentence) boundaries: numbers of the abcissa indicate interword positions, which are allocated according to the sequential distance to the boundary. "0": HV at boundary; positive numbers +p1, +p2, +p3 . . . (right): HV after the start of the clause; negative numbers -p1, -p2, -p3 . . . (left): HV before the end of a clause. Ordinate gives preference strength in γ (see text): high preference ($\gamma \leq 1$) for HV between clauses and among the first few words of a clause; avoidance ($\gamma < 0$) among the last few words of a clause. Capitals indicate data of 5 of the 14 investigated subjects

3. Is there a specific timing of hesitation vowel occurrence at clause boundaries?

In former studies we had found (Todt, 1976) that the distribution of interval length between the vocalic end of a clause and the start of the next word initiating a clause corresponded in one and the same person to the distribution of silent intervals preceding the HV at clause boundaries. The interval formed one maximum in both cases, normally within the range of 800 to 1000 msec. This correspondence implies that the HVs start often particularly at those locations where the first word of the new clause would begin. Based on these findings Todt concluded that the HV may occur instead of a particular word and can be uttered in those cases where only the starting time but not yet the specific quality of the verbal sign is determined.

Proceding on this hypothesis we asked whether and how HV utterances would be integrated into the ongoing speaking process. Would the process continue independently of the uttered HV, or would the HV utterance affect it?

To answer this question we analysed in particular the interval length following the HV. As shown by the distribution inserted in Fig. 2 we found a multimod 1 distribution with the first maximum, predominantly established by intervals < 80 msec, which can be explained by the assumption that HV utterances do not interrupt the process of word determination and vocalisation, in so far HVs are handled as the start of a new clause. The second maximum, formed by classes of lengths equivalent to these establishing the maximum of interval lengths preceding the HV, has to be explained by a different assumption. Presumably, these intervals show, that the HV utterances may affect the speaking process, acting actually as the end of a clause. - At present, further analysis is being carried out. We think that our results are of interest for the elucidation of the process of verbal encoding and production.

References:

1) Boomer, D.S.: Hesitation and grammatical encoding. Language and Speech 8, 148-158 (1965).
2) Brüser, E.: Nicht-verbale Vokalisationen beim Menschen - und ihre verhaltensbiologischen Hintergründe, Staatsexamensarbeit, Berlin (1977).
3) Conrad, B. & Schönle, P.: Speech and respiration. Archives of Psychiatry and Neurological Sciences (1979).
4) Cook, M.; Smith, J.; Lalljee, M.G.: Filled pauses and syntactic complexity. Language and Speech 17, 11-16 (1974).
5) Cook, M.: The incidence of filled pauses in relation to part of speech. Language and Speech 14, 135-139 (1970).
6) Fant, G.: Analysis and synthesis of speech process. In: Malmberg, B.: Manual of Phonetics. Amsterdam and Canada, 173-277 (1968) (1. Aufl.).
7) Goldman-Eisler, F.: Pauses, Clauses, Sentences. Language and Speech 15, 103-113 (1972).
8) Goldman-Eisler, F.: Psycholinguistics. London-New York (1968).
9) Maclay, H. & Osgood, C.E.: Hesitation phenomena in spontaneous English speech. Word 15, 19-44 (1959).
10) MCK Mercer, N.: Frequency and availability in the encoding of spontaneous speech. Language and Speech 19, 129-142 (1976).
11) Rietveld, A.C.M.: Untersuchungen zur Vokaldauer im Deutschen. Phonetica 31, 248-258 (1975).
12) Rosengren, J.: Ein Frequenzwörterbuch der Deutschen Zeiungssprache. Lund (1972).
13) Schank, G.; Schoenthal, G.: Gesprochene Sprache. Tübingen (1976).
14) Thimm, F. et al.: Zeitabhängigkeit von Verhaltensmusterfolgen. J.Comp.Physiol. 93, 55-84 (1974).
15) Todt, D.: Untersuchungen zum Auftreten von Füllauten in spontaner Rede. Nova Acta Leopoldina, Halle (1976) (in press).
16) Todt, D. & Brüser, E.: Hesitation vowels as indicators of discoordinations in speech processing (manuscript ready for print).
17) Townsend, D.J.; Brever, F.G.: Interclause relations and clausal processing. J. of verbal Learning and verbal Behaviour 17, 509-521 (1978).

Inborn Vocalizations of the Human Baby and Communicative Value for the Mother

M. MORATH, Freie Universität Berlin, FRG

Introduction

Babies keep contact with their mothers with a variety of biological signals transmitted to various perception centers. At the visual level signals include locomotory movements, certain positions of the head and extremities, and facial expressions. Tactile signals are communicated with body contact. Research on the acoustic signaling of infants in their first half year of life, and the effectiveness of these signals in auditory perception, was thus far mainly restricted to the study of crying. We can assume that a baby's cry is unique on the grounds that mothers can recognize their own baby's crying (1). Crying especially in the first quarter of the year seems to have a single form unaffected by changes in situations and many vary only in intensity (2). Cry analysis showed differences in cry patterns (3) but they seemed to have no communicative functions for the mother. This is however not the case in preverbal vocalizations, that is, all the acoustic utterances which are not crying or babbling. Until now preverbal vocalizationes of human babies have not enjoyed much attention either from linguists or paediatricians.

Some mentioned a possible function for the mother-child interaction without further evidence (4).

Methods

Ethological methods including audio-visual-tape analysis were employed in sequential analysis of preverbal acoustical behavior.

The subjects in the study reported here were ten infants, females and males, whose parents had agreed to having recordings made at home. All of the children, who were two to three months old were fed on self-demand schedule. Recordings lasted one to three hours, beginning toward the end of a sleep phase and including activities such as feeding, diaper changing, play, or bath, till the start of the next sleep period.

The time of day was varied so that as many different activities were included as possible. The microphone, a very small Lavalier condensor-microphone, was fastened to the infants cloths or hung above it. It was connected to the recorder with thin flexible cable.

Results

So far, data evaluations of the third month of life revealed five patterns of non-crying vocalizations. They were easily differentiated because of their very varied characteristics.

The patterns identified were:

Type I (Fig. 1): A single short vocalization, characterized by a short duration of about 1/10 sec. and covering almost the whole range of frequencies up to 8000 Hz.

Type II (Fig. 1): A repetitive vocalization occurred at the high rate of about 14/sec. with an average of about 3 con-

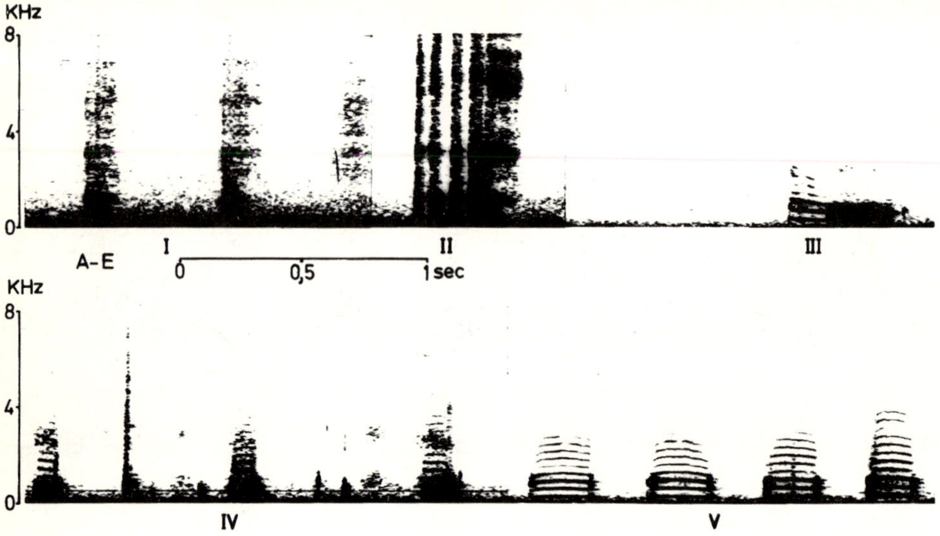

Fig. 1. Sound spectrograms of five different vocalizations of human babies in the third month of life

secutive units, which clearly distinguished it from the other vocalizations. Just as vocalization Type I, it covered the whole range of frequencies similarly to white noise.

Type III (Fig. 1): A single vocalization during sleep lasting about 3/10 sec., that is three times as long as vocalization Type I. It has two characteristeic components, a noise component in the lower range or frequencies up to 3000 Hz and harmonious component in the same range.

Type IV (Fig. 1): A harmonious sounding vocalization in close association with food consumption. The pleasant-sounding frequencies in this vocalization were in the range of up to 3000 per sec. as in the case of the sleep vocalizations. This vocalization uttered while the mother's or bottle's nipple was in the infants mouth, occurred in the same rhythm as the sucking itself (about 1.2/sec.).

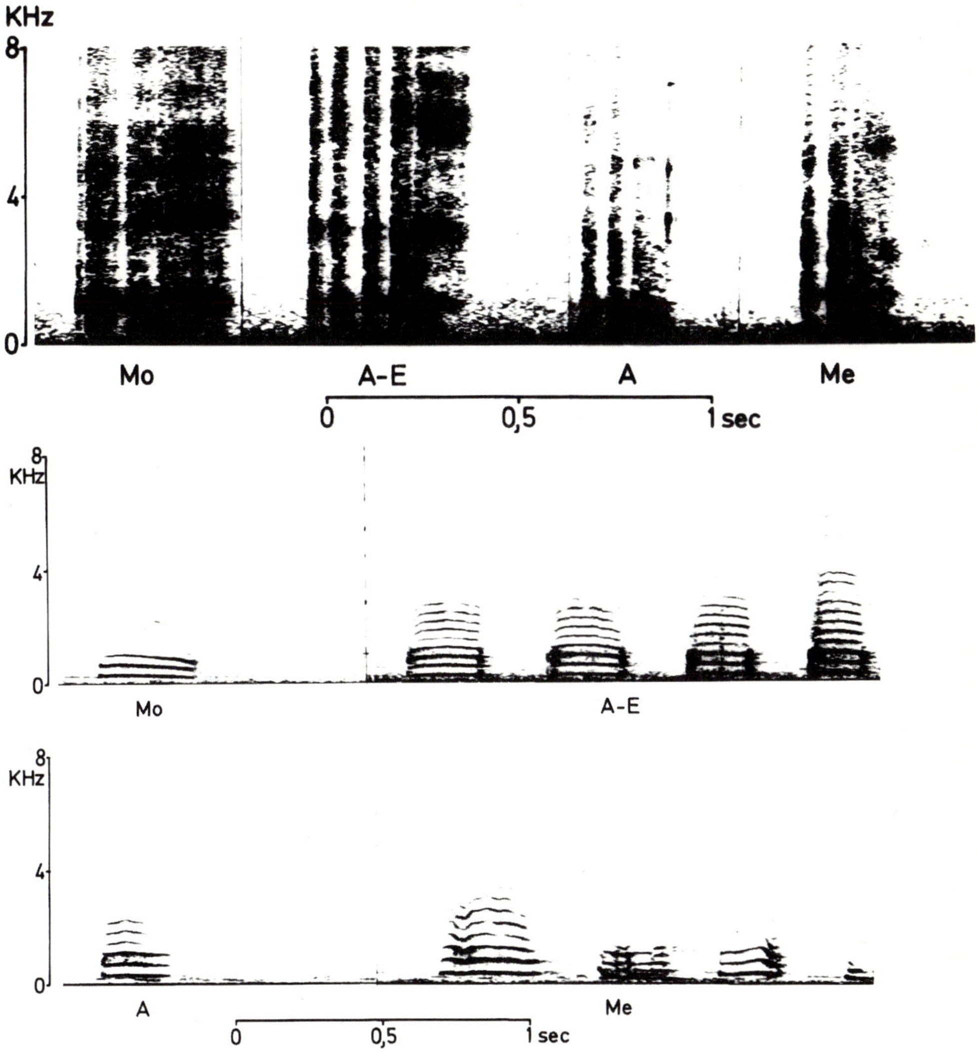

Fig. 2. Sound spectrograms of vocalization type II and V from four babies (three girls, one boy)

Type V (Fig. 1): Another harmonious-sounding vocalization remained almost constant for its duration (up to 3/10 sec.), the main frequency range being up to 5000 Hz. Sometimes this vocalization occurred several times at intervals of 1/2 sec.

All types were observed in all infants, with only minimal inter-individual variation, as to be seen in Fig. 2 with types II and V for four infants.

Discussion

The communicative function of these five vocalization types was indicated by the fact that they occurred only under specific conditions which I will describe here in more detail:
The vocalization Type I often occurred alternately with brief crying, when no one else was present, before sleeping or after awaking. From the ethological point of view this vocalization would serve the function of an attempt to make contact. The appearance of a person usually ended this vocalization. In other cases, if the baby no longer wanted situations continued, this vocalization also serves in a more general way the function to change the situation.

The repetitive vocalization, Type II, was mostly coupled with motor behavior and occurred in a variety of situations, all of which included a brief unpleasant condition (e.g. mouth was wiped, lost pacifier, hindrance of milk flow from the bottle). The communicative significance was evident here in the reaction of the mother: She changed or hurried her ongoing behavior and answered the child, saying: "Yes, I know, you don't like that."
Both types, I and II, of non-crying vocalizations often alternated with crying in the behavior chain. Also, Type II followed Type I more often in the vocalization chain, or vice versa, than did these types follow the other three vocalizations. Because of this relationship these two vocalizations do not

indicate an alarming situation as does the more intensive crying but rather they indicate displeasure to the mother in a way which is faster and more subtle. That allows the baby to follow acoustically very rapidly a change in the situation in which it is involved. The short duration of these broad band sounds, Types I and II, is produced like a burst with air pressure, thus with less energy expense than in crying. A Type III vocalization means that the infants did not remain quiet during sleep but emitted this sound at rather long intervals, of about 10 or 20 min., usually when changing positions. This vocalization could be interpreted biologically as a call to keep contact. It allows the mother to continue her activity without looking at the child, while it signifies that the child is ok, and in a sleeping stage. The other two harmonious-sounding vocalizations communicate a desire for stabilisation and continuation, that is: hold position or situation. The typical situation for Type IV shows the following traits:

a) appetence for food consumption

b) relaxed and undisturbed condition without distraction

c) easy and regular food flow

This drinking vocalization is therefore usually uttered at the beginning of a meal, after the sucking rhythm becomes more regular but no longer at the end of a meal. The drinking vocalization is not necessarily connected with swallowing. It appeared more quickly and more often with breast feeding and was often hindered by bottle feeding as a result of the unavoidable irregular drinking procedure. This vocalization type indicated to the mother that the milk was flowing at an appropriate rate, so she maintained her position with the baby. Type V appeared to indicate satisfaction occurring for example when the infant was satiated of the lap of its mother, playing with her or an object with undivided attention. Both Types, IV and V consist of frequencies in harmonic bands, which obviously indicated satisfaction of needs. With both classes of vocalizations, one indicating displeasure (Types I and II) and the other indicating situations leading to satisfaction of needs (Types IV and V) the baby can easily describe its feelings about the present situation. During an interaction chain with the mother the baby permanently comments on the behavior of the mother, thus manipulating her with its utterances, assuming that the mother is responsive to it. The rapid responsiveness of the baby, within seconds to the change in the situation is shown in Fig. 3 in varying situations.

Finally, I would like to mention that with the discovery of preverbal vocalizations in human infants, a gap is closed between varying statements of linguists on the formation of language and others of biologists on animal utterances. Liebermann (1971) (5) had already proven that the infant's capacity is limited, and that the capability to produce all vowels is not present before the sixth month. Tembrock (1967) (6) described the vocalizations of both chimpanzee and human baby as being similar, and sonographic analysis has proven that identical acoustical patterns do occur in many other primate forms (7). Such identical patterns are also found in human

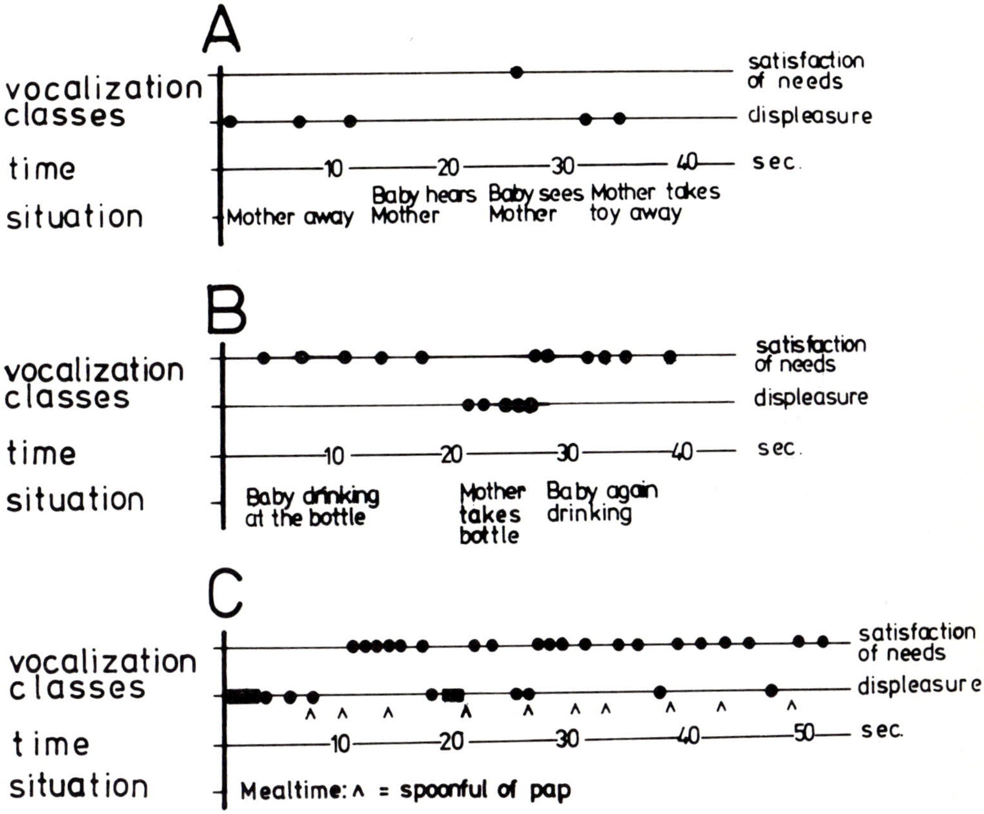

Fig. 3. Human baby, acoustically commenting the changing situation in which it is involved.
Vocalization class "satisfaction of needs" includes vocalization types IV and V. Every vocalization is marked with a •.
Vocalization class "displeasure" includes vocalization types I and II, also marked with a •, in addition crying is marked with a —•

babies albeit in an elementary form, hence increasing evidence for the presence of inborn forms of acoustical communication also in humans.

References:

1) Müller, E. et al.: Perceptral responses to infant crying: Identification of cry types. J.of Child Language 1, 89-95
2) Rieder, Oskar: Die vorsprachlichen stimmlichen Äußerungen. Dissertation Universität Heidelberg (1963).

3) Ringel, R.L.; Kluppel, D.: Neonatal crying: a normative study. Folia phoniatrica 16, 1-9 (1964).
4) Schiefelbusch: Language Perspectives. Acguisition, Retardation, and Intervention. Acta paed. (Uppsala) Supp. 1963, 93 (1965).
5) Lieberman, P. et al.: Newborn infant Cry and nonhuman primate vocalizations. J. of Speech and Hearing Res. 14, 718-727 (1971).
6) Tembrock, G.: Probleme der Phylogenie der Lautgebung der Säugetiere. Zool.Beitr.N.F. 13, 409-439 (1967).
7) Green, Steven: Variation of vocal pattern with social situation in the papanese monkey. In Rosenblum, L.A. (e.d.): Primate Behavior. Vol. 4, (1975). Academic Press, New York 1975
8) Prechtl, H.F.R. et al.: A statistical Analysis of Cry Patterns in normal and abnormal newborn infants. Devel.Med. Child Neurol. 11, 142-152 (1969).
9) Bosma, J.F. et al.: Studies of neo-natal transition: correlated sineradiographie and visual-acoustic observation. Acta paed. (Uppsala) Suppl. 1963, 93 (1965).
10) Stark, R.E. et al.: Features of infant Sounds: The first 8 weeks. J.Child Lang. 2, 205-221 (1975).
11) McNeill, David: The acquisition of language. Harper u. Row, N.Y., 183 (1976).
12) Lenneberg, E.H. et al.: The vocalization of infants born to deaf and to hearing parents. Human Development 8, 23-27 (1965).
13) Bullowa, M.: From non-verbal communication to language. Linguistics 1972, 5-14 (1976).
14) Vogel, C.: Acoustical communication among free-ranging common indian Langurs (Presbytis entellus) in Two Different Habitats of North India. American Journal of Physical Anthropology 38, No. 2 (1973).
15) Jürgens, U.; Ploog, D.: On the Evolution of voice - with special reference to Neurophysiological Aspects. Arch.Psychiat. Nervenkr. 222, 117-137 (1976).

IV) Psychoacoustic Elements in Language

What Acoustic Stimulation can teach us about Physiological Mechanisms Underlying Speech Perception

MANFRED R. SCHROEDER, Drittes Physikalisches Institut, Universität Göttingen, F. R. Germany

The human auditory periphery performs a spectral analysis, mediated by the tuning characteristics of the basilar membrane and further enhanced by other processes in the inner ear. This spectral analysis takes the form of a transformation from frequencies components in the acoustic stimulus to spatial firing patterns of neurons in the eigth nerve.

Much in human speech perception can be accounted for on the basis of this spectral analysis. Certainly vowel sounds can be classified on the basis of their "formant" frequencies in the amplitude spectra of their "waveforms" (sound pressure in front of the lips as a function of time). Other sounds are characterized by their formant transitions in time.

Monaural <u>phase</u> effects play comparatively minor roles in speech perception if we understand "phase" to mean phase in a <u>short</u>-time spectrum. (Phase alterations in <u>long</u>-time spectra can convert speech into an unintelligibel noise - albeit one with a speech-like power spectrum.) However, the quality of synthetic speech can be noticeably degraded if improper or unnatural phase angles are used in the synthesis.

By contrast, binaural phases can have pronounced perceptual effects in auditory localisation ("stereophony") and intelligibility in noisy environments ("binaural masking level differences"). Furthermore, binaural phase can be exploited to make flat-spectrum (unintelligible) speech intelligible - at least for listeners with normal hearing and speech perception. Since higher-level processes must be involved in the decoding of such "speech" signals, a new tool for the study of aphasia may result from the use of such binaural-phase signals (see below).

Among the numerous transformations, based on spectral analysis and subsequent synthesis with altered parameters, that can be realized are changes in pitch and formant frequencies without changing duration (metamorphosis of male into female speech, restoration of "helium speech") and pure changes in duration or speaking rate (without affecting spectral characteristics). While changes in speaking rate (either natural or synthetic) have been used before in the study of aphasia, modern speech processing methods allow speech rate changes by large ratios with no audible degradation (other than the speed change).

The highest quality in synthetic speech can probably be realized by the method of linear prediction analysis-synthesis (LPC), in which the speech signal is described by 12 to 24 "predictor" coefficients and the fundamental frequency ("pitch") or its absence ("hiss"). Once a speech signal has been decomposed into these parameters, synthesis at any desired speaking rate is effected by a simple recursive filter.

Diagnostic and therapeutic problems that can be studied with rate-changed speech are the following:

1. What is the intelligibility as a function of speaking rate for normal vs. abnormal subjects?
2. Can speech comprehension be improved by a training program involving speech at various rates?

An interesting application of accelerated speech occurs in the recorded book program of the American Foundation for the Blind. In 1965, the author and his collaborator R.M. Golden made the design plans of an "harmonic compressor" type speech accelerator available to the Foundation which has used accelerated speech with great success and grateful acceptance by the blind ever since.

By altering the formant bandwidths in synthetic speech, the low spectral resolutions and poor speech perception in some hearing impaired subjects can be simulated in listeners with normal hearing. Preprocessing of speech signals (involving one or both ears) to counteract poor spectral resolution is another possibility (Ainsworth, 1976).

Evidently, one of the problems of old age is poor binaural processing to reduce noise (traffic noise, cocktail party babble, etc.) and reverberation. Again studies with synthetic speech facilitate diagnosis and may hold promise for therapy ("noise stripping", "dereverberation").

One of the more astounding effects that can be elicited by sophisticated signal processing techniques is the following. Consider a speech signal $s(t)$ and samples of its short-time Fourier-transform $S(f_i,t)$ as available at the output of a filter bank. The sum of all filter outputs $S(f_i,t)$ approximates the original speech signal $s(t)$:

$$s(t) = \sum_i S(f_i,t). \tag{1}$$

Add to the output of each frequency-channel a signal with amplitude

$$\frac{S^2(f_i,t)}{\sqrt{S^2_{max}(t) - S^2(f_i,t)}}, \tag{2}$$

with a phase difference of +90° and -90° (see Fig. 1). Here

$$S_{max}(t) = \max_i S(f_i,t). \tag{3}$$

Then limit ("clip") the amplitudes of the two resulting signals $R_1(f_i,t)$ and $R_2(f_i,t)$ to a constant (over frequency) magnitude, namely $S_{max}(t)/2$, to obtain a new set of signals $r_1(f_i,t)$ and $r_2(f_i,t)$. Finally, sum these two sets of signals over all frequencies to obtain the following two "flat-spectrum" signals

$$r_1(t) = \sum_i r_1(f_i,t),$$

and (4)

$$r_2(t) = \sum_i r_2(f_i,t).$$

Each of these signals, if listened to by itself, is an unintelligible buzz of hiss. However, if $r_1(t)$ and $r_2(t)$ are listened to <u>binaurally</u> (over stereophonic headphones), a speech-like signal is perceived inside the head.

A possible explanation for this phenomena is the fact that - under certain conditions of binaural listening - human auditory processing produces a <u>difference</u> between the two binaurally applied signals. And $r_1(t)$ and $r_2(t)$ have been so processed electronically that their difference equals the original speech signal s(t):

$$r_1(t) - r_2(t) = s(t). \tag{5}$$

This can readily be inferred from Fig. 1 by noting that, by construction,

$$\tan \phi_i(t) = \frac{S(f_i,t)}{\sqrt{S^2_{max}(t) - S^2(f_i,t)^2}} \tag{6}$$

and $r_1(f_i,t) - r_2(f_i,t)$, the signal indicated by a double line, equals

$$\frac{1}{2} S_{max}(t) \cdot \sin \phi_i = S(f_i,t). \tag{7}$$

Thus, the final result, Eq. 5, follows immediately.

Needless to say, speech perception under these circumstances presupposes the functioning of certain auditory processes that may be impaired in abnormal listeners. Hence the diagnostic potential of this proposal.

Another potent tool for probing higher nervous centers by signals that elicite speech-like perceptions is the following: Consider the short-time spectrum of an utterance

$$S(f_i,t), \tag{8}$$

and its complement at a selected speech t_o during the utterance

$$C(f_i,t_o) = S_{max} - S(f_i,t_o), \tag{9}$$

where

$$S_{max} = \max_{i,t} S(f_i,t) \tag{10}$$

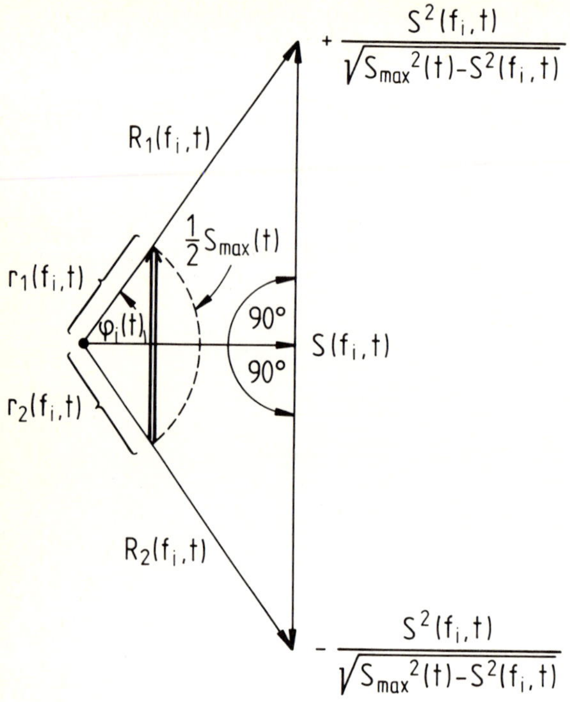

Fig. 1. Construction of pair of binaural signals with flat spectrum (see text)

is the highest spectral power over frequency <u>and</u> time. Thus, the "complement spectrum" $C(f_i,t_o)$ is never negative.

Now present the complement spectrum $C(f_i,t_o)$ (a steady buzz or hiss) to a listener and, after several seconds, add to it the time-varying spectrum $S(f_1,t)$ of the utterance. By construction, at time $t = t_o$ the total spectrum presented to the listener is <u>flat</u>:

$$C(f_i,t_o) + S(f_i,t_o) = S_{max}. \quad (11)$$

Yet, it is precisely at this moment that the listener perceives something aking to the utterance near the preselected time t_o. An astounding effect that is not satisfactorily accounted for by reference to "adaptation"! Here we have another stimulus potentially useful in exploring higher brain functions.

In conclusion, although much has been learned about speech perception, it is apparent that modern signal processing methods hold great promise for generating acoustic stimuli that can probe the human mind in interesting and perhaps yet unforseen ways.

Selected References:

1) M.R. Schroeder: Vocoders: Analysis and Synthesis of Speech-A review of 30 years of applied speech research. Proc. IEEE 54, 720-734 (1966).

2) J.L. Flanagan: Speech Analysis Synthesis and Perception, 2nd ed. Springer, Berlin (1972).

3) J.L. Flanagan, L.R. Rabiner: Speech Synthesis. Dowden, Hutchington & Ross, Stroudsburg (1973).

4) B.S. Atal, M.R. Schroeder: Adaptive Predictive Coding of Speech signals. Bell Syst. Techn. Journal 49, 1973 (1970).

5) J.D. Markel, A.H. Gray,jr.: Linear prediction of Speech. Springer, Berlin (1976).

6) W.A. Ainsworth: Mechanisms of Speech Recognition. Pergamon Press, Oxford (1976).

7) M.R. Schroeder: Models of Hearing. IEEE Proc. 63, 9 (1975).

An Outline of Pitch Analysis in Speech: A Hearing Theory Approach

H. DUIFHUIS, L. F. WILLEMS, Institute for Perception Research, Eindhoven, The Netherlands
R. J. SLUYTER, Philips' Research Laboratories, Eindhoven, The Netherlands

In recent years there has been significant progress in the development of the theory of auditory pitch perception. Many perceptual phenomena are now unified in the framework of a theory which predicts pitch(es) of complex sounds. Basically, all recent theories assume a peripheral auditory frequency analysis, with a limited frequency resolution, followed by some harmonic pattern recogniser (1,2,4,7). Of the theories proposed, Goldstein's (2) is the most quantitative. Therefore it is most suited for an implementation into a pitch-measuring device for speech signals. It can be put into the form of an algorithm which will produce pitch values which have subjective, i.e. psychoacoustical value. We claim that the performance of an algorithm that models human performance is the best that can be achieved, as well as all that is needed in a technical pitch meter. Recently Terhardt (5) has formulated his theory in a more specific way. It now contains some elements that are virtually identical to parts of our procedure.

At this moment the algorithm described has been implemented in software on a non-real-time basis. A real-time hardware implementation, however, is feasible.

General outline of the procedure: In line with the above suggestion the pitch meter consists of the two independent major elements, viz. a spectral analyser and a harmonic pattern recogniser. The analyser detects harmonic components and measures their frequencies. The pattern recogniser produces the optimum fit between the component frequencies and a purely harmonic sequence. Properties of analyser and recogniser are chosen to match what is known of the human observer of pitch. Some compromises are called for, however, by the signal-processing techniques which we used.

Although, on the one hand, it is plausible that the human makes use of expectations of the pitch to be perceived, and although in pitch-measuring algorithms it is common practice to smooth the predicted pitch values accordingly, we have chosen not to include such elements in our procedure at this stage. This avoids the problem of tracking a wrong track, and moreover, our algorithm appears to perform quite well without this feature.

Description of spectral analyser and peak-picker: Analyser and peak-picker will have to model auditory frequency resolution and frequency representation, respectively. Resolution is characterized by the so-called critical band (CB) and should be about 1/2CB. The accuracy of the internal representation of the component frequencies is narrower by about one order of magnitude.

For practical reasons we have used an FFT frequency analysis, which has a constant resolution over the entire frequency range. Therefore a worst-case approach was followed to specify the

FFT-parameters, resulting in an analysis range from 0 to 2.5 kHz and the use of a 256 points FFT. This fixed the resolution Δf at 19.5 Hz and the time window T at 51.2 ms. T was filled with 40 ms of signal, shaped with a Hamming window and supplemented with zeros. So far we used a 12-bit A/D conversion and a floating-point FFT with a mantissa of 23 bits. This proved to be sufficient to cope with regular amplitude variations. The higher accuracy of the internal representation of component frequencies is modelled by the peak-picker which determines the precise location of peaks in the spectrum by parabolic interpolation. In order to qualify as a regular peak, the peak shape as well as the peak level have to meet certain threshold criteria. Once qualified, only the peak frequency information is retained as X_i (for peak number i), and the amplitude information is discarded. The peak-picker starts looking for peaks at the 1f end of the spectrum, and never looks for more than 6 peaks. The nonlinear operation, which the peak-picker performs on the spectrum, is essential. It reduces ambiguities in the final results.

Description of the harmonic pattern recogniser:
A fundamental difference between the problems of finding pitch in speech and finding pitch in a psychoacoustically defined stimulus is that the speech spectrum may contain spurious components which bear no relation to the harmonic signal. Thus, the problem is to find the harmonic pattern which best fits the set of peak frequencies $\{X_i\}$, all (N) components not necessarily being classified. This requires a significant modification of Goldstein's theory, which classifies all components.

Goldstein (2) has shown that the problem of finding the optimum fundamental frequency f_o can be split into two successive steps. The first labels the frequencies X_i with optimum harmonic numbers $\hat{n}_i$, the second determines the maximum likelihood estimate of f_o based on all the classified X_i and the corresponding $\hat{n}_i$. We estimate the harmonic numbers by a new method which we refer to as the *harmonics-sieve* procedure. Then f_o is estimated using the maximum likelihood estimate proposed by Goldstein (2). Below we describe the harmonics-sieve procedure in some detail. In some aspects it turned out to be equivalent to the procedure recently published by Terhardt (5), which looks for near-coincidences of subharmonics of stimulus frequencies.

The harmonics-sieve is a one-dimensional sieve in the frequency domain. The sieve has meshes of a bandwidth $W=W(f)=2\alpha j f_o$ around the harmonic frequencies $f_j=jf_o$, with j=1 . . 11. The sieve procedure amounts to successively setting the sieve to all possible values of f_o, covering the entire range encountered in human speech (50 - 500 Hz). Of course the frequency domain is scanned in discrete steps (index ℓ, ℓ=1 to L), the size of each being taken proportional to f. Obviously the step size should be smaller then W(f) in order not to miss parts of the frequency scale. Minimizing the total number of steps, L, is equivalent to maximizing W(f) or α. In our system we used α=5%, and a step size of 1/24 octave, or approx. 3%.

At each position of the sieve, characterized by the fundamental frequency value of $f_{o\ell}$, a check is made as to which components pass the sieve, thus registering as candidate harmonics. A component X_i passing through mesh j is labelled with the candidate harmonic number $m_{k\ell}=j$. Let the total number of components passing the sieve at position be K_ℓ (k_ℓ runs from 1 to K_ℓ). If more than one component passes through the same mesh, then only the one closest to the centre is labelled, the others are rejected.

The optimum set of harmonic numbers $\{\hat{n}_k\}$ is found from the candidate sets $\{m_k\}_\ell$ with the use of a minimum-distance classifier. It is rather straigthforward to show that minimizing the distance between $\{m_k\}_\ell$ and the ideal harmonic pattern is equivalent to maximizing the quantitiy C_ℓ defined as $C_\ell=K_\ell/(M_\ell + N)$, where N is the number of spectral peaks to be recognised and M_ℓ the highest candidate harmonic number ($=m_{K\ell}$). The harmonics-sieve procedure in combination with the minimum-distance classifier is much more efficient than the straightforward optimum estimation procedure of calculating the least-square error fit from all possible permutations of harmonic numbers.

Performance: We have been able to compare the performance of our pitch meter (in software) directly with a pitch extractor working with an advanced autocorrelation method (6). The latter supposedly ranks amongst the best discussed by Rabiner et al. (3). Performance of the new pitch meter proved superior. Figure 1 gives an example of the raw results for a female Dutch voice.

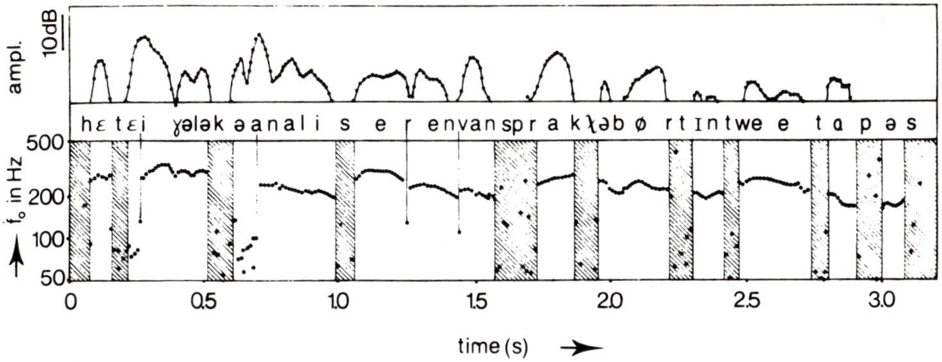

Fig. 1. Unsmoothed f_o measurements in an utterance (in Dutch) by a female speaker. The hatched areas are unvoiced, as judged from amplitude and from respective phonemes. The amplitude contour and phonemic transcription of the utterance are lined up with the f_o-contour

References:

1) de Boer, E.: Pitch theories unified. In: Psychophysics and Physiology in Hearing, E.F. Evans and J.P. Wilson (eds.) Academic, London, 323-334 (1977).

2) Goldstein, J.L.: An optimum theory for the central formation of the pitch of complex tones. J.Acoust.Soc.Am. 54, 1496-1516 (1973).

3) Rabiner, L.R.; Cheng, M.J.; Rosenberg, A.E.; McGonegal, C.A.: A comparative performance study of several pitch detection algorithms. IEEE-ASSP 24, 399-418 (1976).

4) Terhardt, E.: Zur Tonhöhenwahrnehmung von Klängen. Acustica 26, 173-186, 187-199 (1972).

5) Terhardt, E.: Calculating virtual pitch. Hearing Research 1, 155-182 (1979).

6) Vogten, L.L.M.; Willems, L.F.: The formator: a speech analysis synthesis system based on formant extraction from linear prediction coefficients. I.P.O. - Annual Progress Report 12, 47-54 (1977).

7) Wightman, F.L.: The pattern transformation model of pitch. J.Acoust.Soc.Am. 54, 407-416 (1973).

Pitch Determination of Speech Signals – A Survey

WOLFGANG J. HESS, Lehrstuhl für Datenverarbeitung, Technische Universität München, W. Germany

In this short survey, the numerous pitch determination algorithms (PDAs), devices, and methods are grouped into the major classes: time domain PDAs and short-term analysis PDAs. The short-term PDAs leave the time domain by some short-term transform specific to the individual method applied. They provide a sequence of average estimates of fundamental frequency F0 or fundamental period T0 emerging from the short-term intervals (frames). Opposed to this, the time-domain PDAs extract the information of periodicity from the signal directly or after filtering; these PDAs are usually able to track individual fundamental periods.

Fig. 1 presents an overview of the prevailing short-term analysis PDAs. These PDAs are further grouped according to the individual short-term transformation applied. The sequence of operations is quite similar for all these PDAs. After an optional preprocessing step (which can be a moderate low-pass filter or an adaptive center clipper), the signal is subdivided into short segments (frames) whose typical duration ranges between 30 and 50 ms. This value is chosen because most of the short-term transforms (with the only exception of the AMDF, see below) require several pitch periods within a single frame.

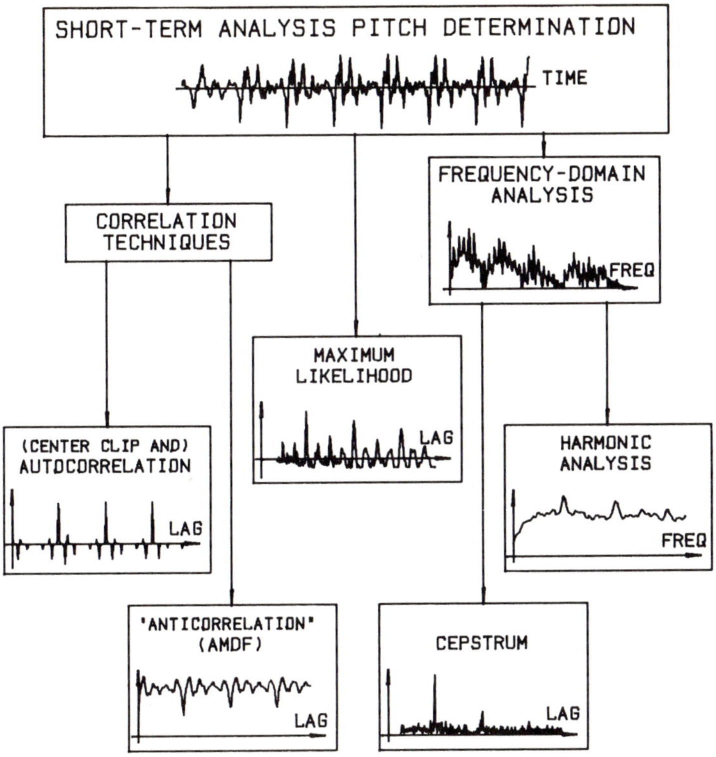

Fig. 1

After the formation of the frames, the short-term transform is performed on every frame individually. This transform is intended to perform in a way that it concentrates all the available information on periodicity into a single principal peak which is then detected by a peak detector and labeled as the pitch estimate for that frame.

For each transform, the figure shows a typical example (computed from the 50 ms frame displayed in the upper part) of the short-term function from which the estimate of pitch is derived. Not all the known short-term transformations, however, behave in the desired way. Among those which do, we find the well-known short-term autocorrelation technique (Rabiner, 1977) whose performance is greatly improved when the signal is preprocessed by center clipping. Its counterpart, the average magnitude difference function AMDF (Ross et al., 1974) is defined by

$$\text{AMDF}(k) = \Sigma |a(n) - a(n+k)|$$

where a(i) represents the signal. The summation is performed over the whole frame which, in this case, is permitted to be quite short. The AMDF reveals a strong minimum at a lag equalling the period T0. The well known cepstrum analysis (Noll, 1967) as well as harmonic analysis (Schroeder, 1968; Terhardt, 1979) are frequency-domain methods. Both are derived from the logarithmic power Fourier spectrum. The cepstrum PDA transforms this spectrum back into time domain, thus generating a large peak at T0. One of the several methods of harmonic analysis is spectral compression. The log power spectrum is compressed along the frequency axis by integer factors k = 2, 3, 4 etc. Adding all these compressed spectra causes the harmonics to contribute coherently to the distinct peak at F0. The maximum likelihood PDA (Friedman, 1977), finally, represents the mathematical procedure of detecting a periodic signal with unknown period T0 in a noisy environment.

Short-term analysis PDAs are unable to track individual periods since the phase relation between the signal and the short-term function is lost during the transform. This loss, however, makes these PDAs insensitive to phase distortions of the signal. Moreover, since they focus the whole information of periodicity into one single peak, they tend to be resistive against noise and signal degradation. The disadvantage of large computing

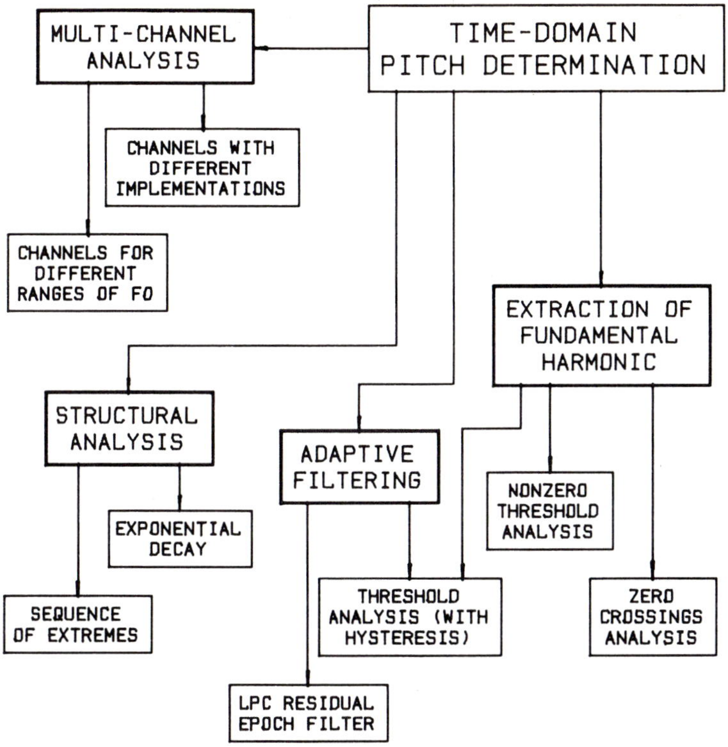

Fig. 2. Principles of time-domain pitch extractors

effort more and more loses its importance because of the current progress in fast digital circuitry.

For the time-domain methods, the grouping provided in fig. 2 is somewhat more arbitrary. Leaving aside the multi-channel PDAs and the special purpose PDAs applying adaptive filtering (e.g. De Mori, 1977), we find most time-domain PDAs somewhat between two extremes: analysis of the temporal signal structure on the one hand and extraction of the fundamental harmonic on the other. In the typical single-channel PDA, we find a (linear or nonlinear) filter as the first step of signal processing. The effect necessary for this filter ranges from zero for structural analysis to extreme low-pass filtering for the PDAs which extract the fundamental waveform from the signal. Contrary to this, the subsequent period detection algorithm range from a simple zero crossings analyzer for fundamental waveform extraction to the highly complicated procedures for structural analysis. Further details on these analyzers are shown in figs. 3 and 4.

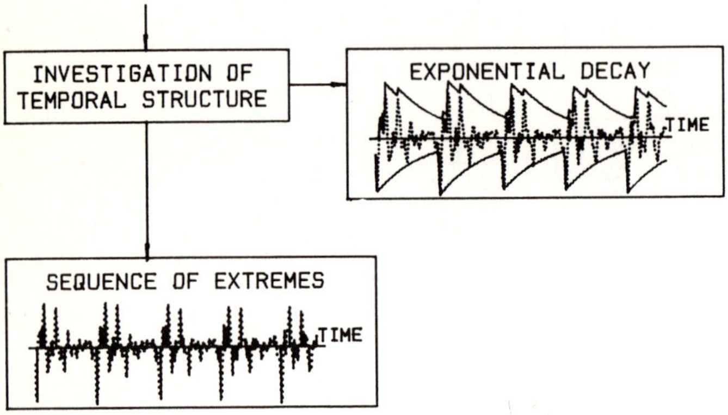

Fig. 3. Time-domain PDAs: Investigation of temporal signal structure. The signals are taken from the example of fig. 1

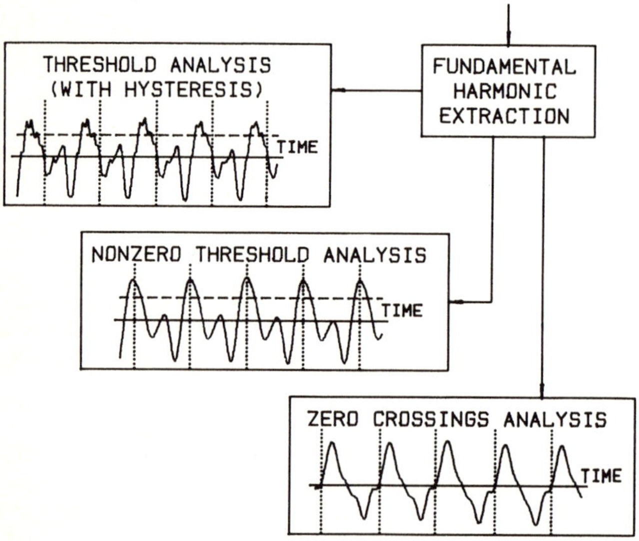

Fig. 4. Time-domain PDAs: Enhancement and extraction of fundamental harmonic. The signals are taken from the example of fig. 1

The structural analyzers use the fact that the speech signal consists of several exponentially damped oscillations (fig. 3). The signal may thus be modelled either as a sequence of extremes, such as maxima, minima, or zero crossings (Tucker and Bates, 1978), or by its envelope in form of a decaying exponential (Filip, 1969). Just this last concept leads to a very simple analog circuit consisting of a diode, a capacitor, and two resistors. The disadvantage of this concept, however, is that it cannot cover the whole range of F0 possible for a multitude of speakers (at least 70 to 500 Hz) without producing significant errors.

At the other end of the scale, we find the PDAs which extract the fundamental waveform (fig. 4). Among these PDAs there are the oldest realizations, and a detailed survey of much of this work is presented by McKinney (1965). The amount of low-pass filtering necessary to realize this concept depends on the subsequent periodicity extractor: the simple zero crossings analysis extractor needs the greatest degree of low-pass filtering, whereas the nonzero threshold analysis extractor, somewhat more complicated due to the need of level normalization or threshold adaptation, can tolerate the presence of higher harmonics to a certain extent. A further step towards tolerating the presence of higher harmonics is made when a hysteresis is incorporated into the threshold analyzer. A single-channel PDA based on this concept, however, cannot cope with all types of signal and all ranges of F0. For instance, the concept of fundamental harmonic extraction requires the first harmonic to be present in the signal. If this does not apply, the first harmonic can be reconstructed by nonlinear distortion of the signal. In doing so, on the other hand, one risks to attenuate this very harmonic when it is strong in the original signal. The only way out, if one intends to process arbitrary signals by the relatively simple time-domain concept, is the implementation of a PDA which contains several channels, and which is provided with the facility to automatically switch between them. These channels may process subranges of F0 with identical implementation (McKinney, 1965), or they may represent different implementations, such as different ways of nonlinear distortion covering the whole range of F0 in each channel (Hess, 1979). These concepts, compared to the corresponding single-channel PDAs, give a considerable improvement in performance.

In spite of the many proposals and different principles, the problem of pitch determination in speech communication is still unsolved (Rabiner et al., 1976). Further research has to be done towards answering the question what kind of errors are most annoying from the perceptual point of view, and by what means a PDA can be optimized in order to produce a minimum number of these errors.

References:

1) De Mori, R.; Laface, P.; Makhonine, V.A.; Mezzalama, M.: A syntactic procedure for the recognition of glottal pulses in continuous speech. Pattern Recognition 9, 181-189 (1977).

2) Filip, M.: Envelope periodicity detection. JASA 45, 719-732 (1969).

3) Friedman, D.H.: Pseudo-maximum-likelihood pitch extraction. IEEE-T-ASSP 25, 213-221 (1977).

4) Hess, W.J.: Time-domain pitch period extraction of speech signals using three nonlinear digital filters. Proc. ICASSP 79, 773-776 (1979).

5) McKinney, N.P.: Laryngeal frequency analysis for linguistic research. Ann Arbor MI: Communic.Sciences Lab., Univ. of Michigan; Res.Rept. 14, 340 (1965).
6) Noll, A.M.: Cepstrum Pitch Determination. JASA 41, 293-309 (1967).
7) Rabiner, L.R.: On the use of autocorrelation analysis for pitch detection. IEEE-T-ASSP 25, 24-33 (1977).
8) Rabiner, L.R.; Cheng, M.J.; Rosenberg, A.E.; McGonegal, A.: A comparative study of several pitch detection algorithms. IEEE-T-ASSP 24, 399-413 (1976).
9) Ross, M.J.; Shaffer, H.L.; Cohen, A.; Freudberg, R.; Manley, H.J.: Average magnitude difference function pitch extractor. IEEE-T-ASSP 22, 353-361 (1974).
10) Schroeder, M.R.: Period histogram and product spectrum: New methods for fundamental-frequency measurement. JASA 43, 829-834 (1968).
11) Terhardt, E.: Calculating virtual pitch. Hearing Res. 1 (1979).
12) Tucker, W.H., Bates, R.T.H.: A pitch estimation algorithm for speech and music. IEEE-T-ASSP 26, 597-604 (1978).

Virtual Pitch and Our Own Voice

J. DROOGLEEVER FORTUYN and R. J. RITSMA, University of Groningen, The Netherlands

In the following pages we wish to discuss the possibility of a causal relationship between the phenomenon of virtual pitch and the process of hearing one's own voice.

In hearing one's own voice one perceives a sound of definite pitch, although in the spectrum of wave-forms emitted by the source and carried through the air to one's ear, the wave-form of the frequency corresponding to that pitch is not present.

The qualification "virtual" with respect to pitch was introduced by Terhardt: it suggests an analogy with the well-known fact that we locate an object in a plane behind a mirror although that object is not physically present at that place. In that sense Terhardt proposes a distinction between spectral pitch (as a physical entity) and virtual pitch (as a psychological entity). The main characteristics of the phenomenon will be described shortly, but first of all in order to facilitate the understanding of the kind of relationship we have in mind we will discuss certain physiological and physical aspects of vocalization.

<u>Vocalization</u>: The instrument which enables us to utter sounds, as in speaking and singing, consists of the vocal cords in the

larynx and the cavities of throat, mouth and nose. During vocalization the cords are moved towards each other and stretched by muscular contraction of variable force.
The pressure of the air which pushes the vocal cords upward and outward determines the loudness of the voice. The tension of the cords determines the frequency of the vibration and thereby the pitch of the sound.

The air above the vocal cords is in strong motion. Vortices and pressure-waves are being transmitted to the walls of the cavities which act as resonators. Resonating media do not add energy to the energy of the source of the sound. Rather the energy produced by vocalization is distributed over the source and the cavities. The end-product which passes the lips is a complex sound i.e. a complex of different wave-forms of various frequencies and amplitudes. In a complex wave we distinguish waves of a fundamental frequency and harmonics (overtones). Differences between vowels are produced by varying the shape of the resonators and the tension of its walls, whereby the distribution of energy over the components of the complex sound is varied. We are able to produce different vowels at the same pitch.

It has long been held that in complex sounds the energy of the fundamental frequency - the determinant of the pitch of that sound - is greater than the energy of the harmonics. However, due to the properties of the resonator and the redistribution of energy the fundamental may be completely absent from the sound that is emitted by the speaker and yet in perception the fundamental is stronger than the overtones. This is known as "virtual pitch" (Terhardt, 1972, 1974), or "the missing fundamental" (Licklider, 1956). During perception of speech and song this situation is the rule.

Absence of the fundamental in the cochlea. Although the missing fundamental is not present at the level of the eardrum the wave form corresponding to the fundamental could originate within the cochlea itself. The interference between frequencies of various harmonics can give rise to difference tones (f2 - f1) or combination tones (2f2 - f1, etc.).

However, considering:

1. the low intensity of combination tones (Schouten, 1938)
2. the absence of beats when a tone is presented of a frequency near the missing fundamental (Schouten, 1938 and 1962)
3. the impossibility to block the fundamental at the level of the basilar membrane (Licklider, 1956) favours the conclusion that the fundamental is represented neither at the level of the eardrum nor in the cochlea.

Houtsma and Goldstein (1972) discovered that the pitch of complex tones can be heard equally well when two-tone sounds are presented either monotically (both constituent tones to one ear) or dichotically (one single tone in each ear). Together with the negative evidence of a peripheral input, this can be considered convincing proof of the central origin of the missing fundamental.

Although there is little doubt concerning the central origin of virtual pitch the mechanisms at work are by no means defined. Parts of the puzzle can be put together. The existence region of virtual pitch coincides with the frequency range of the human voice. This suggests a relationship with human speech. Terhardt proposes a learning process in early life derived from listening to the human voice. One could think of a kind of precursor to learning the mother tongue. However, as we saw in the first part of this paper, the sound leaving the mouth of the speaker and transferred to the eardrum of the listener consists of a complex sound, in which the fundamental frequency is relatively weak compared to the harmonics or absent. The fact that the harmonics must have tone quality in order to contribute to virtual pitch leaves the problem only half-solved. In principle, the listener should hear the individual harmonics. There is no cogent reason to refer these harmonics to one fundamental tone. We now propose a different solution which is, in a sense an extension of Terhardt's theory. The mechanism which lies at the root of the phenomenon of virtual pitch could be the process of listening not to voices of other people, but instead to the perception of the sounds of one's own voice. The sound of our own voice differs from the sounds of other people's voices in three aspects:

a) It reaches the ear both by bone conduction and by air conduction whereas other people's voices are exclusively air conducted.

b) The spectrum of the bone conducted component of our voice is characterised by preponderance of the fundamental frequency, because at the level of the larynx the fundamental is well represented as shown experimentally by Van den Berg (1965), whereas in the air conducted speech sounds the fundamental is relatively weak.

c) The relations of space and time from the source to the cochlea are constant.

We know from experience with band-recorded voices that our own voice sounds distorted, unnatural, tinny. Shortcomings of the recording apparatus could explain distortion. However, our fellow men do not share our surprise. To them our voice sounds natural. Also, other people's recorded voices sound to us acceptably natural. The inference is, that we hear the sound of our own voice differently from that of other people. The distorsion could appear not only because one's voice is bone conducted but also, because the frequency spectrum of the bone conducted component differs from the spectrum at the level of the mouth.

In order to investigate this problem, the following experiment was set up. We produce a spoken sound, record it on a tape and play it back. The recorded sound differs from the sound we uttered. The recorded sound is filtered so that six octave bands can be varied in strength. By changing the amplitudes, the timbre of the voice is being modified and presented to us through earphones. We now alternatively utter the original sound and listen to the modified and recorded version. By manipulating the relative strength of the octave bands the sound of the recorded voice can be transformed so that it becomes very similar to our own voice.

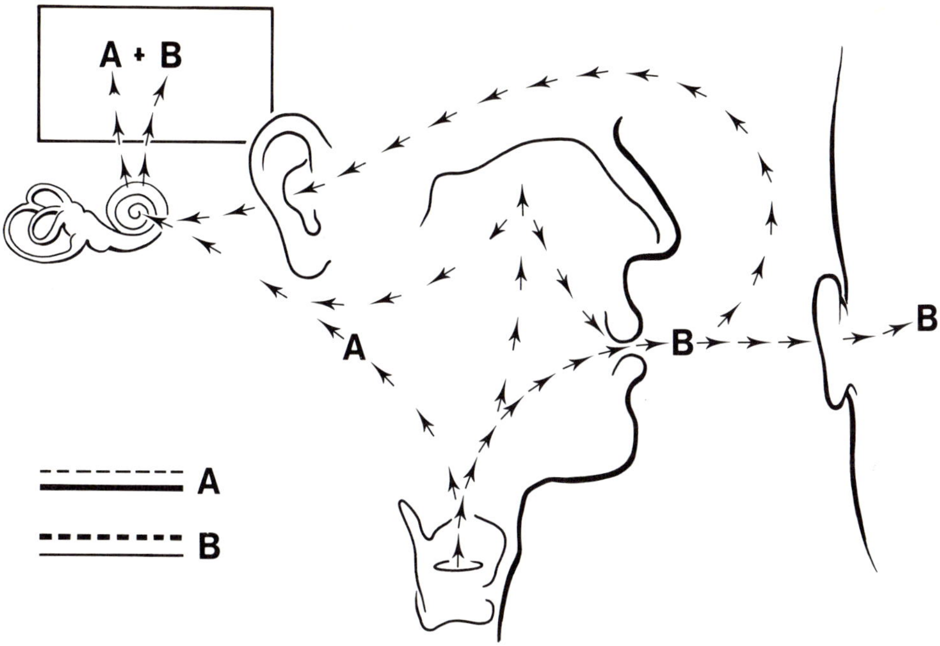

Fig. 1. Spectral composition A differs from B: Fundamental in A well represented, in B reduced. Harmonics in A reduced, in B well represented. Note that the spectrum reaching the eardrum differs from the combination as presented to the nervous system

The transformation consists of a reduction of the higher harmonics, while leaving the fundamental and the first harmonic at the original value. Thus it can be shown that the spectrum of our own voice is characterized by a relative enhancement of the fundamental and first harmonic. This finding should not be too suprising since the situation is comparable to the production of sound in musical string instruments like a piano or a violin. In the spectrum of the vibrating string the fundamental is a major component (Roederer, 1975). The sound of our own voice then, is composed of two fractions, one bone-conducted, one air-borne. In the bone-conducted fraction the lower

frequencies, including the fundamental are more strongly represented than the high frequencies. This bias has two roots:
a) one is due to the conductive properties of bone which favours the lower frequencies.
b) the other is a difference of frequency spectrum between the two sources of the sound, i.e. the larynx and the resonating cavities. The bone-conducted fraction carries the combined frequency spectrum of larynx and resonator. The air conducted fraction carries predominantly the resonating frequencies.

The subjective timbre of our own voice is the result of these differentiating factors. Consequently, the timbre of our own voice differs from the frequency spectrum presented to the eardrum.
According to the theory that we propose a possible link is envisaged between the perceptual experience of our own voice, the phenomenon of virtual pitch and the evaluation of pitch in general. Before presenting arguments in favour of this assumption we wish to draw attention to a few points related to phonation, i.e. the production of sounds.
1. The limits set to the human voice are caused by limitation of <u>production</u> of sound and not by restrictions of the sensory apparatus: the auditory spectrum exceeds the motor capacities at both ends of the spectrum.

2. The production of language implies the mastering of intonation and accentuation. The motor act of phonation is controlled by the sound produced and heard by the speaker: it is part of a motor sensory feed-back loop. As in all voluntary acts the force of contraction of laryngeal and intercostal muscles is

set by innervation of the alpha and of the gammasystem: we produce a force of contraction corresponding to the expected sound effect (Sears, 1977).

Taken together these points characterize phonation as a motor-sensory activity and as a product of learning and practise (Wijke, 1974a,b).

Assuming that the experience of music is related to the production of musical sounds, the evaluation of pitch may be connected to the production of steady sounds. Pitch both produced and perceived is primarily the outcome of centrally controlled processes. The role of the cochlea may be limited to that of a sensor. As is well-known the scale of just noticeable differences of pitch is more precise than the scale of differences of pitch. The cochlea, as a feeler, is better equipped to indicate changes of pitch than absolute values.

We suggest that the sensomotor central apparatus controlling phonation and developed in the course of early life, is the instrument through which the pitch of sounds reaching the eardrum is evaluated, under the condition that the auditory frequencies of that sound lie within the boundaries of our own voice.

Several characteristic features of the phenomenon of virtual pitch are in agreement with this assumption.

a. The existence region of virtual pitch is restricted to the frequency range of the human voice (Ritsma, 1962 and 1967). By "human voice" we understand phonation perceived by the individual.

b. Virtual pitch implies reference of a variety of harmonics to a unique fundamental although the distribution of energy does not necessitate such a reference. During phonation we produce only one tone at a time and thereby the fundamental is privileged.

c. In virtual pitch the tone perceived differs from the auditory frequencies reaching the eardrum. There is a bias towards the fundamental. This situation is identical with the perception of our own voice.

d. Only the harmonics with tonal qualities as produced by phonation contribute to virtual pitch.

e. In the process of evaluation of pitch the sensomotor mechanism operative in phonation functions as calibrator.

This term is used to define a component essential to perceptual judgments although it is not overtly presented in perception. This state of affairs is not exceptional in sensory perception of other modalities, for example in vision. Correctly localising an object in space implies normal motor control of the eyes, although we are not necessarily aware of the position of the eyes. Thus motor control is an essential element of the ultimate perceptual judgment. By the same token components which are not as such present in direct experience might well contribute to the outcome of evaluation of pitch.

I mention two components of this kind:

1. The first is phonation itself, which is neither a purely motor nor a purely sensory event. Phonation is the outcome of a control mechanism, in which, as in all feed-back loops we find a blending of outgoing and incoming impulses. We listen to our voice through this mechanism. What we hear is the result of a complicated network of activities and additional

transformations. We know that the pitch perceived is not equivalent to the physical properties of the sound-waves impinging on the eardrum.

2. The second factor is as powerful as it is unnoticed. Indeed, it is powerful because it is unnoticed.

Its importance can be gathered from a difficulty inherent in the theory as proposed so far. By a complex process we transform the effect of one physical spectrum into the effect of a different one, i.e. a fundamental frequency, not present in the peripheral sense organ is present in perception. The acceptance of this theory creates a new problem. Why do we hear our own voice distorted when played back to us? The reason might be the following: since early life we treated our own voice and other people's voice indiscriminately: we put them all in the same class, although the frequency spectrum is not the same. This lack of distinction is carried over into adult life by a process of learning or habituation. Shortcomings of spectral differentiation are by no means exceptional in auditory perception: we might easily fail to identify the pitch of two voices one octave apart. Our own voice, however, is presented to us in two different ways, one in its original state, the other in recorded, i.e. reduced form. We suggest that our own voice, played back to us, sounds unusual, unnatural not only because the physical characteristics are different but also because we are now in the position to compare two different presentations of the same voice, in a unique experimental situation, since we are unable to appreciate the experience of others listening to their own voice. This line of reasoning brings us back to there where we made the remark that the peripheral sense organ is exquisitely fitted to record differences, but not to evaluate pitch.

The theory presented in this paper differs in certain respects from contemporary theories, as proposed by Terhadt and Goldstein.

Our theory follows Terhardt's suggestions: It is, in a way an extension of the presumable link between virtual pitch and the perceptual experience of human language. Restriction of this experience to the own voice makes the theory more precise and more cogent.

Our differences with Goldstein are of a general kind. They consider the relationship between pitch as a physical entity and as a psychological entity. As is often the case, the terminology used betrays certain theoretical assumptions. Goldstein (1973) discusses the perceptual mechanism in terms of a pitch-processor, whereas Schouten et al. (1962) speak of a pitch-extractor. The former formulation allows a theoretical construction whereby a physical entity is presented to a sense-organ, at which stage it is transformed into a code, transported through the brain and finally decoded. The organism is thought to be more or less transparent to a pre-existing entity: it perceives a tone because this tone was present in the outside world. Pitch extraction requires more activity from the side of the organism.

Perhaps it would be more correct to say that pitch is not processed nor extracted but evoked. In the case of virtual pitch the perception is present whereas the corresponding wave-form in the outside world is completely lacking.

If the mechanism of virtual pitch is similar to perception of pitch in general, then pitch is evoked under all circumstances.

The role of the cochlea in this process is complex and in some cases ambiguous (Schouten et al., 1962). Goldstein's assumption of analysis by the cochlea of complex tones into pure tones may not be a necessary condition of perception of pitch. The role of the cochlea may be that of a feeler indicating changes and differences rather than absolute values. As in other modalities the sense-organs might help to update our perceptual world rather than be the exclusive source of "sense-data".

References:

1) Van den Berg, J.W.: Physica van de stemvorming met toepassing. Thesis. Uitgeverij Excelsior, 's-Gravenhage, The Netherlands (1956).
2) Goldstein, J.L.: An optimum processor theory for the central formation pitch of complex tones. J.A.S.A. 54, 1496-1516 (1973).
3) Houtsma, A.J.M. and Goldstein, J.L.: The central origin of the pitch of complex tones: evidence from musical interval recognition. J.A.S.A. 51, 520-529 (1972).
4) Licklider, J.C.R.: Auditory frequency analysis. In: Information Theory C. Cherry (ed.), Academic Press, New York (1956).
5) Ritsma, R.J.: Existence region of tonal Residue. J.A.S.A. 34, 1224-1229 (1962).
6) Ritsma, R.J.: Frequencies dominant in the perception of the pitch of complex sounds. J.A.S. 42, 191-198 (1967).
7) Roederer, J.G.: Introduction to the physics and psychophysics of music. Springer Verlag, Berlin-Heidelberg-New York (1975).
8) Seebeck, A.: Beobachtungen über einige Bedingungen der Entstehung von Tönen. Annalen der Physik u. Chemie 53, 417-437 (1841).
9) Seebeck, A.: Über die Sirene. Annalen der Physik u. Chemie 60, 449-481 (1843).
10) Schouten, J.F.: The perception of subjective tones. Proc. K.Ned.Akad.Wet. 41, 1086-1093 (1938).
11) Schouten, J.F.; Ritsma, R.J. and Lopes Cardoze, B.: Pitch of the residue. J.A.S.A. 34, 1418-1424 (1962).
12) Sears, T.A.: Some neural and mechanical aspects of singing. In: Music and the Brain Ch. 6, Macdonald Critchley and R.A. Henson (eds.) W. Heinemann Med. Books, London (1977).

13) Terhardt; E.: Zur Tonhöhewahrnehmung von Klängen. Acustica 26, 173-186 (1972).
14) Terhardt, E.: Pitch, consonance and harmony. J.A.S.A. 55, 1061-1069 (1974).
15)Wijke, B.D.: Laryngeal myotatic reflexes and phonation. Folia-phoniatrica 26, 249-264 (1974a).
16) Wijke, B.D.: Laryngeal neuromuscular control systems in singing. Folia phoniatrica 26, 295-302 (1974b).

On the Perception of Spectral Information in Speech

E. TERHARDT, Institute of Electroacoustics, Technical University München, Germany

Evaluation of that part of information which is conveyed by the energy spectrum of quasi-steady speech elements is probably the most basic and "simple" problem of speech perception. The present contribution is intended to convey an idea, and sketch an outline, of how that problem may be approached quantitatively on the basis of established psychoacoustic facts and principles. The evaluation of perceptually significant features such as certain auditory attributes and difference limens may be accomplished by using quantitative representations of the *psychoacoustic excitation pattern* and the *spectral-pitch pattern*.

The psychoacoustic excitation pattern

Probably, the most adequate representation of a steady speech signal is the psychoacoustic excitation pattern as defined by Zwicker (19,20). It is usually represented by the *excitation level* L_E as a function of frequency or critical-band-rate (*Tonheit*, cf 18). Although the excitation level is operationally well defined by masking thresholds, its theoretical determination from a given sound spectrum is not yet completely and universally specified. Thus the following approach to a quantification of the excitation pattern may be suitable.

Essentially, speech is a sequence of either harmonic complex tones (the voiced segments) or random-noise spectra (the unvoiced segments). Hence two different and specific algorithms may be used for establishing the corresponding excitation patterns. In the case of random-noise spectra (i.e. fricatives and stops), the procedure is largely identical with that suggested by (20).

The excitation level $L_E(f)$ is approximately equal to the critical-band level $L_G(f)$, where both $L_E(f)$ and $L_G(f)$ are continuous functions of frequency. $L_G(f)$ is the sound-pressure level which is found in a bandpass-filter of bandwidth Δf_G (critical bandwidth). $L_G(f)$ can be obtained from the spectral-density pattern by integrating over that bandwidth. The formula

$$\Delta f_G = [\,0.23(x-1) + 0.32\exp(-2x/3)]\ \text{kHz}\ \ (x = f/\text{kHz}) \qquad (1)$$

provides a reasonable approximation to f_G for center frequencies up to about 10 kHz. L_E differs from L_G at those frequencies where the slope of $L_G(f)$ exceeds certain values, which are not followed by $L_E(f)$. The maximal positive slope which may occur in $L_E(f)$ is about 27 dB/Bark, while the maximal magnitude of negative slope is between about 25 dB/Bark at low L_G and about 5 dB/Bark at high L_G values. It is both the integration of spectral energy over critical bandwidth and the constraints on the slope of spectral transitions by which the $L_E(f)$ pattern is smoothened in comparison with a high-resolution power spectrum. Therefore, several spectral peaks and dips which may occur in a particular power spectrum may be invisible in the corresponding $L_E(f)$ pattern, proving them to be perceptually irrelevant.

In the second type of speech spectra, i.e. harmonic complex tones (essentially vowels and nasals), a suitable estimate of the excitation pattern can be obtained by a specific application of the principles developed by (9, 20).

To each spectral component (harmonic) there corresponds a "virtual excitation pattern" which may be considered with sufficient approximation as triangular in shape if displayed as a function of critical-band-rate (*Tonheit*), z. z is a nonlinear function of frequency which can be specified by

$$z = 13.3 \arctan(0.75x) \text{ Bark (approximation for } 0 < f < 4 \text{ kHz)}, \tag{2a}$$

or

$$z = [12.82 \arctan(0.78x) + 0.17x^{1.4}] \text{ Bark (for } 0 < f < 16 \text{ kHz)} \tag{2b}$$

Here, as in all following formulae, x is the frequency in kHz. The "virtual excitation level" of the ν-th component is thus specified by

$$L_{E\nu}(z) = L_\nu + \sigma(z-z_\nu), \text{ where } L_\nu = \text{SPL of } \nu\text{-th harmonic, and} \tag{3}$$

$$\sigma = 27 \text{ dB/Bark if } z \leq z_\nu; \tag{4a}$$

$$\sigma = (-24-0.23/x + 0.2L_\nu/\text{dB}) \text{ dB/Bark if } z > z_\nu. \tag{4b}$$

The $L_E(f)$-pattern of the whole complex tone is obtained by a superposition of the individual contributions which in principle is nonlinear. As a suitable estimate, *amplitude addition* is suggested (16), yielding

$$L_E(f) = 20\log \sum_{\nu=1}^{N} 10^{L_{E\nu}/20\text{dB}}. \tag{5}$$

Here $L_{E\nu} = L_{E\nu}(f)$ is the "virtual excitation level" of the ν-th harmonic, taken at frequency f. N is the number of components.

In Fig. 1 the amplitude spectra, and the excitation patterns calculated by this formular are shown of a harmonic complex tone with a flat spectrum (left column of diagrams), and of the synthesized vowel /i:/ (right column). Some more examples are shown in Fig. 2. As is apparent, the excitation pattern of a particular voiced speech segment exhibits a specific general shape and a certain "fine structure", i.e. a number of fine peaks. While the general shape reflects more or less clearly the formant structure, the fine peaks are representative of certain individual harmonics.

The spectral-pitch pattern

The fine peaks of the excitation patterns of voiced speech segments indicate an important perceptual phenomenon: The corresponding harmonics can actually be "heard out" as indi-

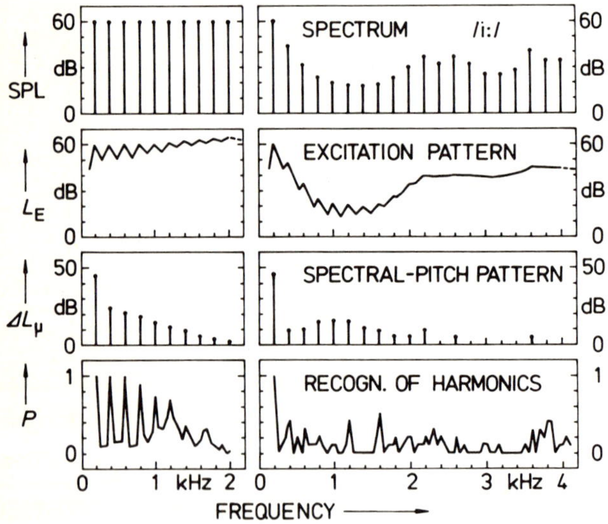

Fig. 1. Amplitude spectra, excitation patterns, spectral-pitch patterns, and relative No. of positive decisions on "hearing out"individual harmonics, P. Left column of diagrams: harmonic complex tone with equal amplitudes (60 dB) of all harmonics. Right column: synthetic vowel /i:/

vidual pure tones (8,10). Although, in normal speech perception, one is not aware of hearing individual harmonics (but rather perceives the spectral pattern as a holistic entity), it is suggested that the *spectral-pitch pattern* which is established by those individual components provides a significant contribution to the final auditory percept, in addition to the general spectral shape which normally is considered only.

To take appropriate account of the perception of individual harmonics (and thus of the excitation pattern's fine peaks), the spectral-pitch pattern is formally represented by the *SPL-excess* of the individual harmonics, i.e. the difference between every individual harmonic's SPL and that SPL which corresponds to the masking effect of all the other harmonics. Taking account of the absolute threshold of hearing as well, the SPL-excess ΔL of the μ-th harmonic is specified by

$$\Delta L\mu = L1 - 10\log\left[\left(\sum_{\nu=1}^{\mu-1} 10^{L_{E\nu}/20dB} + \sum_{\nu=\mu+1}^{N} 10^{L_{E\nu}/20dB}\right) + 10^{L_{HS}/10dB}\right] \text{ dB} \tag{6}$$

Here $L_{E\nu} = L_{E\nu}(f)$ is the "virtual excitation level" of the ν-th harmonic, taken at the frequency of the μ-th harmonic, f_μ . L_μ is the SPL of the μ-th harmonic. L_{HS} represents the absolute threshold of hearing:

$$L_{HS} = [3.64x^{-0.8} - 6.5\exp\{-0.6(x-3.3)^2\} + 10^{-3}x^4] \text{ dB} \tag{7}$$

(for details see (16)).

The spectral-pitch patterns of a complex tone with flat spectrum and of the vowel /i:/ are shown in Fig. 1. Some more examples are depicted by Fig. 2.

The perceptual relevance of the spectral-pitch pattern is

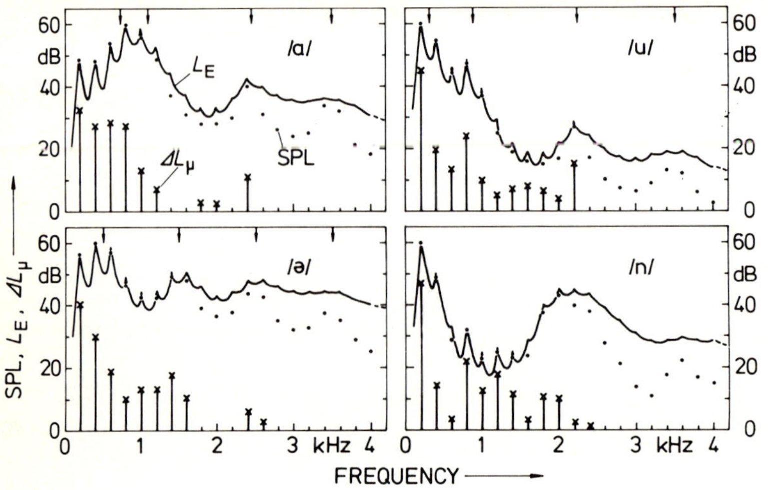

Fig. 2. Amplitude spectra (dots), excitation patterns (solid curves) and spectral-pitch patterns (crosses) of /a/, /u/, /ə/, and /n/ (examples). Fundamental frequency Fo=200 Hz. Vertical arrows indicate formant frequencies

demonstrated by some preliminary results of an experiment on the audibility of harmonics (Fig. 1, bottom). In that experiment, the complex tone (flat spectrum, and vowel /i:/, respectively) with 200 Hz fundamental frequency was presented in alternation with a single pure tone and the subjects had to decide whether or not a component with the same pitch as the pure tone's was heard in the complex tone (3 subjects). In successive presentations, the pure tone's frequency was randomly changed while the complex tone's parameters were kept constant. The relative number of positive decisions, P, is displayed at the ordinate as a function of the pure tone's frequency (abscissa). The resulting pattern shows peaks and dips similar to, and correlated with, the peaks and dips of the corresponding excitation patterns.

A significant item of the "P-patterns" is, that the peaks which correspond to high harmonics show a tendency to be somewhat horizontally shifted. This effect was expected, since it is known that the pitch of a pure tone is affected by additional, adjacent spectral components (13). For example, in Fig. 1 (bottom, left) it can be seen that the pitch of the 9th harmonic actually is increased to a value which corresponds to about the "9.5th harmonic". It is probably due to this pitch-shift effect that Plomp and Mimpen (11) were not able to find detection of harmonics beyond the 7th with "flat complex tones"; by the particular experimental method used by them, the possibility to account for pitch shifts was excluded.

Evaluation of auditory attributes

Loudness is typical of those auditory attributes which are dependent on the excitation pattern. Its quantitative evaluation has been established since many years (7, 17, 20).

Pitch. A considerable number of psychoacoustic observations indicate that the perceived pitch of voiced speech sounds (called *virtual pitch*) is dependent on the individual pitches of resolved harmonics, i.e. the spectral-pitch pattern. The determination of virtual pitch (or equivalent "fundamental frequency") from the stimulus parameters has been described elsewhere (14, 16).

Timbre. The evaluation of timbre as yet is established to a much smaller extent than is the case with loudness and pitch. The influence of the general shape of the amplitude spectrum (i.e. the spectral envelope) has been investigated (12, 3, 2).

Probably, a more accurate description of timbre can be accomplished by considering the general shape of the excitation pattern *and* the spectral-pitch pattern as well. Recently, an approach to such a "bimodal concept" of timbre has been realized by Benedini (1).

Roughness. Though the sensation of roughness is typical of the perception of temporal fluctuations, thus in principle requiring consideration of the phase spectrum, several helpful predictions can be made on the basis of the amplitude spectrum alone, cf. (15).

Evaluation of difference limens (DL's)

The L_E-pattern and the spectral-pitch pattern are very suitable to yield reliable estimates of the DL's of several speech parameters. The DL of any parameter which primarily affects the amplitude spectrum can be found by determining that parameter change which produces a 1 dB-change of L_E at any frequency (20). As examples, the DL's of fundamental frequency and of formant frequency are considered.

DL of fundamental frequency, Fo. Using the L_E-pattern, the DL of Fo of a particular voiced speech sound may be obtained by determining that Fo-change which produces a 1 dB-change of L_E at any frequency, while the spectral envelope is kept constant. From the excitation patterns shown in Figs. 1, 2 it is apparent that a given Fo-change will produce maximal L_E-changes in the vicinity of the fine peaks which correspond to individual harmonics. To obtain a general estimate, the maximal slope of the excitation pattern may be considered as independent of the particular speech sound, its magnitude being about 27 dB/critical band. Taking into account the dependence of critical bandwidth on frequency (Eq. 1), one finds that a frequency shift of a particular peak of 3 - 4 Hz will be detectable if that peak is situated below 500 Hz, while a shift of 0.4 - 0.6% (i.e. a constant *relative* change) will be detectable of peaks situated beyond about 500 Hz. Hence the sensitivity to frequency shifts of harmonics is maximal in the region beyond 500 Hz. Provided, that at least one peak does exist in that region (which usually will be the case, cf. Figs. 1, 2), the DL of Fo will be also 0.4 - 0.6%, since the relative change of every harmonic is equal to that of Fo. This estimate agrees well with experimental data (6).

The frequency DL's of individual harmonics obtained in this way correspond well to the experimentally observed frequency DL's of single pure tones (20, 9). Therefore one may also obtain the DL of Fo more directly by considering the spectral-pitch pattern and the theory of virtual pitch: Since the voice pitch is identical with a common subharmonic of the spectral pitches of the "dominant frequency region" beyond 500 Hz, its relative DL will naturally be equal to that of single pure tones in that region, i.e. 0.4 - 0.6%.

DL of formant frequency, Fn. The DL of a particular formant frequency Fn may be obtained by determining that Fn-change which produces a 1 dB-change of L_E at any frequency, while Fo is kept constant. This can be theoretically accomplished by using Fant's theory of vowel production (4). Using an algebraic approximation of the frequency-dependent formant-bandwidth, Fant's formula specifying the SPL of vowel envelope is modified into

$$L(f) = [(2.16x^2+0.023x^4)]\ dB + 20\log\ [x/(1+100x^2)]\ dB - \sum_{n=1}^{4} 10\log\ [(1-x^2/X_n^2)^2 + 2.5\ 10^{-3}(x+0.1x^4)^2/X_n^4]\ dB \qquad (8)$$

($L(f)$ = relative SPL, i.e. undefined reference; X_n = frequency of the n-th formant, in kHz).

When a suitable constant SPL is added to L(f) such that the desired absolute SPL is obtained, and Fo is specified, Eq. 8 yields the discrete amplitude spectrum corresponding to any formant-frequency combination. As examples, the individual changes of F1 and F2 of the vowel /ə / (F1 = 500 Hz; F2 = 1500 Hz; F3 = 2500 Hz; F4 = 3500 Hz; Fo = 125 Hz; SPL = 60 dB) which produce a 1 dB-change of L_E were calculated, yielding a DL of F1 of 25 Hz (5%) and a DL of F2 of 20 Hz (1.3%). These results agree well with experimental data (5).

Conclusion

Though the present approach to quantitative perceptual evaluation of speech spectra as yet is somewhat preliminary, it appears to produce realistic and helpful results and thus deserves further development and elaboration.

References:

1) Benedini, K.: Psychoakustische Messung der Klangfarbenähnlichkeit. Thesis Tech. Univ. München (1978).
2) Bismarck, G.v.: Timbre of steady sounds: a factorial investigation of its verbal attributes. Acustica 28, 146-159 (1974).
3) Bismarck, G.v.: Sharpness as an attribute of the timbre of steady sounds. Acustica 28, 159-172 (1974).
4) Fant, G.: Acoustic Theory of Speech Production. Mounton, The Hague (1970).

5) Flanagan, F.L.: A difference limen for vowel formant frequency. J.Acoust.Soc.Am. 27, 613-617 (1955).
6) Flanagan, J.L. and Saslow, M.G.: Pitch discrimination for synthetic vowels. J.Acoust.Soc.Am. 30, 435-442 (1958).
7) Fletcher, H. and Munson, W.A.: Relation between loudness and masking. J.Acoust.Soc.Am. 9, 1-10 (1937).
8) Helmholtz, H.: Die Lehre von den Tonempfindungen; Vieweg, Braunschweig (1863).
9) Maiwald, D.: Ein Funktionsschema des Gehörs zur Beschreibung der Erkennbarkeit kleiner Frequenz- und Amplitudenänderungen. Acustica 18, 81-92 (1967).
10) Plomp, R.: The ear as a frequency analyzer. J.Acoust.Soc. Am. 36, 1628-1636 (1964).
11) Plomp, R. and Mimpen, A.M.: The ear as a frequency analyzer II. J.Acoust.Soc.Am. 43, 764-767 (1968).
12) Plomp, R.: Timbre as a multidimensional attribute of complex tones: In: Plomp, R. and Smoorenburg, G.F. (eds.) "Frequency Analysis and Periodicity Detection in Hearing", Sijthoff, Leiden (1970).
13) Terhardt, E.: Pitch shifts of harmonics, an explanation of the octave enlargement phenomenon. Proc. 7. ICA, Budapest, 3, 621-624 (1971).
14) Terhardt, E.: Zur Tonhöhenwahrnehmung von Klängen, I., II. Acustica 26, 173-199 (1972).
15) Terhardt, E.: On the perception of periodic sound fluctuations (roughness). Acustica 30, 201-213 (1974).
16) Terhardt, E.: Calculating virtual pitch. Hearing Research 1, 155-182 (1979).
17) Zwicker, E.: Über psychologische und methodische Grundlagen der Lautheit. Acustica 8, 237-258 (1958).
18) Zwicker, E.: Subdivision of the audible frequency range into critical bands (Frequenzgruppen). J.Acoust.Soc.Am. 33, 248 (1961).
19) Zwicker, E.: Masking and psychological excitation - consequences of the ear's frequency analysis. In: Plomp, R. and Smoorenburg, G.F. (eds.) "Frequency Analysis and Periodicity Detection in Hearing", Sijthoff, Leiden (1970).
20) Zwicker, E. and Feldtkeller, R.: Das Ohr als Nachrichtenempfänger; Hirzel, Stuttgart (1967).

Perceptual Difference Limens in Pair-Comparison of Complex (Speech-Related) Signals

S. MEHRGARDT, Drittes Physikalisches Institut, Universität Göttingen, W-Germany

Difference limens of nearly any kind of small changes in signals have already been studied during the last decades. For simple signals, like pure tones or noise, therefore the difference limens can be computed from known models. But for more complex sound signals, for example speech, it is usually not possible to compute the difference limens precisely. A model for calculating such difference limens for stationary sounds, using the known psychoacoustic properties of the human ear, is described in the following.

The starting point is the power spectrum E(f) of a signal at the outer ear. It is modified by the transfer function of the outer and the middle ear H(f), which may also include any other linear influence that can be written as a transfer function. Now the power spectrum P(f) at the entrance of the inner ear is

$$P(f) = E(f) \cdot H(f)$$

Next, the excitation pattern $B_o(z)$ of the basilar membran is computed:

$$B(z) = \int_{0.5}^{24} P(f(z')) \cdot C(z-z')\,dz' + B_o(z)$$

First the power spectrum has to be transformed into a place

spectrum, using the place-to-frequency transformation f(z). The z denotes the coordinate on the basilar membrane in units of the critical bandwidth. The place spectrum then is convolved with the excitation pattern C(z) of a pure tone. On the z- or Bark-scale this function is of triangle shape and depends only little on the frequency of the pure tone. The low-frequency side of C has a slope of approximately 25 dB/Bark, independent of the sound pressure level. The high-frequency side has a slope of 10 dB/Bark. This value decreases for higher sound pressure levels, down to 5 dB/Bark at 100 dB. Finally a function B_o is added, which reflects the threshold of hearing.

Given two signals, the subjective difference ΔB is defined on the basis of the related basilar membrane excitations B_1 and B_2:

$$\Delta B = \int_{0.5}^{24} (\log B_1(z) - \log B_2\ (z))^n \, dz \qquad (n \text{ even})$$

Because the ear is more sensible to relative than to absolute changes in the sound pressure, the difference of the logarithm of the B's is taken, raised to an even power and integrated over the whole z-range. The model now predicts a noticeable difference between the signals, if ΔB is greater than a critical, yet to be determined, constant.

Fig. 1 shows the frequency difference limen of a pure tone at 70 dB sound pressure level. The dashed line was computed with the model. It agrees very well with experimental data obtained by Zwicker (1), if the critical threshold of ΔB is suitably chosen. For the following computations this value will now be

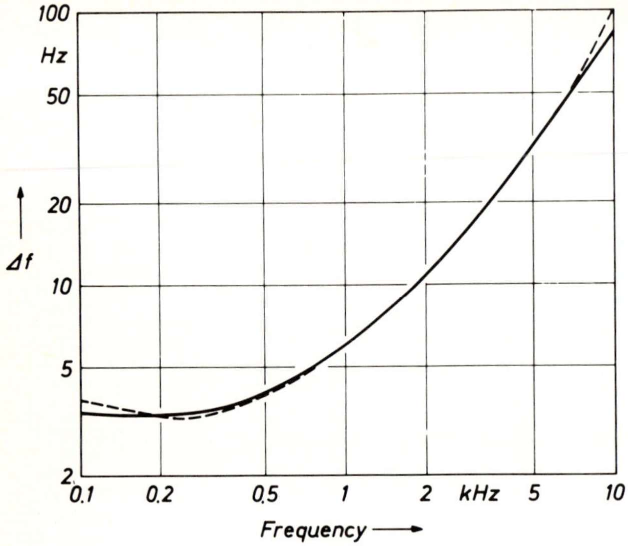

Fig. 1. Frequency difference limen for a pure tone at 70 dB SPL (-Subjective data, Zwicker 1967; ---model)

kept constant. The little deviations at very low and at very high frequencies are due to the fact that the model uses a constant shape of C (the excitation pattern of a pure tone) in contrast to reality.

Difference limens of more complex signals were measured in experiments. The signals consisted of 50 harmonics with a fundamental frequency between 100 Hz and 200 Hz. The amplitudes of the harmonics had a slope of 6 dB/octave, starting with 60 dB for the first harmonic. These signals were presented to the subject three times, once with small changes in amplitude or phase of one or more harmonics. The duration of each signal was 500 msec, which can be considered as stationary. Fig. 2 shows the difference limen for the change of one harmonic (left) or three harmonics (right). The experimental results (small crosses) agree very well with the solid line obtained

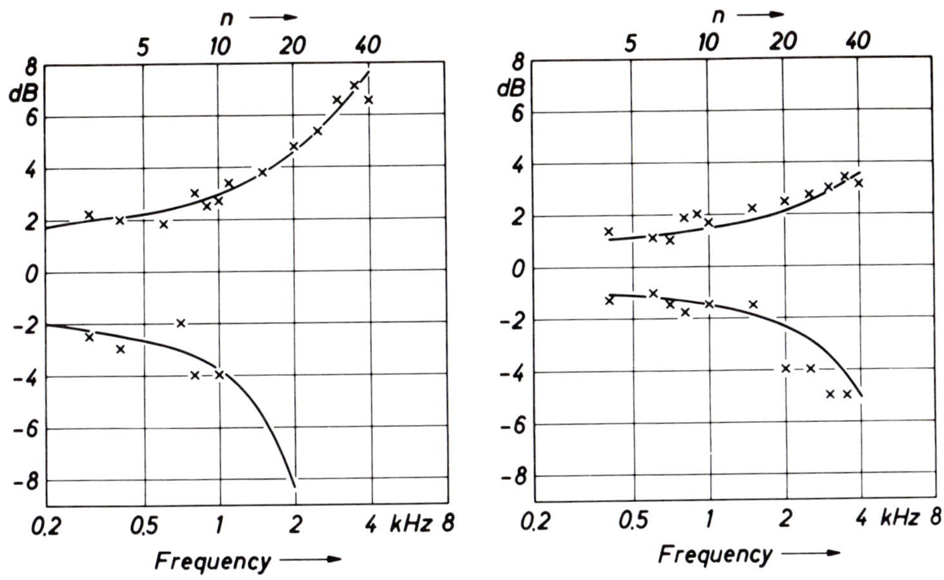

Fig. 2. Amplitude difference limen of one harmonic n(left) and three harmonics n = 1, n, n + 1 (right). Fundamental frequency 100 Hz (x experimental result, - model)

by the model. Only for negative dB-values, larger deviations were observed. They are due to the fact that, for higher harmonics, even a complete removal of a harmonic is hard to hear, and the subject therefore cannot be conditioned sufficiently.

The experiment was repeated for different situations: changing of the amplitude of more than 3 harmonics, different fundamental frequencies or different spectral slopes of the amplitudes of the harmonics. The experimental result always agreed very well with the values obtained by the model. Concluding, in the case of pure tones or more complex stationary signals, the model yields difference limens which are in good agreement with subjective data.

Although the model does not consider any phase effects, phase changes of the harmonics of complex signals are noticeable (2), and even small changes in the phase of only one harmonic of the signal described above can be heard. The experimental result for the phase difference limen is shown in Fig. 3. The limens are rather asymetrical for positive and negative phase changes of the same harmonic, very pronounced at example for harmonic number 8. The difference limen depends strongly on the harmonic number n, whereas the difference of positive and negative limen is such more constant and seems to decrease for higher frequencies. These effects are even more pronounced, if 2 or 3 harmonics are changed at once. In contrast the phase difference limens reported in the literature are usually said to be symmetrical (3).

Changing of the signal duration yields a rather complicated behavior of the difference limens. The amplitude difference limen of single harmonics (same signal as in Fig. 2) is shown

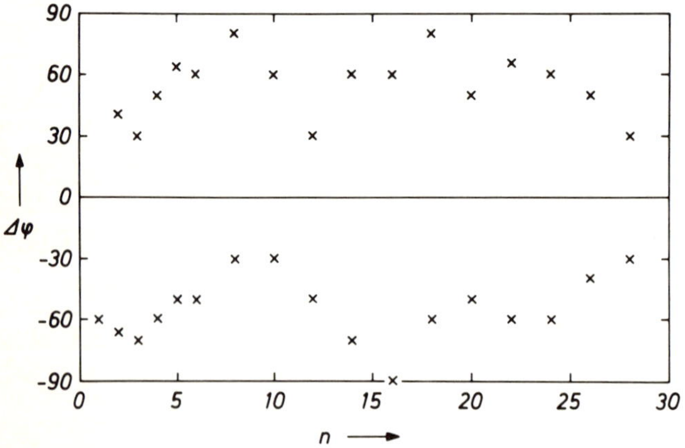

Fig. 3. Phase difference limen of harmonic n. Fundamental frequency 200 Hz

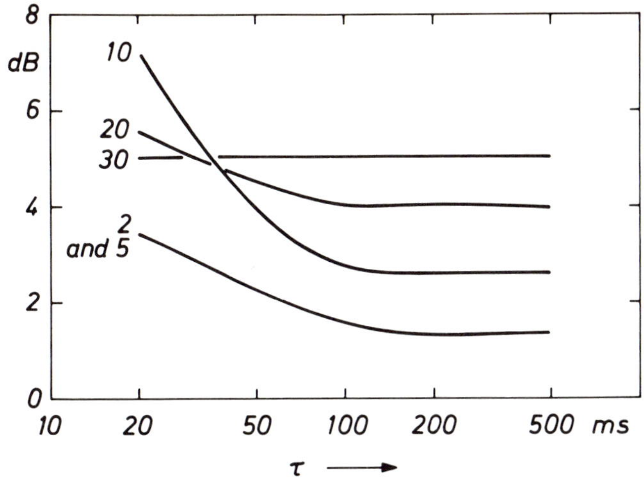

Fig. 4. Amplitude difference limen of single harmonics. Fundamental frequency 200 Hz

in Fig. 4. The limen of the high harmonic number 30 is not influenced by any shortening of the signal duration, even down to 20 msec: this harmonic, at a frequency of 6 kHz, corresponds to a critical band with a bandwidth of approximately 1 kHz. Thus a pulse with a duration of 20 msec is not yet distorted.

On the other hand, at the low harmonics 2 and 5 with corresponding frequencies of 400 Hz and 1 kHz the filtering of the cochlea with a bandwidth of approximately 100 Hz yields a broadening of the harmonics and thus complicates the perception of an amplitude change, resulting in a slight increase of the amplitude difference limen at signal increase of the amplitude difference limen at signal durations below 100 msec.

In contrast, the harmonic number 10 (2 kHz) shows a significant increase of the amplitude difference limen for a shortening of the signal duration. The slope reaches 10 dB per decade of signal duration, a value also found in experiments on subjective loudness (1). This behavior could be explained, if the critical bandwidth would decrease to approximately 50 Hz at 2 kHz center frequency, instead of the 300 Hz found in reality. It is likely that this effect is due to a more complex mechanism of perception, which has still to be explored.

References:

1) Zwicker, E. and Feldtkeller, R.: Das Ohr als Nachrichtenempfänger. S. Hirzel Verlag, Stuttgart (1967).
2) Schroeder, M.R.: New results concerning monaural phase sensitivity. J.Acoust.Soc.Am. 31, 1579A (1959).
3) Fleischer, H.: Untersuchungen zur Hörbarkeit von Phasenänderungen. Doctoral dissertation, München (1976).

V) Linguistic Elements in Speech Perception

Aspects of Categorical Processing of Speech Sounds in Man: On the Determinants of Phonetic Category Boundaries

PETER J. BAILEY, Department of Psychology, University of York, U. K.

The perceptual process for speech must transcend considerable stimulus variability, arising from different phonetic contexts, talkers of different sizes, and a wide range of suprasegmental variables, to make rapid and accurate judgements of phonetic identity. During perception of running speech these judgements are undoubtedly influenced by supraordinate factors like the listener's awareness of syntactic, semantic, and emotional constraints on the content of the message, but, as Klatt (1979) has argued, an efficient and sophisticated mechanism for phonetic categorisation of acoustic patterns must form an early stage of the speech perception process. The comments which follow will be concerned with a significant part of the characterisation of phonetic perception - a specification of the determinants of phonetic category boundaries.

It is reasonable to suppose (with others, for example, Kuhl and Miller, 1978) that the evolution of phonetic categories is constrained by at least two factors. First, languages should avoid the futility of selecting phonetic categories whose acoustic specification renders them beyond the resolving capacity of the auditory system. Secondly, languages should take advantage of phonetic categories whose articulatory specification minimises the acoustic concomitants of variation in vocal tract size and in articulatory precision (Stevens, 1972). Clearly, many other factors conspired to produce the phonemic ranges characteristic of different languages, but in establishing a rationale for the acoustic form of the boundaries between adjacent phonetic categories in a given language, it is particularly desirable to identify the relative contributions of these auditory and articulatory constraints on boundary placement.

Distinct auditory and articulatory constraints on the location of phonetic category boundaries imply the need for a specialised 'speech mode' of perceptual processing. Early interest in the phenomenon of categorical perception - where discrimination performance is good between exemplars of different categories, but poor or absent between two exemplars of the same category (see Liberman et al. 1957) - arose from the supposition that it was speech-specific and indicative of processing in 'speech mode' (Liberman et al. 1967). Despite subsequent demonstrations that categorical perception is not restricted to speech (for example, Cutting and Rosner, 1974; Miller et al. 1976), there may still be good reasons for maintaining the distinction between a generalised mode of auditory processing accorded to all acoustic inputs, and a specialised mode of phonetic processing for speech sounds. Not least is the obvious point that the process of primary auditory transduction, common to all inputs, is a necessary precursor to the 'neural spectrogram' (Licklider, 1952) upon which all subsequent perceptual processes must act. It may be pertinent, although outside the scope of the present discussion, to speculate about the extent to which the characteristics of the neural spectrogram, determined by the actual tuning and dynamic range of cochlear fibres, will differ from those of the representation typically assumed to simulate it - the output of a sound spectrograph (see Klatt, 1979). Differences between actual and assumed auditory representations will have consequences for the interpretation of another supposed indicant of speech mode processing - its apparent insensitivity to allophonic variation (Liberman et al. 1967), although it is noteworthy that the extent to which the acoustic properties of speech sounds are, in fact, contextually non-invariant is a live issue (Stevens and Blumstein, 1978; see below).

Whether auditory and phonetic perceptual processes are nonetheless distinct is an empirical matter; to maintain the distinction it is necessary to apply Lloyd Morgan's canon and show that a putatively phonetic process cannot be understood in terms of constraints imposed by the normal process of auditory perception. In other words, it must be established whether, and under what circumstances, auditory and phonetic category boundaries are coincident. This dictum argues for care in the interpretation of data from speech identification experiments where significance is attached to the location of category boundaries on the underlying stimulus dimension.

It has been demonstrated, using a habituation-dishabituation technique, that very young infants discriminate between synthetic stop consonants from different adult voicing categories ([ba]-[pa]) but fail to discriminate two exemplars of the same voicing category which differ on the voice onset time (VOT) stimulus dimension by the same amount (for example, Eimas et al. 1971; Lasky, Syrdal-Lasky and Klein, 1975; Streeter, 1976). The inference that, with minimal exposure to speech, infants are revealing an awareness of phonetic categories which suggests their perception is essentially phonetic can only be drawn legitimately if it can be shown that the determinants of adult voicing category boundaries are linguistic in origin. Provoking demonstrations that voicing boundaries may be at least partly auditory in origin are given by Miller et al. (1976), Pisoni (1977), and Kuhl and Miller (1978).

In Pisoni's (1977) experiment, following a brief training procedure, adult listeners categorised the members of a non-speech analogue of a voicing (VOT) series formed by varying the temporal onset asynchrony of two simple tones to generate a tone onset time (TOT) continuum. The location of category boundaries on the TOT dimension was broadly similar to the location of phoneme boundaries on a VOT dimension. The similarity of TOT and VOT category boundaries could reflect a common underlying constraint on processing auditory events which are close together in time. When two auditory events are separated in time by less than about 20 msec their temporal order cannot be resolved and they are perceived as simultaneous (see also Hirsh, 1959). Pisoni argued that this limit on temporal resolution applies whether the auditory events in question are non-phonetic pure tone onsets or the speech-related events of a consonant closure release burst and the appearance of periodic energy associated with glottal activity.

Support for the view that voicing category boundaries are determined by general properties of the auditory system also comes from the remarkable similarities between the identification functions for stop voicing of human and chinchilla listeners (Kuhl and Miller, 1978). An intriguing feature of these data is the close correspondence of animal and human voicing category boundaries at the three places of stop articulation. The tendency for perceived voicing boundaries to lie at longer values of VOT for more dorsal places of articulation has been rationalised by assuming that phonetic perception makes use of the articulatory knowledge that produced VOT varies inversely with the rate at which the vocal tract constriction is released. Kuhl and Miller' results undermine this account. An explanation for the similarities between human and chinchilla data which respects the acoustic concomitants of articulatory constraints is that the temporal resolution of auditory events is influenced by the spectral relationship between those events (see Summerfield and Haggard, 1979; Divenyi and Danner, 1977). These simple notions hardly do justice to a phonetic distinction as complex as voicing, for whose acoustical ramifications adults have a broad range of perceptual sensitivity. The foregoing argument does, however, lend substance to the suggestion that, initially at least, a major determinant of the location of phoneme boundaries on the voicing dimension could be the temporal resolving power of the auditory system.

Similar explanatory principles may not be so forceful in consideration of phonetic distinctions other than voicing, particularly place of articulation. Traditionally, place of articulation was seen as a highly encoded dimension (Liberman et al. 1967) for which the special speech decoder was required to resolve the perceptual problems imposed by contextual non-invariance of the acoustic patterns representing a particular phone. Since articulatory targets are typically less influenced by context than are their concomitant acoustics, the process of phonetic perception has been supposed to be mediated in part by articulatory knowledge, particularly for highly encoded distinctions (for example, Liberman et al. 1967; Stevens and Halle, 1967). Furthermore, there have been many studies of phonetic categorisation of schematic synthetic syllable series varying in place of articulation (by virtue of systematic change in second and higher formant transitions) which show that place category boundaries do not coincide with any obvious acoustic discontinuity in the parametric specification of the stimulus dimension (for example, Delattre et al. 1955; Pisoni, 1971; Mattingly et al. 1971). An awareness of articulatory targets on the part of the listener provides a convenient rationalisation of the location of place category boundaries in these series of syllables; place boundaries should correspond to the mid-point between canonical exemplars of place categories in a particular vocalic context. This notion was captured neatly in the concept of acoustic loci for stop consonants produced at different places of articulation (Delattre et al. 1955); the loci correspond to the resonant frequency of a vocal tract constricted at a given place. However, since acoustic loci are not entirely independent of vocalic context (Stevens and House, 1956), the concept loses some force as an organising principle for phonetic perception.

More recently the claim that place categories do not coincide with auditory categories has been subject to close scrutiny.

Stevens and Blumstein (1978) have argued that, when the range of acoustic consequences of normal consonant articulations is widened to include release bursts in addition to formant transitions, an invariant acoustic pattern associated with each place of articulation can be identified by a short-time spectrum analysis of the interval immediately following consonant release, or preceding consonant closure. The distinctive spectral properties are described as diffuse-rising (or grave) for /b/, diffuse-falling (or acute) for /d/, and compact-spreading for /g/. These descriptions are inadequate for characterising perception of synthetic two- and three-formant patterns with no release bursts, for which category boundaries do not relate to such simple spectral properties. However, children are said to learn, during development of speech perception skills, about secondary, context-dependent cues like formant transitions, which co-occur naturally with the invariant spectral properties described above, and which assist in disambiguating schematic stimuli in speech perception experiments (see also Simon and Fourcin, 1978). This account implies that young infants, who have presumably had little chance to learn about secondary cues, should not be expected to discriminate schematic stimuli differing in place of articulation in adult-like ways. However, both Eimas (1974) and Miller and Morse (1976), using different experimental designs and measurement techniques, have reported that infant and adult place category boundaries do coincide on a three-formant [dae - gae] stimulus series. The boundary stimulus pair are apparently not distinguished any more obviously than non-boundary stimulus pairs by the spectral property compact/diffuse (see Figure 1). Clearly a spectrum analysis of the onsets of these stimuli will be required to resolve the issue. Infants' discriminative capacity for place of articulation is improved by addition of explicit release bursts to transition-cued stimuli (Williams and Bush, 1978), but it remains to be determined whether infants are detecting the coherence of these bursts and transitions, or merely responding to the increase in discriminative acoustical information.

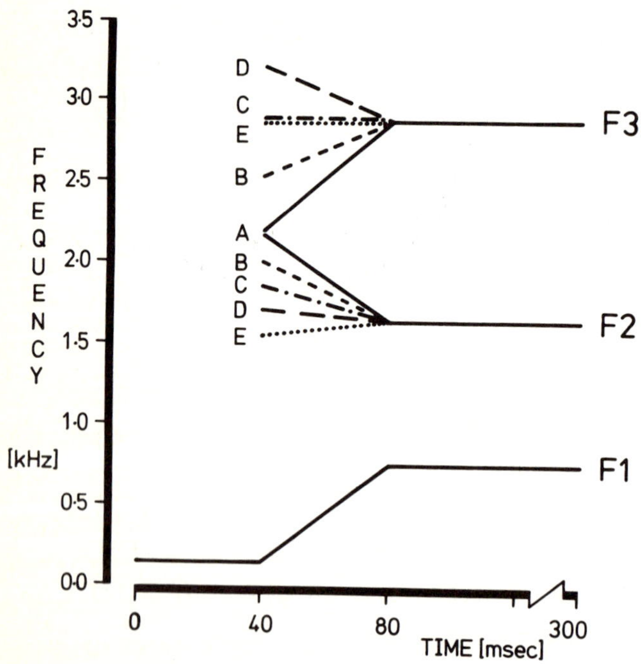

Fig. 1.

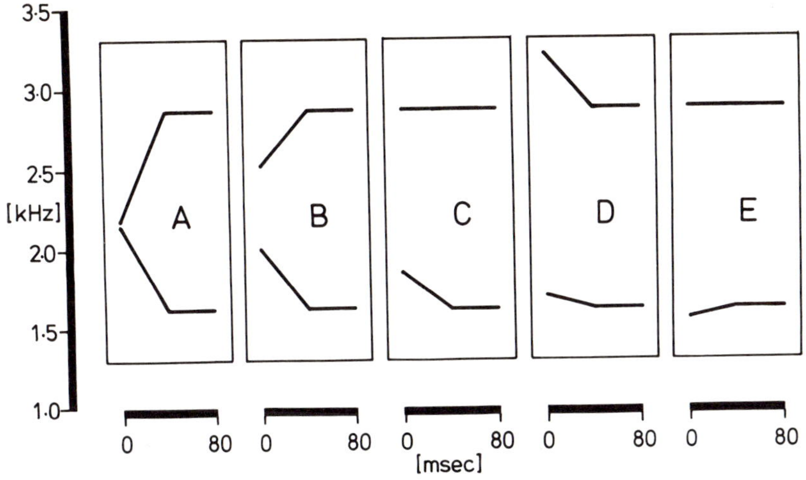

Fig. 1. Schematic spectrograms of the five stimulus patterns from Pisoni (1971) used by Eimas (194) and Miller & Morse (1976). The lower panel shows the second and third formant transitions in the five patterns individually. For clarity the transitions are represented here as linear segments while in the actual stimuli they were parabolic. English-speaking adults identify patterns A and B as [gae] and patterns C, D, and E as [dae]. Eimas showed with a non-nutritive sucking measure of habituation-dishabituation, that infants discriminated patterns B and C but not patterns D and E. Miller and Morse used a heart-rate measure in a within-subjects design to show that infants discriminate patterns B and C but not patterns A and B or C and D

There are other reasons for not accepting too readily the notion that the process of speech perception relies upon assimilation of invariant spectro-temporal properties from the signal at specific points in time. As one example from many (for example, Repp et al., 1978), Bailey and Summerfield (1978) have shown that place and manner information, to which listeners are sensitive, is distributed in time around and within the period of closure associated with a consonant. Listeners' attunement to information dynamically distributed in the speech signal by the events of articulation is more consistent with a perceptual process which can attend directly to change over time, than one which samples the spectrum at abrupt onsets or offsets of energy. As Stevens and Blumstein (1978) acknowledge, a final conclusion that place category boundaries are determined by simple non-phonetic invariant spectral properties must await further investigation of place identification, preferably by animal as well as human listeners.

It was noted above that a technique which proved informative about perception of stop voicing was the use of stimulus series which modelled some aspects of the speech pattern that was supposed to carry phonetic information, but which were not heard as speech-like, did not require a phonetic response, and were assumed to receive only general auditory processing (for example, Miller et al. 1976; Pisoni, 1977). Tractable stimulus series with these properties are not easely devised if it is desired to generate anything more than a minimally complex analogue of speech, because the phonetic percept is often hard to avoid, even in highly schematic signals. However, a potentially informative candidate for investigating perception of place of articulation was introduced by Cutting (1974). He created non-speech stimuli by replacing the formant structure of speech sounds by pure tones with the same frequency and relative amplitude as the formant peaks. We have extended this modelling technique in an attempt to compare directly categorisation of stimulus continua having phonetic and non-phonetic quality (Bailey, Summerfield, and Dorman, 1977). In one experiment, two series of consonant-vowel syllables heard as [bo - do] and [bɛ - dɛ] (see Figure 2) were modelled with pure

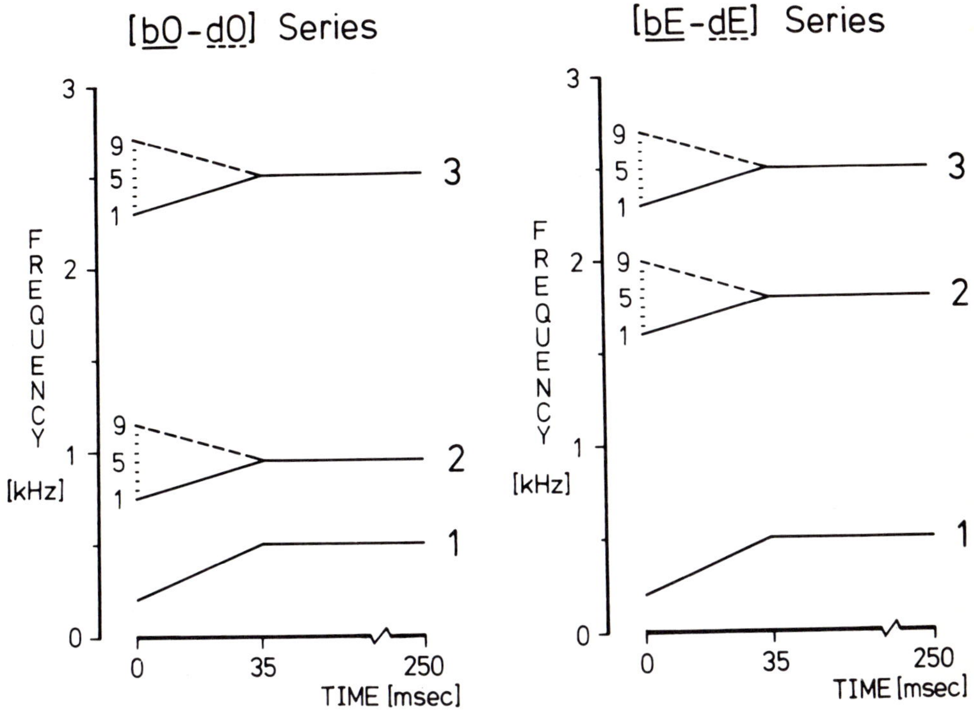

Fig. 2. Schematic spectrograms of the stimuli used in the tone analogue experiment. The formant series were synthesised with an OVE IIIc serial resonance synthesiser and the tone analogues with a software tone generator. All stimuli were low-pass filtered at 3.2 kHz and digitised with a sampling rate of 10 kHz

tones whose frequencies and relative amplitudes were set to be equal to those of the spectral peaks corresponding to the formants. The two vowels differed only in the second formant, and were chosen so that the location of category boundaries on the two formant series would tend to be asymmetrical in opposite directions. Using an identification technique not requiring overt labelling, in which members of the series had to be judged as more like one or the other series end-point, six listeners furnished identification functions for the two formant series and the two tone series.

During pilot studies we had observed that a notable feature of the tone stimuli was their tendency to be heard initially as whistles but, after exposure, as whistles preceded by a consonant-like event with clearly identifiable place of articulation. It was of particular interest, therefore, to establish whether any change in category boundary location accompanied this change from non-phonetic to phonetic percept. Thus, identification functions for the tone series were obtained twice: once in the first testing session, and once again in a third testing session after the formant series had been heard in the second session and after the relationship between formant and tone series had been explained to the subjects. In this final session, the subjects all agreed that the tone stimuli admitted a phonetic percept with bilabial or alveolar place of articulation.

A comparison of the identification functions obtained for the tone stimuli before and after they were heard as having a phonetic quality (see Figure 3) reveals that, in the latter condition, tone series tended to be judged as more asymmetrical and categorical, with identification functions similar to those found for formant series. A broadly similar result has been obtained in a second experiment which modelled a single more asymmetrical stimulus series in a between-subjects design where subjects were assigned to a non-phonetic or phonetic group according to their report of the tone stimulus percept.

Much remains to be learned about subjects' strategies in this type of experiment before the results can be used as a basis for extensive theorising. For example, these experiments have

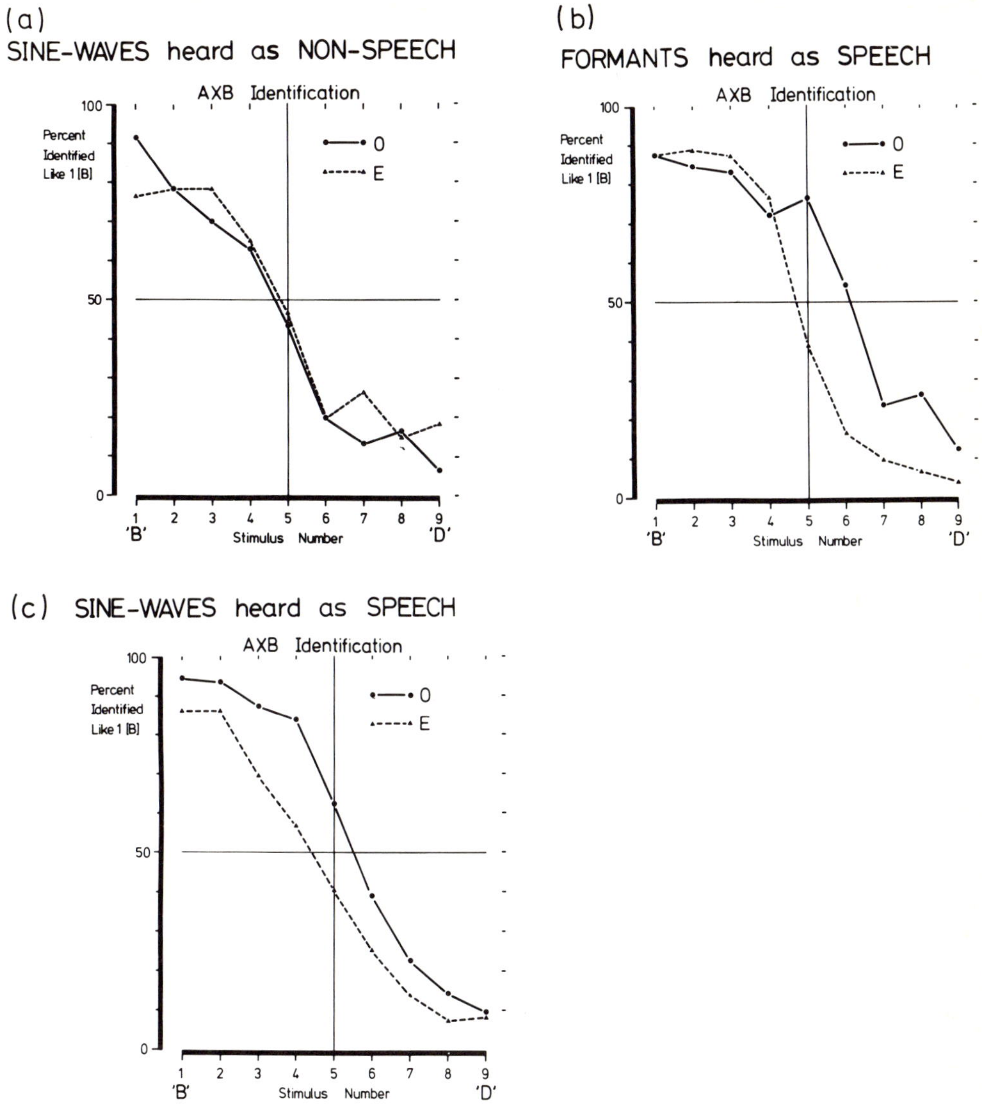

Fig. 3. (a) Top panel: Identification functions for the tone series in the first session when the tone stimuli were not perceived to have phonetic quality.
(b) Middle panel: Identification functions for the formant series in the second session.
(c) Bottom panel: Identification functions for the tone series in the third session when the tone stimuli were perceived to have onsets with identifiable place of articulation

not dissociated factors such as absence of frequency change and mid-point of stimulus series as determinants of the location of the category boundary on tone series. However, the results do illustrate some properties of phonetic categorisation rather directly. For example, it would seem that phonetic processing is not inevitably engaged by some speech-specific physical attribute or 'trigger feature' of the signal, since there is no change in the tone stimuli associated with the change to a phonetic percept (for further discussion of this point see Summerfield and Bailey, 1979). It is noteworthy that listeners reported that the change to a phonetic percept for the tone stimuli was not easely reversible, and tended to be accompanied by an increase in the 'clarity' of the signals, with a concomitant easing of the difficulty of the identification task and increase in the slope of the identification functions. Taken together, the results encourage the speculation that the change in perceptual processing which underlies the change in tone stimulus percept is a strategic modification of attention to the organisation inherent in the stimulus pattern. Thus it is tempting to suppose that for naive listeners in the first session of our experiment, the tone patterns were not perceived as specific to any natural identifiable event; in contrast, during the later session they were perceived as characteristic, if schematic, specifications of the event of speech production at a particular place of articulation (see Bailey, Summerfield, and Dorman, 1977).

These results do not necessarily favour the conclusion that, unlike voicing categories, the characteristics of general auditory processing play no part in the specification of category boundaries for place of articulation. They argue for continued research effort to investigate the psychophysics of acoustic signals having properties comparable with those of speech sounds. The results of such investigations will be essential pre-requisites to some resolution of the apparent differences between the major determinants of voicing and place category boundaries, and to advancing our understanding of phonetic as distinct from auditory processing in general.

Acknowledgement: My thanks to Quentin Summerfield for many discussions of these issues, and to Quentin Summerfield and Chris Darwin for their comments on a draft of this paper.

References:

1) Bailey, P.J. & Summerfield, Q.: Some observations on the perception of [s]-stop clusters. Haskins Laboratories Status Report on Speech Research SR53 (Volume 2), 25-60 (1978).
2) Bailey, P.J., Summerfield, Q., & Dorman, M.F.: On the identification of sine-wave analogues of certain speech sounds. Haskins Laboratories Status Report on Speech Research SR51/52, 1-26 (1977).
3) Cutting, J.E.: Two left-hemisphere mechanisms in speech perception. Perception & Psychophysics 16, 601-612 (1974).
4) Cutting, J.E. & Rosner, B.S.: Categories and boundaries in speech and music. Perception & Psychophysics 16, 564-570 (1974).
5) Delattre, P.C., Liberman, A.M., & Cooper, F.S.: Acoustic loci and transitional cues for consonants. J.Acoust.Soc.Am. 27, 769-773 (1955).
6) Divenyi, P.L. & Danner, W.F.: Discrimination of time intervals marked by brief acoustic pulses of various intensities and spectra. Perception & Psychophysics 21, 125-142 (1977).
7) Eimas, P.D.: Auditory and linguistic processing of cues for place of articulation by infants. Perception & Psychophysics 16, 513-521 (1974).
8) Eimas, P.D., Siqueland, E.R., Juscyk, P.W., & Vigorito, J.M.: Speech perception in infants. Science 171, 303-306 (1971).
9) Hirsh, I.J.: Auditory perception of temporal order. J. Acoust.Soc.Am. 31, 759-767 (1959).
10) Klatt, D.H.: Speech perception: A model of acoustic phonetic analysis and lexical access. In: R.A. Cole (ed.), Perception and Production of Fluent Speech. New Jersey: Erlbaum Associates (1979).

11) Kuhl, P.D. & Miller, J.D.: Speech perception by the chincilla: Identification functions for synthetic VOT stimuli. J.Acoust.Soc.Am. 63, 905-917 (1978).
12) Lasky, R.E., Syrdal-Lasky, A., & Klein, R.E.: VOT discrimination by four to six and a half month old infants from spanish environments. J.Exp.Child Psychol. 20, 213-225 (1975).
13) Liberman, A.M., Cooper, F.S., Shankweiler, D.P., & Studdert-Kennedy, M.: Perception of the speech code. Psych.Rev. 74, 431-461 (1967).
14) Licklider, J.C.R.: On the process of speech perception. J.Acoust.Soc.Am. 24, 590-594 (1952).
15) Mattingly, I.G., Liberman, A.M., Syrdal, A., & Halwes, T.: Discrimination in speech and non-speech modes. Cog.Psychol. 2, 131-157 (1971).
16) Miller, C.L. & Morse, P.A.: The 'heart' of categorical speech discrimination in young infants. J.Speech Hear.Res. 19, 578-589 (1976).
17) Miller, J.D., Wier, C.C., Pastore, R., Kelly, W.J., & Dooling, R.J.: Discrimination and labelling of noise-buzz sequences with varying noise-lead times: An example of categorical perception. J.Acoust.Soc.Am. 60, 410-417 (1976).
18) Pisoni, D.B.: On the nature of categorical perception of speech sounds. Ph.D. thesis, University of Michigan. (Suppl. to Haskins Laboratories Status Report on Speech Research) (1971).
19) Pisoni, D.B.: Identification and discrimination of the relative onset time of two component tones: Implications for voicing perception in stops. J.Acoust.Soc.Am. 61, 1352-1361 (1977).
20) Repp, B.H., Liberman, A.M., Eccardt, T., & Pesetsky, D.: Perceptual integration of acoustic cues for stop, fricative, and affricate manner. J.Exp.Psychol.: Human Percep. & Perf. 4, 621-637 (1978).
21) Simon, C. & Fourcin, A.J.: Cross-language study of speech-pattern learning. J.Acoust.Soc.Am. 63, 925-935 (1978).
22) Stevens, K.M.: The quantal nature of speech: Evidence from articulatory-acoustic data. In: E.E. David & P.B. Denes (eds.), Human Communication: A unified view. New York: McGraw-Hill (1972).
23) Stevens, K.N. & House, A.S.: Studies of formant transitions using a vocal tract analog. J.Acoust.Soc.Am. 28, 578-585 (1956).
24) Stevens, K.N. & Halle, M.: Remarks on analysis-by-synthesis and distinctive features. In: W.Wathen-Dunn (ed.), Models for the Perception of Speech and Visual Form. Cambridge: MIT Press (1967).
25) Stevens, K.N. & Blumstein, S.E.: Invariant cues for place of articulation in stop consonants. J.Acoust.Soc.Am. 64, 1358-1368 (1978).
26) Streeter, L.A.: Language perception of 2-month-old infants shows effects of both innate mechanisms and experience. Nature 259, 39-41 (1976).
27) Summerfield, A.Q. & Haggard, M.P.: On the dissociation of spectral and temporal cues to the voicing distinction in initial stops. J.Acoust.Soc.Am. 62, 435-453 (1977).

28) Summerfield, A.Q. & Bailey, P.J.: What tells us that speech is speech? Invited contribution to the Ninth International Congress of Phonetic Sciences, Copenhagen (1979).
29) Williams, L. & Bush, M.: Discrimination by young infants of voiced stop consonants with and without release bursts. J.Acoust.Soc.Am. 63, 1223-1225 (1978).

Selective Adaptation of Acoustic and Phonetic Feature Sensitive Detectors

W. A. AINSWORTH, Department of Communication and Neuroscience,
University of Keele, England

Since the discovery by Eimas and Corbit (1) that the position of phonetic boundaries could be shifted by selective adaptation, there has been much discussion as to whether the cause of this phenomenon is the fatiguing of detectors sensitive to acoustic features or of detectors sensitive to phonetic features. Bailey (2) has demonstrated that acoustic features are involved by showing that the effects are less when the spectral overlap of the adapter and test stimuli are reduced. Attempts to show that phonetic features are involved have been made by Diehl (3), Ganong (4) and Ainsworth (5). The technique employed was to adapt with a stimulus containing a burst and no formant transitions and test with a stimulus having transitions and no burst but having phonetic features in common with the adapting stimulus. Further experiments by Blumstein et al. (6), however, employing adapters with bursts appropriate to one phoneme and transitions appropriate to another, suggested the presence of integrated feature detectors sensitive to both bursts and transitions. The presence of these detectors can explain the results of the previous experiments without recourse to the phonetic feature detector hypothesis.

At some stage in the human speech recognition mechanism, a

process of vocal tract normalisation probably takes place. This is necessary if the speech of men, women, and children, who have different sized vocal tracts and, therefore, different ranges of formant frequencies, is to be understood by the same mechanism. If phonetic feature detectors exist they must be sited after the mechanism responsible for vocal tract normalisation.

Miller (7) has shown that if the fundamental frequency of some vowel sounds is doubled, the perceived identity of the vowel may change. The object of the present experiments was to locate such a vowel sound, and to employ it as an adapter. If adaptation were purely acoustic, changing the identity without changing the formant frequencies should not change the direction of the perceptual boundary shift. On the other hand, if it were purely phonetic the direction of the shift should be reversed.

Method:

An analysis of the formant frequencies, amplitudes, and fundamental frequencies of vowels produced by men, women, and children was made by Peterson and Barney (8). If the first formant frequency (F1) is plotted against the second formant frequency (F2) of the vowels /ʋ/ and /ae/, an approximate straigt line results (Ainsworth (9)).

$$F2 = 2F1 + 260 \text{ Hz}$$

A series of vowel sounds in which F2 was related to F1 by the above equation was generated by a parallel formant speech synthesiser (Holmes et al. (10)). The duration of the sounds was 180 msec with the intensity increasing during the first 30 msec and decreasing during the last 30 msec.

Nine listeners were presented with the vowels binaurally via headphones and asked to identify the vowels as /ʌ/ or /æ/ and press a switch labelled UH or AE.

The first experiment was designed to discover which vowel sounds change their identities as a function of fundamental frequency. Twelve sounds were generated with F1 ranging from 550 Hz to 880 Hz in 30 Hz steps. These were presented 10 times with the fundamental frequency (F0) at 86 Hz, and then 10 times at 320Hz.

The results are shown in Fig. 1. The boundary at which half of the responses were UH and half AE occurred at 670 Hz with the low F0 and at 730 Hz with the high F0. A sound having F1 at

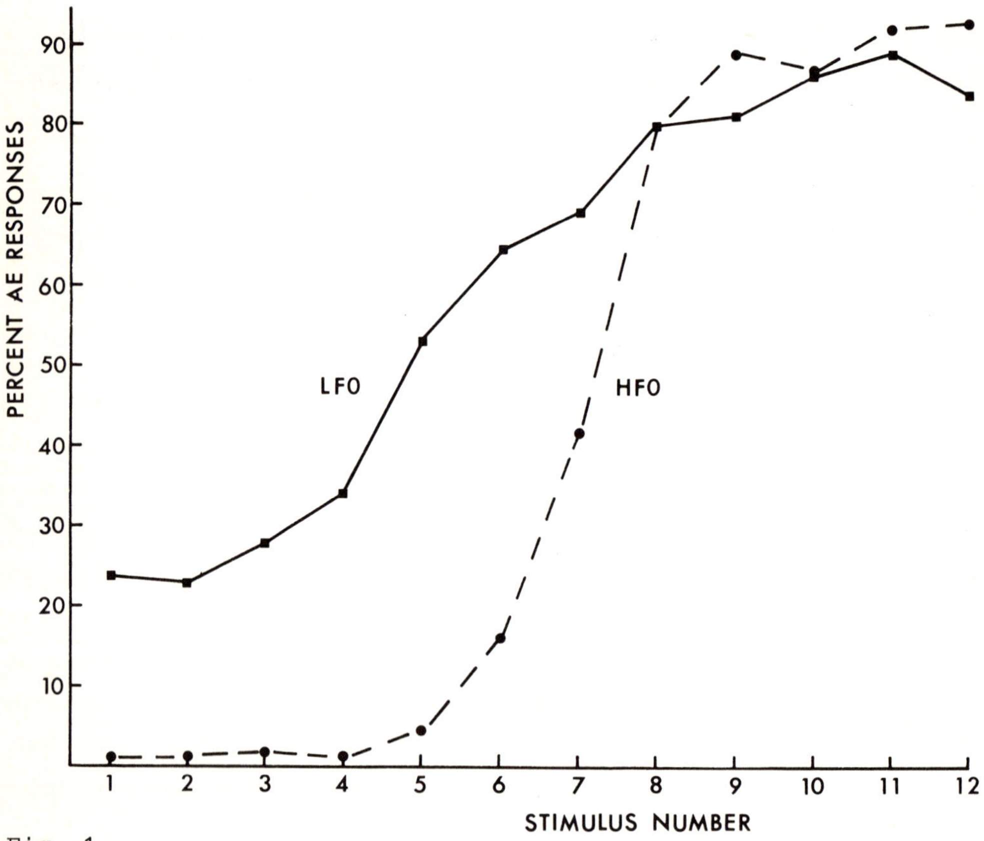

Fig. 1.

700 Hz and F2 at 1660 Hz should thus sound like /æ/ at 86 Hz and /ʋ/ at 320 Hz.

In the second session, F1 of the test stimuli ranged from 580 Hz to 700 Hz in 30 Hz steps, whilst F2 ranged from 1420 Hz to 1660 Hz. F0 remained constant at 86 Hz. The position of the unadapted boundary was determined first by representing each of the stimuli 10 times. The experiment was then repeated, but each test stimulus was preceded by an adapter (AH) having F1 at 700 Hz, F2 at 1660 Hz and F0 at 320 Hz repeated 20 times. Next the experiment was repeated with the adapter (AL) having F0 at 86 Hz.

In the third session, the test stimuli were the same as in the second session. The position of the unadapted boundary was determined first, then an adapter (UL) with F1 at 580 Hz, F2 at 1420 Hz, and F0 at 86 Hz was employed. Finally F0 of the adapter (UH) was changed to 320 Hz. In each case the adapter was repeated 20 times before each test stimulus.

Results:

The mean values and standard errors of F1 at the boundaries for each of the conditions are shown in Table I.

The difference between the unadapted conditions was 1.5 Hz which is not statistically significant with a t-test. The shift caused by AL was 37.5 Hz which is significant at $p<0.01$, but the shift caused by AH was only 3.0 Hz which is not significant. The shift caused by UL was -12.6 Hz ($p<0.01$) and that caused by UH was -10.2 Hz ($p<0.01$).

Table I. Position of the F1 boundary for various adaptation conditions

Adapter	F1	F2	FO	F1 boundary	S.E.
None	---	----	---	634.3	4.4
AH	700	1660	320	637.3	3.8
AL	700	1660	87	671.8	2.7
None	---	----	---	632.8	4.1
UL	580	1420	87	620.2	2.4
UH	580	1420	320	622.6	3.5

Discussion:

Both of the low F0 adapters produced a shift of the perceptual boundary. The high F0 adapter AH produced no significant shift, but UH did. The reason why AH produced no shift cannot, therefore, be due solely to its F0 being different from that of the test stimuli. As AH was acoustically similar to AL in all respects except this, the apparent lack of shift must be due to its being perceived as /ʋ/ instead of / æ / .

There is no reason to suppose that the acoustic sensitive detectors were not adapted by AH, so the results might be explained by an acoustically related shift in one direction being almost cancelled by a phonetically related shift in the other direction.

References:

1) Eimas, P.D., Corbit, J.D.: Selective adaptation of linguistic feature detectors. Cognitive Psychol. 4, 99-109 (1973).
2) Bailey, P.J.: Perceptual adaptation for acoustical features in speech. Speech Perception 2, University of Belfast, 29-34 (1973).
3) Diehl, R.L.: The effect of selective adaptation on the identification of speech sounds. Percept. Psychophys. 17, 48-52 (1975).
4) Ganong, W.F.: An experiment on 'Phonetic Adaptation'. Q.P.R. MIT Res.Lab.Electronics 116, 206-210 (1975).

5) Ainsworth, W.A.: Some effects of adaptation on phoneme boundaries. Acustica 40, 205-206 (1978).
6) Blumstein, S.E., Stevens, K.N., Nigro, G.N.: Property detectors for bursts and transitions in speech perception. J. Acoust.Soc.Amer. 61, 1301-1313 (1977).
7) Miller, R.L.: Auditory tests with synthetic vowels. J. Acoust.Soc.Amer. 25, 114-121 (1953).
8) Peterson, G.E., Barney, H.L.: Control methods used in a study of the vowels. J.Acoust.Soc.Amer. 24, 175-184 (1952).
9) Ainsworth, W.A.: Influence of fundamental frequency on perceived vowel boundaries in English. Speech Communication Seminar 3, 123-129, Stockholm (1974).
10) Holmes, J.N., Mattingly, I.G., Shearme, J.N.: Speech synthesis by rule. Language and Speech 7, 127-143 (1964).

Speech Sounds in Relation to Speech Processing

M. P. HAGGARD, MRC Institute of Hearing Research, Nottingham University, UK

Properly-controlled experiments designed to restore normal loudness contours by multi-channel amplitude compression of speech have been unsuccessful in enhancing intelligibility for the hearing impaired (HI) (Barfod, 1976; Lippman, 1978) although with more severely HI listeners and considerable amplitude fluctuations in the test materials (Villchur, 1973) they may give benefit over simple schemes. Evans (1978) has demonstrated how abnormal loudness growth may arise as a secondary consequence of degraded frequency resolution of the type found in animal models for deafness-causing conditions. Parsimony therefore dictates that compression be considered primarily as enabling patients to tolerate beneficial gain levels which comfort would otherwise preclude (cf. Posner and Ventry, 1977). The enhancement of intelligibility as such will have to be sought within a less limited framework for speech-processing than negative-feedback variable-gain amplifiers, and probably through approaching more directly the root problem of degraded frequency resolution.

Human frequency resolution is measured in many forms, through JNDs, masking and critical bandwidths in various tasks. Not all such measures demonstrate a consistent degradation for sensory

HI listeners; and the relationships between them in pathology remain obscure; however, there is enough sufficiently diverse evidence to state that significant numbers of the HI have such difficulties (Scharf, 1978; Tyler, 1979). Pick et al. (1977) have shown correlations of the order of 0.70 between hearing loss and resolution. Using synthetic speech-like signals and a discrimination task, Pickett and his colleagues (eg. Danaher and Pickett, 1975) have demonstrated in several experiments on the severe-to-profoundly HI a particular proneness to simultaneous upward spread of masking as well as forward and backward masking. This is inferred from a marked release from masking with formants fed to different ears (DSFMR). In our own laboratory (Haggard, 1977) we have done several experiments on normal listeners at normal absolute and relative formant levels to develop DSFMR as a laboratory model for intelligibility enhancement in the hearing impaired. Turek et al. (1979) using synthetic speech showed abnormalities in both biasing and sensitivity parameters of /b,d,g/ identification by the HI; though present, DSFMR was less marked than in Pickett's investigation.

The present experiments, were directed at a scheme readily realisable and miniaturisable in the near future, unlike formant tracking and splitting. Combfiltering can be realised with a simple delay line. It profits from the principle that a given total bandwidth is most effective if divided and spaced across the spectrum (Kryter, 1960). Furthermore Brandauer et al. (1959) showed negligible deterioration on PB words when alternate bands of the spectrum were sent to different ears.

Thus if upward spread of masking is what underlies DSFMR in normal and HI, the resolution of energy pattern change within one narrow band of the comb should be facilitated by the attenuation on the same ear of the immediately lower (and higher) band in a comb filter.

Conditions for experiments

One pilot experiment (b) established various parameters for the main experiment and one (a) furnished additional data for the conclusions. They shared the same method and stimuli. Rather than use natural speech a 2-choice word identification "bud"/"dub" was chosen which could be reduced schematically to a discrimination of F_2 frequency trajectory. The stimuli are shown in Fig. 1, which depicts a family of three rising/falling (ie. "bud" versus "dub") trajectory contrasts in F_2; these different centre frequencies were used, to correspond to different average locations on the lobes of the comb filters, and F_0 trajectory was also varied. The level of F_2 & F_3 was lowered by 38 or 43 dB with respect to F_1, to lower intelligibility and enhance the effects of upward spread of masking (Rand, 1974). Linear comb filters were achieved with a CCD delay line giving 20 dB peak-to-valley ratio. A spectral periodicity (p) of 400 Hz was employed in four conditions; $1-\cos(2\pi f/p)$, $1+\cos(2\pi f/p)$, diotic sum (ie. flat), dichotic sum; dichotic sum for p=800 Hz was used also. Formal identification testing with 10 subjects gave no significant differences, save that between single combs and summed combs. This indicated that neither specific relations between filter lobes and spectral cue information and F_0 value nor lobe-width were

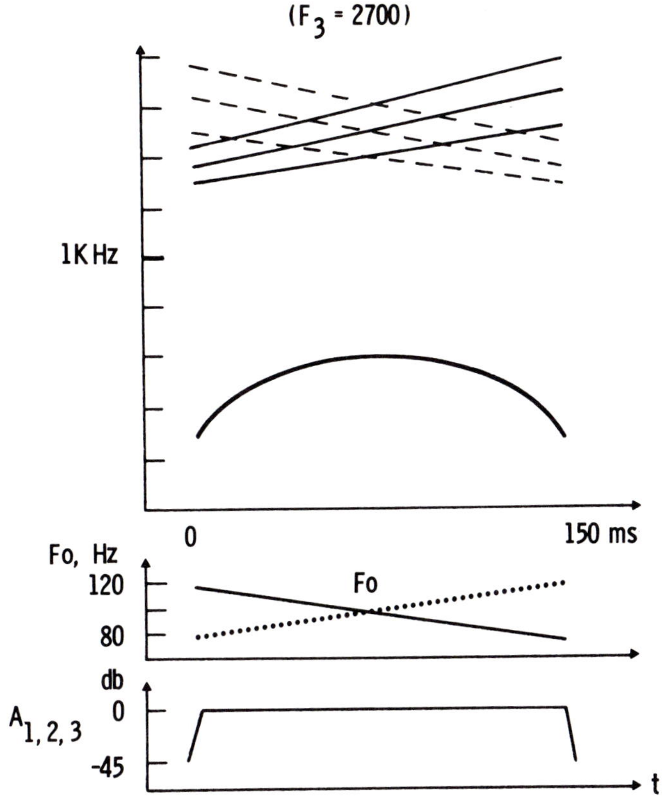

Fig. 1.

likely to be critically important. The fact that dichotic sum did not differ from diotic sum indicated that, with cosine ripple in linear power, attenuation in stop bands might be insufficient to confer benefit for patients.

The main experiment had three aspects, comparison of filter forms for p=800 Hz on normals; comparison of patients and normals on comb filters, and comparison of patients and normals on two high pass filtering conditions. For <u>all</u> subjects a 'hearing loss' was artificially created or increased by presenting speech against an absolutely calibrated masking noise of spectrum determined in preliminary trials to give masked thresholds identical to the mean better ear hearing losses of a national sample of 1143 adults with sensorineural hearing loss. Stimuli were closed-set 4-alternative consonant items of the rhyme test type from a new test ("FAAF") to be described elsewhere. 100 items were used per condition. 16 sensory HI people heard these in counterbalanced order at individual predicted most comfortable loudness (MCL), given by T + 0.67 (ULL-T) (Stephens et al., 1977) where ULL and T respectively are the uncomfortable loudness level and the detection threshold in dB for speech materials. This gave an average of 92.5 dB SPL. The level for normal subjects (81 dB SPL) was determined in pilot work to give a similar %-correct to the patients. The patients were homogeneous as to age (M = 53) but heterogeneous as to HL, averaging 38 dB at 0.5 - 4 KHz and ranging from 5 to 70 dB in their better ears.

The filters shown in Fig. 2, and their complements were programmed on a 12-bit digital FIR filter. This allowed linear and log power scaling also linear and log frequency characteristics as shown. The logarithmic spacing function is 2/3 octave with lobe width matching that of the linear function at 1.6 KHz. The remaining functions are an abrupt 20 dB high-pass (HP) for frequencies above a transition region at 1.0 KHz, and a similar HP for frequencies above 2.4 KHz; the former were presented diotically, the latter only dichotically with the former. Flat spectrum was always incorporated as a control condition.

Results and discussion

Comparison of the comb conditions on normals showed no effect

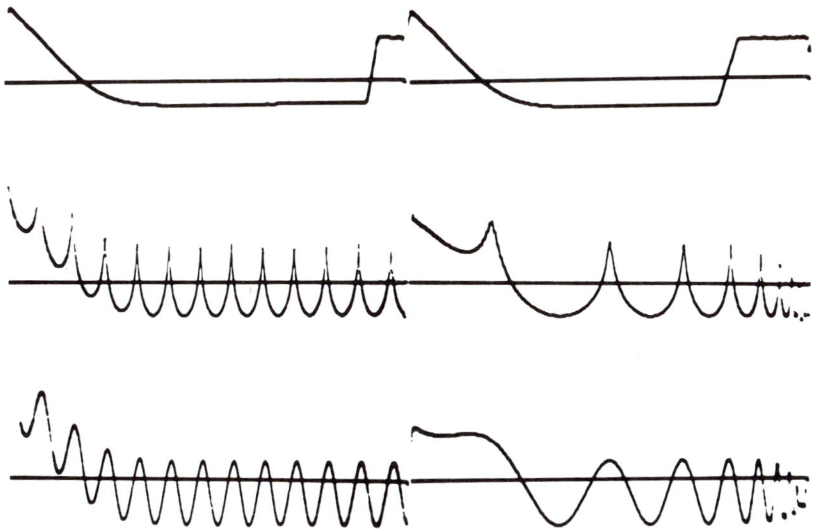

Fig. 2.

This result forces a reassessment of the upward spread of of spacing type but a substantial effect of power scale; as before linear power scaling gave insufficient degradation from flat spectrum to offer hypothetical advantages for patients. The main result with log power scaling (Table 1a) showed that patients perform relatively better than normals on comb filters but still absolutely worse than with flat spectra. The same is true for the dichotic HP conditions (Table 1b). Our conclusion is that such conditions do display some relief from masking for

Table 1a

COMB FILTER EFFECTS
(FAAF % correct)
p = 800Hz at 1.6K, Log Power

	Log f	Linear f	Flat
8 normals	63.0← ns →64.1		82.6
16 patients	76.6← ns →78.2		84.7
	└——— p < .001 ———┘		

Patient disadvantage smaller (p < .001)

Table 1b

DIFFERENTIAL HP CHARACTERISTICS
(FAAF % correct)

L. Ear	+ 20db at 1.0K	+ 20 db at 2.4K	Flat
R. Ear	"	+ 20 db at 1.0K	Flat
8 normals	73.5 ← p < 0.01 →	67.6	82.6
16 patients	85.3 ← p < 0.01 →	82.1	84.7

Patient disadvantages smaller (p < 0.01; p < 0.02)

patients, though perhaps at over 90 dB SPL normals would also display more masking and masking release. More important, however, is that release from masking is offset by a greater loss of intelligibility due perhaps to loss of binaural fusion in the dichotic conditions. This is contrary to the null results of Brandauer et al., a discrepancy we attribute to greater sensitivity of materials or control of conditions in our experiment. It is not due to learning as a subsequent experiment showed no improvement on diotic or dichotic summation with log frequency, log power combs after 2 1/4 hours listening through them. This makes the comb filter limited as an aid scheme for the majority of patients.

This result forces a reassessment of the upward spread of masking, consistent with Pickett's suggestion of a dynamic component. Haggard (1977) invoked the acoustic constraints on speech spectra whereby F_1 changes as the vocal tract opens and closes; the F_1 skirt movement modulates higher frequencies with broad-spectrum amplitude variation (Fant, 1960) obscuring the fine local amplitude variations due to F_2 and F_3 that cue place of articulation. With a normally precise frequency and amplitude analyser this overlaid mapping may offer a useful source of secondary cues, but in sensory hearing loss it will entail inability to register F_2 and F_3 changes, because only the broad spectrum variations are registered by an analyser with degraded frequency resolution.
Some evidence for this hypothesis comes from contrasting the pilot experiments. In Experiment (a) the signal was synthesised with parallel formants and either mixed before filtering

and presentation to different ears or not so mixed. In both (a) and (b) there was a further condition with high pass and low pass at 1.0 KHz fed to different ears. The crucial factor is not filtering, which gives small and inconsistent relief from conventional upward spread of masking. The crucial factor is formant mixing arrangement: splitting gives a DSFMR as large as could be reliably measured (Table 2). I interpret this as indicating that amplitude co-variation, not masking, is being 'released' in dichotic conditions. Hence if a miniaturisable yet accurate way to track formants and extract them by dynamic inverse filtering can be found it will promise well as an aid for the severely impaired. We have not yet tested this on patients. In so doing it will be necessary to take account of the fact that in both normals and patients (Turek et al., 1979) identification is based upon habitual input patterns from binaural conditions and that the initial biases due to transformed input in dichotic conditions may obscure potential longer term advantages.

Acknowledgements: J. Trinder designed and built the filters, Q. Summerfield and J. Foster set up the conditions of the experiments; R. Spencer and L. Wood ran subjects and analysed data.

Table 2

DICHOTIC ADVANTAGES OVER DIOTIC

Relative level of F_2, F_3 to F_1

	Experiment a		Experiment b
	- 53dB (5Ss)	- 43dB (5Ss)	- 38dB (10Ss)
Filtering HP/LP	-2.6%	+ 12%	- 18%
Splitting $F_1/F_2\,F_3$	+41.1%	+ 41.3%	

References:

1) Barford, J.: Multichannel compression hearing aids: effect of recruitment on speech intelligibility. Acoustics Lab. Tech. Univ. Naerum Denmark. Report No. 11 (1976).
2) Brandauer, C.M., Reilly, N.B. and Liberman, A.M.: Combined spectral and temporal segmentation of speech. Paper to Acoust. Soc.Am.Cleveland, Ohio, (1959).
3) Danaher, E.M. and Pickett, J.M.: Some masking effects produced by low-frequency vowel formants in persons with sensorineural hearing loss. J.Sp.Hearing Res. 18, 261-271 (1975).
4) Evans, E.F.: Peripheral auditory processing in normal and abnormal ears. Scand.Audiol.Suppt. 6, 9-48 (1978).
5) Fant, C.G.M:: Acoustical theory of speech production. The Hague: Mouton (1960).
6) Haggard, M.P.: Mechanisms of formant frequency discrimination. In E. Evans and J.P. Wilson: Psychophysics and physiology of hearing. London: Academic Press (1977).
7) Kryter, K.D.: Speech bandwidth compression through spectrum selection. J.Acoust.Soc.Am. 32, 547-556 (1960).
8) Lippman, R.P.: The effect of amplitude compression on the intelligibility of speech for persons with sensorineural hearing loss. Unpublished PH.D. Thesis MIT (1978).
9) Pick, G.F., Evans, E.F. and Wilson, J.P.: Frequency resolution in patients with hearing loss of cochlear origin. In E.F. Evans and J.P. Wilson (Eds.) Psychophysics and physiology of hearing. London: Academic Press (1977).
10) Posner, J. and Ventry, I.M.: Relationships between comfortable loudness levels for speech, and speech discrimination in sensorineural hearing loss. J.Speech Hear.Dis. 42, 370-375 (1977).
11) Rand, T.C.: Dichotic release from masking for speech. J.Acoust.Soc.Am. 55, 678-680 (1974).
12) Scharf, B.: Comparison of normal and impaired hearing II - frequency analysis, speech perception. Scand.Audiol.Suppt. 6, 81-103 (1978).
13) Stephens, S.D.G., Blegvad, B. and Krogh, H.J.: The value of some suprathreshold auditory measures. Scand. Audiol. 6, 213-221 (1977).
14) Tyler, R.S.: Masking in the hearing impaired. Unpublished Manuscript (1979).
15) Turek, S. Van de G., Dorman, M.F., Franks, R. and Summerfield, A.Q.: Identification of synthetic /bdg/ by hearing-impaired listeners in monotic and dichotic listening conditions. Unpublished Manuscript (1979).
16) Villchur, E.: Signal processing to improve speech intelligibility in perceptive deafness. J.Acoust.Soc.Am. 53, 1646-1657 (1973).

Perceptual Grouping of Speech Components

C. J. DARWIN, Laboratory of Experimental Psychology, University of Sussex, England

How does the perceptual system decide which frequency components originate from the same speaker? Is it able to group sounds appropriately using constraints that are purely acoustic (applicable to sounds in general), or must it also invoke those constraints which are specific to speech? The question has important implications for modelling selective attention in man, and also for designing speech recognition systems which must operate in noisy environments.

A number of criteria have been proposed as candidates for grouping together sounds which originate from a common source (see Bregman, 1978). Perhaps the most powerful, and the easiest to justify in terms of how sounds are produced, is that frequencies that start and stop together, belong together. When one tone of a complex changes frequency it stands out from its unchanging contemporaries and when the constituent tones of a complex come on at sufficiently different times, it is much easier subsequently to hear each individual tone than when they all start simultaneously. Bregman & Pinker (1976), for example, have shown that a tone is more likely to join with another to give a complex timbre if the two tones are simultaneous than if they are temporally staggered. A second equally plausible principle is that sounds originating from the same spatial location are more likely to be from a common source than those that are not.

A less general criterion may be applied to sounds that are periodic, a category that includes many of the sounds of speech and music. Here, frequencies which are integral multiples of the same fundamental are likely to be from a common, complex oscillation. If a periodic sound is band-passed (for example to produce a formant for synthetic speech) the frequencies of the harmonics wihin the band will all be integral multiples of the period of the original sound. Having harmonics derived from the same fundamental within different formants that have been led to opposite ears can give a powerful illusion of a single sound source despite the fact that different frequency bands are arriving at different ears (Fletcher, 1929; Broadbent & Ladefoged, 1957; Rand, 1974; Darwin, Howell & Brady, 1978). Techniques for the automatic separation of the voiced components of one speaker from a competing speech background have exploited the harmonic constraint on periodic sounds and have also used another property of voiced sounds - that their pitch tends to change slowly (Parsons, 1976; Darwin & Bethell-Fox, 1977).

The psychological value of grouping together harmonics from a common fundamental as a criterion for the formants of a single speaker has been questioned by Cutting (1976). Cutting, following Rand (1976), asked subjects to identify the initial stop-consonant of a syllable whose formants had been split between the two ears, the first formant going to one ear and the second and third to the other. When the two ears received formants whose harmonics were derived from the same periodic sources, Cutting's subjects, as expected, reported hearing a single item and had no difficulty in identifying the consonant. When the formants going to different ears had harmonics derived from sounds with different periodicities, two items were heard, but again and surprisingly, subjects had no trouble identifying the initial consonant. His result suggested to Cutting that while a common periodicity may be important for determining how many sounds are heard, a common periodicity is not important for grouping sounds together for analysis of their speech category. In support of Cutting's conclusion, but using binaural or monaural presentation, Bregman & Pinker could find no evidence that harmonically related tones are more likely to group together into a single timbre than are harmonically unrelated ones, and indeed Plomp (1964) found unrelated tones as difficult as harmonic ones to hear out of a tonal complex.

Cutting's experiment had failed to include an appropriate control; he did not ask his subjects to identify the stop-consonant from the second and third formants alone. He thus left open the possibility that fusion of information from the two ears was not essential for the identification task asked of his subjects. I have recently carried out a variant of Cutting's experiment using four different two-formant diphthongs. These diphthongs were chosen so that they could be synthesised by combining two different first formant patterns with two different second formants. In this way I hoped to obtain a better indication of whether subjects were really hearing a timbre that was jointly determined by both formants. For example, the rising first and second formant patterns which together produce the diphthong /uə/ sounded separately like /iə/ and /oə/ respectively. The experimental question was whether the number of fused, /uə/ responses would decrease when the two formants were led to different ears and/or excited by sources with different periodicities. Eight subjects listened to a tape containing five examples each of a number of different sounds, including the four individual formants played binaurally and the four different pairings of these formants played either binaurally or dichotically and on the same or on different pitches. They were asked to identify on each trial which of four diphthong labels best described each of the speechlike sounds they heard. They were instructed to indicate the same diphthong twice if they heard two tokens of the same category and to indicate at least one diphthong on each trial. They were also told to write down the total number of sounds that they heard on each trial.

To my surprise, and in support of Cutting, I found that neither presenting the formants dichotically, nor playing them at different periodicities, nor doing both these things, reduced the probability that at least one fused response would be made on a trial. Table 1 shows these probabilities as percentages together with the average total number of sounds heard on each trial and the number of fused responses as a percentage of the total number of diphthong responses made per trial. The results confirm Cutting's findings and support his conclusion that a difference in periodicity between dichotic formants does

Table I. Average responses of eight subjects to two-formant diphthongs

	Pitch of formants	Average No. of sounds heard	"Fused" responses as % of total	% trials with at least one "fused" response
Binaural	Same	1.07	87.7	92.8
	Different	1.33	78.1	94.1
Dichotic	Same	1.06	87.0	91.3
	Different	1.92	7o.1	9o.6

not preclude them from combining to give a fused percept in terms of the speech category heard, although it does lead to a definite impression of two sounds.

Although my experiment has confirmed Cutting's conclusion for sounds that, like his, were rather short (mine were 140 ms), I have made further informal observations on longer sounds, consisting of the basic /uə/ pattern followed by its temporal mirror-image and this whole repeated a number of times. I found with dichotic presentation on different pitches that after about two repetitions of the basic pattern (about 0.5sec) the initial percept of /uəuə/ gives way to /iəiə/. This is what one would expect to happen if the predominant perceptual category was initially determined by both ears but subsequently only by one (in this case the more speech-like first formant). That some time is required to separate timbres on different pitches at the two ears is reminiscent of Bregman's (1976) finding that sequences of alternating high and low tones are more likely to split perceptually into two tunes (one high and one low) the more tones the sequence contains. Bregman has suggested that the auditory system is biassed towards hearing a single source and only subdivides sound into two or more sources when the evidence becomes compelling. My own observations support that general conclusion with the qualification, derived from Cutting, that two distinct sound sources may be heard, at least one of which is initially a composite, incorporating elements from what subsequently become two entirely separate auditory streams.

The eventual separation of timbres played at different pitches occurs very much less readily (according to my own informal observations) when the two-formant patterns are heard binaurally rather than dichotically. Only after prolonged listening to a continuously repeating binaural diphthong pattern have I been able to hear out the timbre appropriate to each formant. It is not clear whether such resistance to fission is due to the patterns making plausible speech sounds. Parallel experiments with speech and arbitrary timbres are needed to resolve the question. Ecologically it is perhaps appropriate that we should be able to integrate timbres from a common location despite differences in their periodicity. The characteristic timbre of a bell, for instance, arises in part from the presence of two distinct periodicities, while in speech itself it is common to find the higher formants predominantly noise-excited and the lower ones predominantly excited by a periodic source (Holmes, 1973; Makhoul et al. 1978). An heuristic that grouped only harmonically related tones together would fail to include components from the same speaker for a substantial portion of what is conventionally regarded as voiced speech as well as for all whisper, friction and aspiration. It is perhaps not surprising then that the auditory system is prepared to tolerate differences in harmonic structure provided that they originate from a common location; and since even prolonged listening to dichotic formants on the <u>same</u> pitch failed to abolish the fused percept, the auditory system is also apparently prepared to tolerate a difference in location if sounds share a common periodicity.

While such auditory grouping principles may provide useful heuristics to apply at an early stage of processing speech, they produce, at best, candidates for the components of a speaker, they do not define the voice. An intriguing demonstration of the inadequacy of <u>auditory</u> grouping principles for separating speech from contemporary sounds is described by Liberman & Studdert-Kennedy (1977) and was performed in the early days of research on the Pattern Playback. The painted spectrographic formant pattern for a sentence was "masked" by additional spurious formant tracks, whose movements, though quite unspeechlike, nevertheless started and stopped at the same time as the speech formants. The resultant jumble appears to the eye unintelligible; it is not possible using visual grouping principles to decide which formant tracks are part of the speech sound and which are not. But when the pattern is converted to sound, separation is readily made; the original sentence can be heard against a "loud background of variously pitched whistles". Additional knowledge is being used to sort formants on the same pitch, from the same location, and with the same starting and stopping times into those that could have been produced by a human vocal tract and those that could not. But whether successful separation requires the listener to know what or who he is listening for rather than simply that he is going to hear some speech is not yet clear. It is likely though that assignment of speech components to a particular voice is an integral part of the speech recognition process rather than a reliable and isolable preliminary.

References:

1) Bregman, A.S.: Auditory stream formation: an evidence processing system. Paper presented at World Congress of Psychology, Paris (1976).
2) Bregman, A.S.: The formation of auditory streams. In: J. Requin (ed.), Attention and Performance VII. Hillsdale, N.J.: Lawrence Erlbaum Associates (1978).
3) Bregman, A.S., Pinker, S.: Auditory streaming and the building of timbre. Canad.J.Psychol. 32, 19-31 (1978).
4) Broadbent, D.E., Ladefoged, P.: On the fusion of sounds reaching different sense organs. Journal of the Acoustical Society of America 29, 708-710 (1957).
5) Cutting, J.E.: Auditory and linguistic processes in speech perception: inferences form six fusions in dichotic listening. Psychological Review 83, 114-140 (1976).
6) Darwin, C.J., Bethell-Fox, C.E.: Pitch continuity and speech source attribution. Journal of Experimental Psychology: Human Perception and Performance 3, 665-672 (1977).
7) Darwin, C.J., Howell, P., Brady, S.A.: Laterality and localisation: a "right ear advantage" for speech heard on the left. In: J. Requin (ed.) Attention and Performance VII. Hillsdale, N.J.: Erlbaum Associates (1978).
8) Fletcher, H.: Speech and Hearing. New York: Van Nostrand.
9) Holmes, J.: The influence of glottal waveform on the naturalness of speech from a parallel formant synthesizer. IEEE Trans. Audio Electroacoust. 21, 298-305 (1973).
10) Liberman, A.M., Studdert-Kennedy, M.G.: Phonetic Perception. Haskins Laboratories SR-50, 21-60. To appear in Handbook of Sensory Physiology VIII "Perception". Ed. R. Held, H. Leibowitz and H.L. Teuber. Heidelberg: Springer-Verlag (1977).
11) Makhoul, J., Viswanathan, R., Schwartz, R., Huggins, A.W.F.: A mixed-source model for speech compression and synthesis. J.Acoust.Soc.Amer. 64, 1577-1581 (1978).
12) Parsons, T.W.: Separation of speech from interfering speech by means of harmonic selection. J.Acoust.Soc.Amer. 60, 911-918 (1976).
13) Plomp, R.: The ear as a frequency analyser. J.Acoust.Soc. Amer. 36, 1628-1636 (1964).
14) Rand, T.C.: Dichotic release from masking for speech. J.Acoust.Soc.Amer. 55, 678-680 (1974).

Aspects of the Temporal Relationship Between Speech and Word-Recognition Processes

W. MARSLEN-WILSON, Max-Planck-Institut für Psycholinguistik, Nijmegen, The Netherlands

Recent experimental research shows that spoken words can be recognized very soon after their temporal onset, and usually well before all of the word has been heard. This evidence has lead to a new and precise theory of spoken word-recognition, based on the concept of the "word-initial cohort". This is the set of words in the language beginning with a particular sound-sequence, and some new evidence shows that the time it takes to to recognise a word can be accurately predicted by determining the point at which that word becomes uniquely distinguishable (going from left-to-right through the word) from the other members of its initial cohort. This evidence also shows that speech sounds are analysed in terms of their cohort-membership properties from the first phoneme of the word, with apparently great precision and rapidity. The implications of this for the traditional separation between speech analysis and lexical analysis will be discussed.

The Acquisition of Grammar

H. C. LONGUET-HIGGINS, F. R. S., University of Sussex, England

Studies of speech perception are ultimately aimed at the construction of theories of how we understand spoken language. But the most obstinate fact about language comprehension is that we can only understand a speaker if we have learned his language; so it may be appropriate, at this point in the Workshop, to address the problem of language acquisition - of how a person can "pick up" a language from hearing it spoken around him.

A central issue in the theory of language acquisition is whether or not semantic information is used in the acquisition of syntax. There seems no alternative to the view that the meanings of most <u>words</u> can only be discovered by hearing them uttered in circumstances where the meaning is apparent; but although there is strong experimental [1,2] and theoretical evidence[3,4] that people have great difficulty in learning the syntax of a language unless they are provided with semantic clues, it is by no means clear exactly how these clues might be used in inducing the rules of the <u>grammar</u>. For this reason Dr. R.J.D. Power and I decided to write a computer program which would exploit semantic information in the acquisition of natural languages - or rather, of their numeral systems. We chose numeral systems for study because (i) most languages supply ways of naming the natural numbers, (ii) numeral systems display an interesting variety in the ways in which they represent numbers (cf. *ninety seven* and *quatre vingts dix sept*), (iii) they have been thoroughly studied and well documented by linguists[5,6] and (iv) their semantics is exceptionally clear: it is beyond dispute that *neun und zwanzig* stands for the sum of the number denoted by *neun* and that denoted by *zwanzig*.

In fact we succeeded in writing a program which would learn any one of a variety of uninflected numeral systems from a series of representative number/numeral pairs such as (21, *twenty one*) presented in an appropriate order. The details of this work are described in[7]; here there is only space to describe some of the problems that arose, and the solutions which we ultimately adopted.

Like other semantic entities the numbers are divided by a given language into two sets: a small set in which each number has a single-word name such as *sechs* or *tausend*, and a much larger set in which the name is composite (e.g. *sechs tausend* or *sechs tausend und sechs*). Such a name reveals that the number is represented semantically as the sum or product (or difference) of two other numbers which may or may not have single-word names. It is therefore natural to specify a numeral system by (i) a *lexicon*, which lists all the single-word names and the numbers for which they stand and (ii) a set of grammatical *rules*, which indicate what arithmetic expressions are available for the representation of other numbers, and the associated syntactic forms (e.g. < p > *und* < n >, where < p > and < n > denote the names of the larger and the smaller term in a sum of two numbers). The utility of this scheme rests upon various general facts about numeral systems, and various language-independent principles of grammar. Information of both kinds must be assumed to be available to the learner in advance, or it would be impossible for him to draw any inductive generalisations from particular examples. To illustrate this point, consider the number/numeral pair (21, *ein und zwanzig*), presented to a learner who knows the meanings of *ein* and *zwanzig*, but is unfamilar with *und*. If (as he may assume) the numeral signifies an arithmetic combination of 1 and 20, then this combination must be a sum, because the answer is given as 21. So the word *und* must be a mere conjunction, and he can enter the "rule" [20 + 1, < p > *und* < n >] in the grammar. If the next pair he meets is (29, *neun und zwanzig*) he can add the entry [20 + 9, < p > *und* < n >] and now - so we assume - is in a position to "interpolate", arriving at the wider rule [20 + (1,...,9), < p > *und* < n >] which enables him to name all the numbers lying between 21 and 29, and to interpret their names. But he can only perform these logical operations if he can do arithmetic; and this illustrates the point that the acquisition of a language may well be impossible unless the learner already possesses certain cognitive skills - unless he can already handle the ideas that he is attempting to put into words, or to extract from the utterances of the people around him.

Among the problems which we had to face in writing the program were two which must arise in the formulation of any general theory of language acquisition. The first concerned the manner in which grammatical rules should be represented - whether as "data structures" or as "procedures". It has been fashionable in the artificial intelligence literature[8] to recommend that all the general knowledge which is available to an information-processing system should be cast in the form of functions or routines for arriving at decisions in any given circumstances. Such an approach would seem to suggest that the grammar of the language under acquisition should be represented by a growing set of functions for the production and the interpretation of well-formed utterances. The task of writing a program which would compose such sets of functions was a forbidding prospect; but after further reflection we decided to attack the problem in a different way - by representing the learner's language-specific knowledge not as a set of functions but as a developing data-structure, to be updated and consulted by quite general language-independent procedures. It would, of course, be absurd to try to dispense entirely with procedures in the construction of a language-acquisition device; the problem was simply to avoid having to compose, for each new language, special parsing and production routines. We were therefore gratified to discover a language-independent parsing algorithm which assigns semantic interpretations to many-word numerals on the basis of limited information about the numeral system being learned. The algorithm involves searching the numeral for interpretable substrings, and attempting to combine the corresponding numbers to form the result given by the operator. The details are a little complicated, but the unexpected success of the algorithm in this limited domain does suggest that in the acquisition of a language the learner may indeed use "universal" procedures for parsing and interpreting the utterances that he hears, though in order to do this he will need to consult, and may need to update, what he knows about the grammar of the language to which the utterances belong.

There were, of course, many other problems which arose in the course of constructing the program. Could we, for example, take account of the fact that some of the evidence presented to the learner is unreliable or positively misleading, and specify adequate grounds for rejecting it? This proved to be possible if semantic information was presented; thus a misleading example such as (22, twenty one) could be thrown out because neither addition, multiplication nor subtraction can unite 20 and 1 to give 22. Was it possible, furthermore, to model the process of induction by syntactic analogy? Yes, because the occurrence of a familiar syntactic form is likely (but not certain) to indicate a semantic construct known to be associated with that form. Guesses based on syntactic analogy were therefore revealed as such by the printing of a question mark, as in the exchange

(operator:) hundert und vier und zwanzig?
(program:) 124?
(operator:) Yes.

-after which the guess would be regarded as confirmed.

Finally, it may be useful to make a few quite general points about the relevance of such work to the current theory of language acquisition.

First, we would not wish our program to be regarded as embodying a detailed theory of how *children* first learn to count. If it has any direct relevance to human performance, it is more likey to describe how adults pick up the numeral system of unfamiliar languages from the kind of information typically supplied in dictionaries. But secondly, we do want to suggest that the program is faithful to human performance in making essential use of semantic information in the process of language acquisition. Though numeral systems supply a particularly simple example of how this can be done, there are other important kinds of semantic relation (e.g. the relation between subject and predicate in a proposition) whose syntactic counterparts might well be discovered in the same general way.

Thirdly, the experience of teaching the program to count in various languages confirms one's expectation that the rate at which a language can be acquired depends critically on the order in which the examples are presented by the teacher. Fourthly, we feel that there is much to be gained by regarding a grammatical rule as a specification of a syntactic form which may be used *for expressing a given type of semantic construct*, rather than merely as a permissible arrangement of words or phrases. And lastly, we think that the concept of "universal grammar", as defined by Chomsky is most naturally viewed as a set of cognitive skills - some linguistic and some non-linguistic - and modelled in a formal theory as a set of procedures for comparing what people say with what they evidently mean, and using the comparison to build a model of the grammar of their language.

This "special lecture" concluded the original program of the meeting.

References:

1) Miller, G.A.: The psychology of communication. Allen Lane, London: Penguin Press (1967).
2) Moesner, J.D. & Bregman, S.A.: The role of reference in the acquisition of a miniature artificial language. J. Verbal Lang. Verbal Behav. 11, 759 (1972).
3) Gold, E.M.: Language identification in the limit. Inf. Control, 10, 447 (1967).
4) Anderson, J.R.: Computer simulation of a language acquisition system - a first report. In: Information processing and cognition (ed. R.L. Solso) Hillsdale, New Jersey: Erlbaum (1975).
5) Hudson, R.A.: English complex sentences. Amsterdam: North Holland.
6) Stampe, D.: Cardinal number systems. In: Proceedings of the 12th Annual Conference of the Chicago Linguistics Society. Chicago: University Press.
7) Power, R.J.D. & Longuet-Higgins, H.C.: Learning to count: a computational model of language acquisition. Proc.R.Soc. Lond. B. 200, 391 (1978).
8) Winograd, T.: Understanding Natural Language. Edinburgh University Press (1972).

VI) Receptive Defects of Linguistic Elements in Aphasia

Auditory Agnosia After Lesions of the Superior Temporal Gyrus in Monkey and Man

D. PLOOG, Max Planck Institute for Psychiatry, Munich, Federal Republic of Germany

After Wernicke's discovery (1874) that the destruction of the posterior part of the superior temporal gyrus of the dominant hemisphere results in sensory aphasia, numerous studies on auditory discrimination were carried out to investigate the effect of the auditory cortical lesions in cats, dogs, and monkeys. Discriminations studied included frequency, intensity, duration and more complicated temporal cues, complex spectral differences, vowel sounds, and changes in temporal patterning. It became clear that animals with total ablation of the auditory cortex are still able to discriminate between pure tones of different pitch, duration, and intensity. What is lost is the capacity to discriminate continuous from intermittent white noise, some human vowels, simple sequences of tones, and especially auditory patterns (for review see Neff et al., 1975).

In none of these studies was species-specific vocalization employed. Therefore we set up an investigation in which the test stimuli were species-specific calls normally used between conspecifics (Hupfer et al., 1977). The results lend themselves to a discussion of auditory perceptual disorders in the monkey at higher levels of cerebral organization, and their relationship to comparable disorders in man. Does the monkey need its auditory cortex to understand the vocal signals of its own species, and if so, how much of the cortex is necessary?

Methods

The subjects were 11 adult squirrel monkeys from Peru. They were trained in a special test apparatus which consisted of a large cage with a perch above a barred window and a small cage adjacent to the window. The window could be closed automatically with an opaque screen. The experimental animals were kept in social isolation for 5-15 hours prior to each session. They were trained to jump from the perch to the bottom of the large cage whenever they heard a species-specific call played on a tape recorder. During testing there was another monkey in the adjacent cage. Its vocal cords had been coagulated so that it was unable to vocalize. Correct responses were reinforced by lifting the screen for 30 sec. so that visual and tactile contact with the mute partner were possible. This method of social reinforcement produced significantly more rapid learning than shock avoidance. Within one session 10 species-specific and 10 non-specific sounds were presented in random order.

In a Go/No-Go test procedure the monkey was trained to respond positively to any squirrel monkey call regardless of whether or not this call type had been presented before and to stay put on the perch if it heard any other sounds. There were 57 Go stimuli and 75 No-Go stimuli with different degrees of similarity to natural sounds. During the total training phase, in which the animal learned to discriminate between natural and artificial sounds, any given stimulus was presented only twice.

The task was therefore not simply to relate a certain stimulus to a certain behavior but to generalize and to distinguish all natural sounds from all artificial ones. The criterion was reached when the animal responded correctly at least 75% of the time on 3 successive days. After the criterion was reached the animal was not tested again for 2 weeks. Then it was retested for retention. After it had again reached criterion the ablation of the temporal cortex was carried out in two stages, with retesting after both the unilateral and bilateral operations.

Results

The test criterion was reached in an average of 155 trials (20-220), i.e. within 8 sessions. Fig. 1 shows the training curves. Each short horizontal line segment represents a session of 20 trials. The graphs on the right show the performance of the ablated animals 6-11 before the first operation and after the second. Animals 1-5, on the left, are the controls. For the controls "pre" means learning and first retraining phase, and "post" means all following sessions.

Unilateral lesions produced no significant effects.

Bilateral lesions:

The animals with medium-sized lesions (Nos. 6-9) showed a significant retention deficit ($p < 0.01$). With the exception of the animal with the smallest lesion (No. 6), none of these animals reached criterion during retraining, but all performed between 69% and 73%, significantly above chance. Fig. 2A shows a representative brain from this groups. The destruction of the lateral convexity of the superior temporal gyrus is quite extensive and the temporal opercular cortex is partly damaged.

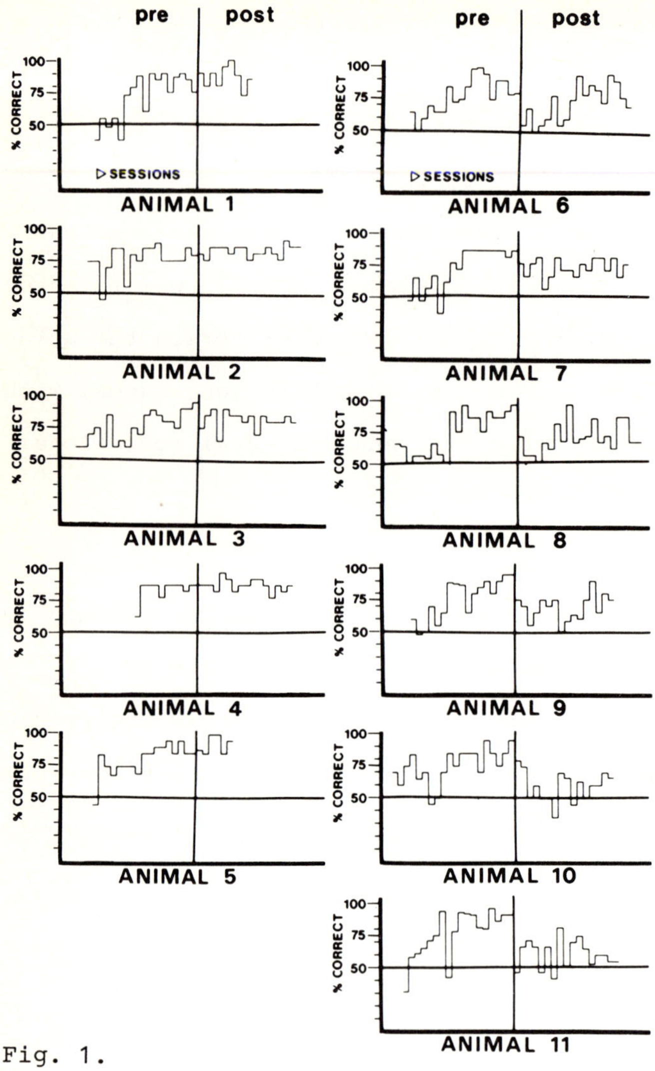

Fig. 1.

The medial geniculate nuclei show heavy, but not total, degeneration of the rostral (a) and intermediate (c) parts of the parvocellular region.

The largest and most complete ablation of the auditory cortex was carried out on animals 10 and 11. The histology (Fig. 2B) shows almost total loss of the auditory association cortex with only small remnants of primary cortex. In the parvocellular

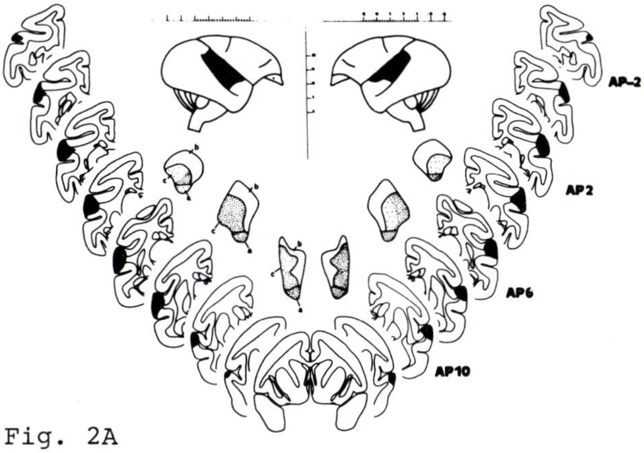

Fig. 2A

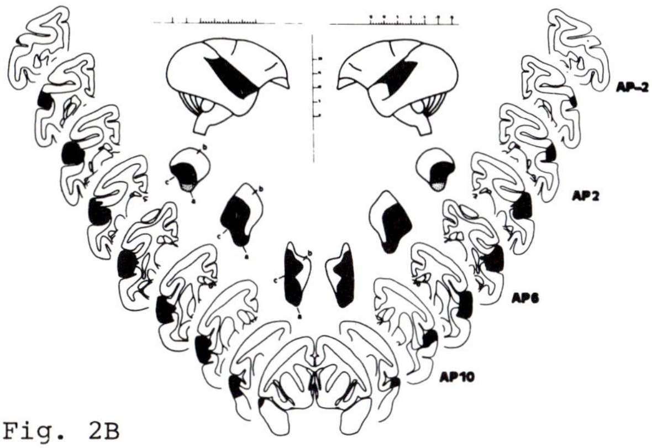

Fig. 2B

part of the medial geniculate body the retrograde degeneration is almost total.

During the whole post-operation training phase with 320 trials the performance of these severely lesioned animals remained at chance level.

There was another important difference between animals with mediumsized lesions and those with large lesions. Two animals from each group were tested with a simple discrimination test. In this task a single pair of stimuli was used: The yapping call was positively reinforced whereas white noise of equal duration and intensity was not; the frequency ranges of both stimuli were similar. The animals with the medium-sized lesions reached criterion within 20 and 40 trials, respectively. The animals with the large lesions could not learn this task within 200 trials. They could, however, easily learn to jump when calls were presented and to refrain from jumping in the inter-trial interval.

Discussion

We can conclude from these experiments that after almost complete ablation of the auditory cortex the animals were unable to discriminate species-specific vocalization from other sounds. That this deficit cannot be explained by a simple hearing loss or loss of memory for the task is proven by the fact that the animals performed perfectly on a task in which only go-stimuli were presented. The animals with medium-sized lesions, which were able to learn the simplified task, namely to discriminate between yapping and white noise, were also able to perform above chance on the generalization task. On the other hand, the animals with large lesions, which were unable to retain the generalization ability, also lost the ability to perform the two-stimuli task. Thus these animals could recognize whether there was a sound or no sound, but they were no longer able to discriminate further.

Precisely this inability to discriminate complex auditory stimuli of any kind is known in humans. This specific impairment is called auditory agnosia (Freud, 1891). About 30 cases have been reported. In each case where the pathology was available large bilateral lesions (mostly infarctions) of the auditory cortex were found. These patients were neither able to understand spoken language nor to identify musical instruments, animal sounds, melodies or noises of any other kind. One of Lhermitte's patients commented on her disability: "Je n'entends rien. C'est toujours le même bruit."

Auditory agnosia is clearly separable from Wernicke's aphasia. The patients can speak in a meaningful way, and they can read aloud and follow written instructions, although they cannot understand spoken language. In a sensory aphasia-like deficit in the monkey one would expect that the animal would fail to identify the calls of its own species but would still be able to discriminate other complex sounds. Yet our study has shown that auditory discrimination was lost for all complex sounds.

References:

1) Freud, S.: Zur Auffassung der Aphasien. Wien: Deuticke (1891).
2) Hupfer, K.; Jürgens, U.; Ploog, D.: The effect of superior temporal lesions on the recognition of species-specific calls in the squirrel monkey. Exp. Brain Res. 30, 75-87 (1977).
3) Lhermitte, F.; Chain, F.; Escourolle, R.; Ducarne, B.; Pillon, B.; Chedru, F.: Étude des troubles perceptifs auditifs dans les lésions temporales bilatérales. Rev.neurol. 124, 329-351 (1971).
4) Neff, W.D.; Diamond, I.T.; Casseday, J.H.: Behavioral studies of auditory discrimination: central nervous system. In: Handbook of Sensory Physiology, W.D. Keidel; W.D. Neff (eds.), Berlin: Springer, Vol. V/2, 307-400 (1975).
5) Wernicke, C.: Der aphasische Symptomenkomplex. Eine psychologische Studie auf anatomischer Basis. Breslau: Max Cohn & Weigert (1874). Reprinted by Springer-Verlag, Berlin-Heidelberg-New York (1974).

Selective Impairment of Perception of Articulatory Place in a Case of Cortical Auditory Disorder

G. MICELI and G. GAINOTTI, Clinica Neurologica,Universita Cattolica, 00168 Roma, Italy

A long credited view (1) considered all comprehension disorders in aphasic patients to stem from a phonemic hearing disorder. This standpoint has been now almost completely discarded (2,3), but the fact remains that some aphasics do have problems in phonological processing, even if the relevance of these problems to the genesis of comprehension disorders is far from clear. The distinctive feature framework (4) has been given renewed attention by neuropsychologists as a model to the study of phonological impairment in aphasia. Some studies (2,5-7) have shown that, among distinctive features, place of articulation seems to be more affected than voicing in patients with aphasic symptoms. This has been tentatively attributed to a more linguistic nature of feature place and to a more acoustic nature of feature voice. However, most often <u>both</u> features are impaired in aphasia (even if to a different degree), so that one is left with the doubt as to whether voice and place are two distinct psychological realities or rather an overimposed artifact. For these reasons it may prove useful to report on a case of cortical auditory disorder in which a selective impairment of feature place was found.

CASE REPORT

The patient is a 54-years old high-school teacher of mathematics. She suffered from two hemispheric strokes in Sept 1974 and Feb 1977, which caused a large right and a smaller left temporal infarction respectively, seen by CT-scan. Neuropsychological examination was made on Jan 1978. Mild neurosensory hearing loss was shown by standard audiometric tests. Language was nearly normal, with few phonemic and very few semantic paraphasias and word-finding pauses. Comprehension on visual data was normal. Auditory comprehension was severely impaired. Music and meaningful sounds could not be either named or recognized satisfactorily in multiple-choice tests. Speech sounds were somewhat better perceived. Dichotic listening tests ruled out the hypothesis of a disconnection syndrome; whenever an asymmetry was noted, it was due to a right ear advantage.

The symptoms shown by the patient could then be defined as a mixed cortical auditory disorder, with an almost total auditory agnosia and a very severe word deafness.

MATERIALS AND METHODS

1) Natural speech sounds

Only stop consonants will be reported. The 6 stops can be contrasted in voicing (/p t k/ are voiceless, /b d g/ are voiced), in place of articulation (/p b/ are bilabial, /t d/ are alveolar, /k g/ are velar) or in both. Thus, for each phoneme, one voice error, two place errors and two voice+place errors are possible (e.g. for /p/, /b/ is the voice error, /t k/ are the place errors, /d g/ are the voice+place errors).

The examiner read aloud one stimulus at a time. His lips were hidden from the patient's eyes. The patient had to point to the syllable she had perceived. The test syllables were written in large characters on cardboards. Stimuli were repeated, if necessary, until the patient had confidently chosen a syllable. Each of the three tests has been administered in ten blocks of 60 stimuli each. No more than two sessions each day were made.

a) Consonant-Consonant-Vowel-Constant (CCVC) Identification Test. Stimuli were/ prin trin krin brin drin grin/. Each stop was presented 100 times.

b) Consonant-Vowel (CV) Identification Test. Each of the 6 stops was followed by each of 5 vowel sounds /a e i o u/. Stimuli were 30 (/pa pe pi po pu ba be.../). In a screening test the patient had had no problems in vowel identification. Since the proportion of errors on stops did not vary according to the vowel in second position, it was decided to group together the responses according to the consonant,without considering the vowel. Each of 30 stimuli was repeated 20 times; then, each stop was presented 100 times, as in the previous test.

c) Vowel-Consonant (VC) Identification Test. The same phonemes as in b) were used, but their order was inverted. Stimuli were /ap ep ip op up ab eb.../. For the same reasons as in b), account was taken of stops only. Each stop was presented 100 times

2) Semisynthetic speech sounds.

a) Voice-Onset Time (VOT) Identification. Test I.

b) Voice-Onset Time (VOC) Identification. Test II.

c) Voice-Onset time Discrimination Test.

Other authors (3,2) have used test a) and tests b) and c). For fuller details the reader is referred to these papers. Suffice it to say here that the subject is asked to identify or to discriminate semisynthetic stimuli varying along a voicing continuum from /da/ to /ta/.

d) Place Identification Test. Stimuli whose formant transitions varied along a continuum were presented to the patient, who was asked to point to the syllable she had identified. Normal controls perceive these stimuli as voiced stops (/ba da ga/).

e) Place Discrimination Test. Each of the stimuli used in d) was paired either with itself or with the stimulus next along the continuum. The patient had to say whether the two syllables were identical or different.

Fig. 1. Results obtained by the patient on the natural speech sounds identification tests. At the top, the confusion matrix (CCVC, CV, VC) is shown. Stimuli are reported in the rows, patient's responses in the columns. At the bottom, the errors and their distribution according to the ill-perceived feature(s) are shown

PERFORMANCES OBTAINED BY THE PATIENT ON THE THREE NATURAL SPEECH SOUNDS TESTS

CCVC	B	D	G	P	T	K
B	80	12	7	1		
D	27	69	3	1		
G	18	54	28			
P	7			48	29	16
T				1	71	28
K				1	4	95

CV	B	D	G	P	T	K
B	39	52	7	2		
D	4	94	1		1	
G		26	74			
P		7	1	36	32	24
T		2			84	14
K	1		1			98

VC	B	D	G	P	T	K
B	32	55	6	6	1	
D		89	10		1	
G	1	7	91			1
P	2	3	6	29	25	35
T		1		2	93	4
K			12			88

	CCVC	CV	VC
Errors:	209 (34.8%)	175 (29.2%)	178 (29.6%)
Place Errors:	200 (95.7%)	160 (91.4%)	145 (81.5%)
Voice Errors:	8 (3.8%)	6 (3.5%)	23 (12.9%)
Voice + Place Errors:	1 (0.5%)	9 (5.2%)	10 (5.6%)

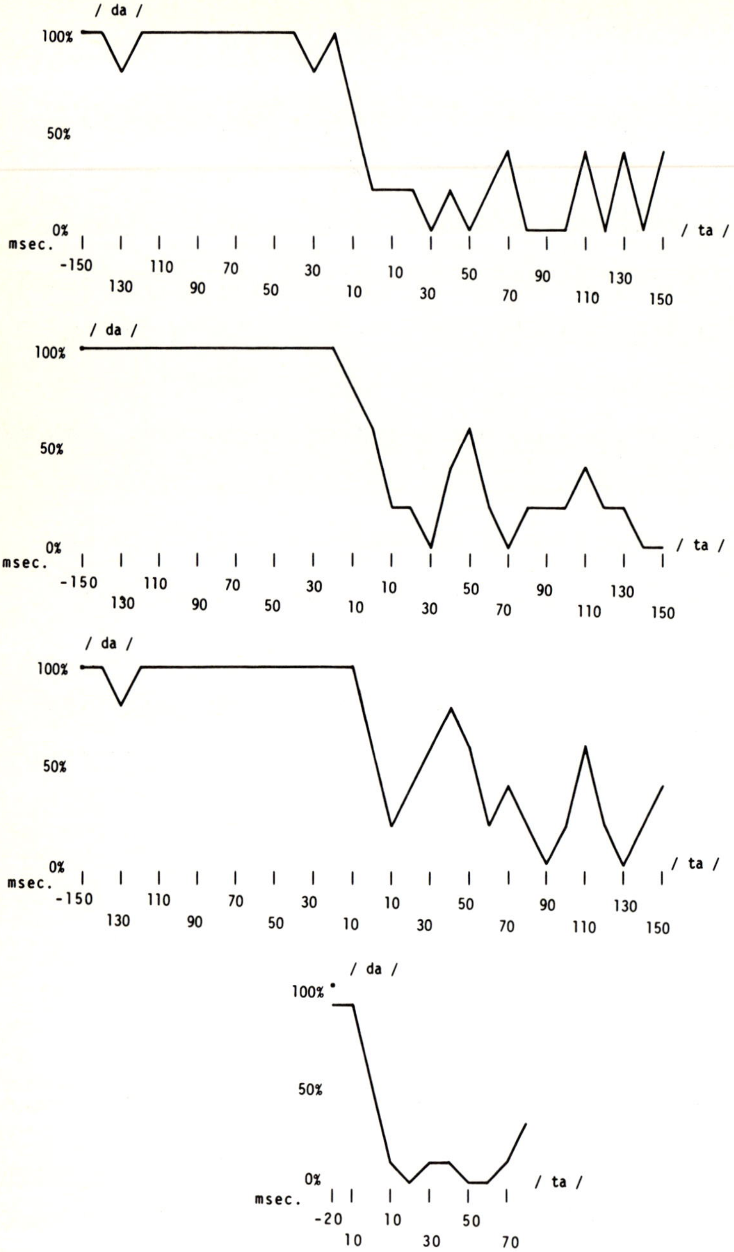

Fig. 2. Semisynthetic CV syllables tests. Results obtained by the patient on VOT Identification Test I (upper three diagrams) and Test II (lower diagram)

RESULTS

1) Natural speech sounds.

Results are shown in Figure 1. According to what has been said in the previous section, a chance distribution of errors would result in a (voice):(place):(voice+place) ratio of 1:2:2. It can be seen, on the contrary, that place errors (ranging from 95.7% of total errors in CCVC test to 81.5% in VC test) dramatically outnumber both voice (from 12.9% in VC to 3.5% in CV) and voice+place errors (from 5.6% in VC to 0.5% in CCVC).

2) Semisynthetic speech sounds.

VOT Identification tests, as shown in Figure 2, show a good preservation of the identification of stimuli in the voiced range, while voiceless stimuli were often incorrectly perceived. The patient performed at chance level on VOT Discrimination. Both Place tests yielded very poor results, with chance distribution.

DISCUSSION

A gross phoneme recognition disorder was revealed in our patient. A clearcut dissociation was found between a good preservation of the processing of feature voice and a very disturbed perception of feature place. It does not mean, of course, that phonological impairment is the only cause of word deafness, or that such an impairment is found in all cases of cortical auditory disorder. In other cases with damage to auditory perception in which the phonological level has been explored, either a pre-phonetic disorder has been found, equally involving both voice and place perception (8,9), or only a trend was noted for place errors to outnumber voice errors (10,11), but never was a dissociation between the two features seen. Many reasons can explain such discrepancies. Among patients with cortical auditory disorders, very few have pure auditory agnosia, some have pure word deafness and most a combination of the two. Furthermore, the disorder results sometimes from a single left temporale lobe damage, other times from bilateral cerebral infarctions successively involving both hemispheres (and the sequence of the strokes is also of relevance to the clinical features shown by the patient (12)).

Lastly, in some cases a disconnection syndrome is found, while in others the extension of cortical damage seems to be most critical. For these reasons, one cannot be too surprised in finding such different performance.

However, in our case of mixed cortical auditory disorder the presence of phonological impairment cannot be disputed. It may have played a relevant (though not absolute) role in the pathogenesis of auditory comprehension damage. Even if obtained from a single-case study of a patient with a very peculiar disorder the pattern of phonological impairment must be stressed. The finding that the processing of place of articulation was selectively impaired, while feature voice was well-preserved is not simply the confirmation of previously reported data (2,5-7). It is also a convincing evidence in favor of voicing and place of articulation being separate psychological realities, and lends further support to the distinctive feature hypothesis.

References:

1) Luria, A.: Traumatic aphasia. Mouton, The Hague (1970).
2) Blumstein, S.E; Baker, E.; Goodglass, H.: Phonological factors in auditory comprehension in aphasia. Neuropsychologia 15, 19-30 (1977).
3) Basso, A.; Casati, G.; Vignolo, L.A.: Phonemic identification defect in aphasia. Cortex 13, 85-95 (1977).
4) Jakobson, R.; Halle, M.; Fant, G.: Preliminaries to speech analysis. M.I.T. Press, Cambridge (1962).
5) Blumstein, S.E.: A phonological investigation of aphasic speech. Mouton, The Hague (1973).
6) Oscar-Berman, M.; Zurif, E.B.; Blumstein, S.E.: Effects of unilateral brain damage on the perception of speech sounds. Brain and Language 2, 345-355 (1975).
7) Miceli, G.; Gainotti, G.; Caltagirone, C.; Payer-Rigo, P.: Discrimination of voice versus place contrasts in aphasia. Brain and Language 6, 47-51 (1978).
8) Denes, G.; Semenza, C.: Auditory-modality anomia: Evidence from a case of pure word deafness. Cortex 11, 401-411, (1975).
Saffran, E.M.; Marin, O.S.M.; Yeni-Komshian, G.H.: An analysis of speech perception in word deafness. Brain and Language 3, 209-229 (1976).
10) Consoli, S.: Performance d'un groupe d'aphasiques àun test de discrimination phonémique. Journal de psychologie normale et pathologique, 66, 325- 348 (1975).
11) Chocholle, R.; Chedru, F.; Botte, M.C.; Lhermitte, F.: Etude psychoacoustique d'un cas de "surditéverbale". Neuropsychologia 13, 163-172 (1975).
12) Ulrich, G.: Interhemispheric functional relationships in auditory agnosia. An analysis of the preconditions and a conceptual model. Brain and Language 5, 286-300 (1978).

Phonemic Auditory Discrimination and Articulatory Defects in Aphasia

J. DEROUESNE, B. SAILLANT, Laboratoire de Neuropsychologie, INSERM U. 84, Hôpital de la Salpêtrière, Paris, France

For a long time, it was thought that patients suffering from an articulatory defect had little or no trouble in the auditory processing of language. However, some recent research has shown that certain subjects suffering from an articulatory defect following a cortical lesion may also have a real defect in the auditory processing of phonemes (1,2,3,4). These last results provoke 2 questions. Firstly, is there a specific relation between an articulatory defect and a defect in the auditory processing of phonemes? In our opinion, these researches do not enable us to answer this question. On the one hand, the characteristics of the processing impairment were similar when subjects had articulatory defects or other defects such as phonemic paraphasias (4,5). On the other hand, the patients suffering from an impairment in the auditory processing of phonemes often had severe aphasia in which several defects have been observed. This made it impossible to decide whether their impairment in the auditory processing of phonemes was actually related to their articulatory defect or to some other defects. Secondly, what kinds of articulatory defect are related to an impairment of the auditory processing of phonemes? For in the researches mentioned, some subjects having articulatory defects also showed impairment of the auditory processing of phonemes, whereas others did not.

The main aim of the present study is to answer the first question concerning the specific relation between articulatory defects following a cortical lesion and a defect in the auditory processing of phonemes. The second aim of the study is to identify a category of articulatory defects associated with a defect in the auditory processing of phonemes. This will allow a partial answer to the second question.

METHOD:

1) Phonemic auditory discrimination

In order to show the relation between some articulatory defects and a defect in the auditory processing of phonemes, an experimental variable thought to correspond to the role of articulation in the auditory discrimination of phonemes was chosen. Then, we researched the question if the phonemic discrimination defect in some aphasic subjects suffering from an articulatory impairment was affected by this variable.

Experimental variable

The variable was the proprioceptive cue provided by articulatory movements. Such cues are more or less perceptible according to the phonemes to be discriminated. Two kinds of phoneme-pairs were compared. In the first pair-category, the proprioceptive cues were not very perceptible to the subject: the phonemes differed in the presence or absence of vibration in the vocal cords (for example b and p). In the second pair-category the proprioceptive cues were very perceptible; the phonemes differed according to their place of articulation: front or middle (for example p and t) and middle or back (for example n and ŋ).

Phonemic auditory discrimination test (P.A.D. test). The test was composed of 120 pairs of syllables (a constant followed by the vowel "ə"). In 60 pairs, the two consonants were the same. In 60 other pairs, the two consonants were different: 30 pairs included two consonants the articulation of which provides non-perceptible proprioceptive cues for their discrimination; the other 30 pairs included two consonants the articulation of which provides very perceptible proprioceptive cues for their discrimination.

2) Analysis of articulatory defects

The subjects suffering from articulatory defects effected a repetition-test. The results of this test made it possible to specify the nature of their articulatory impairment. This test, described in a previous research (5), enables one to distinguish two types of articulatory disturbance, already evoked by Jakobson (6) and Luria (7) in reference to kinesthesic and kinetic aphasia: one in the production of phoneme (disturbance of the simultaneous articulatory component) and the other in the production of successive phonemes (disturbance of the successive articulatory component). Articulatory defects in phoneme-production varied according to the articulatory complexity of the phonemes to be produced, whereas they did not vary with the number of phonemes to be produced. Conversely, defects in the production of successive phonemes varied with the number of phonemes and did not vary with their articulatory difficulty.

3) <u>Subjects</u>

The study was carried out on 3 non-fluent aphasic patients who had articulatory impairment. In order to be sure that the effect of the experimental variable was not simply due to degree of difficulty, 3 aphasic control subjects suffering from phonemic paraphasias also performed the P.A.D. test.

RESULTS

P.A.D. test

Impairment in the phonemic auditory discrimination of subjects A,B,C having an articulatory defect (table 1) was severe when the proprioceptive cues were perceptible, and slight when these cues were not perceptible. The results of control subjects D, E,F, suffering form phonemic paraphasias were the reverse.

Table 1. Test of phonemic auditory discrimination: number of errors according as proprioceptive cues are perceptible or not

		Proprioceptive cues non-perceptible (30 pairs)	Proprioceptive cues perceptible (30 pairs)	Comparisons
Subjects with articulatory defect	A	2	11	$X^2_1 = 6,64$ $P = .001$
	B	2	17	$X^2_1 = 15,78$ $P < .001$
	C	2	11	$X^2_1 = 6,64$ $P = .001$
Control subjects	D	15	1	$X^2_1 = 15$ $P < .001$
	E	17	3	$X^2_1 = 14,6$ $P < .001$
	F	18	2	$X^2_1 = 19,2$ $P < .001$

Repetition-test

The articulatory impairments suffered from by the 2 subjects A and B were clearly affected by articulatory complexity and not by length (table 2). The articulatory impairment suffered from by the subject C was affected by both variables.

Comments

1) The results clearly indicate that aphasic subjects suffering from an articulatory defect may have an impairment in the auditory processing of phonemes which is directly linked with their articulatory defect: their impairment in the auditory discrimination of phonemes was severe or slight according to whether or not articulation provided proprioceptive cues for this discrimination. These results were not obtained because pairs of phonemes with proprioceptive cues are more difficult than pairs of phonemes with few proprioceptive cues. Indeed, the results of the 3 subjects suffering from phonemic paraphasias were the complete reverse of those of the 3 subjects suffering from an articulatory defect.

2) Another aim was to identify a kind of articulatory defect which is linked with a phonemic auditory discrimination defect.

Table 2. Test of repetition: percentage of errors according to articulatory complexity and length of stimuli

	Articulatory complexity			Length		
	easy	difficult		easy	difficult	
A	6%	16%	$P < .001$	11%	10%	N.S.
B	23%	35%	$P < .01$	31%	28%	N.S
C	46%	59%	$P < .01$	44%	57%	$P < .01$

In this study, 2 out of 3 subjects (subjects A and B) had a single defect in phoneme-production; it is therefore possible to conclude that this category of articulatory defect is linked to an impairment of the auditory discrimination of phonemes. And 1 subject (subject C) showed a defect both in phoneme-production and in the production of successive phonemes. Yet he manifested the same discriminatory defect as the other two subjects. It would therefore seem that the correct auditory discrimination of some aphasics with anterior left hemisphere lesions is linked with the fact that their articulatory disturbances stem from a disturbance of the production of successive phonemes and not of the production of phonemes.

References:

1) Assal, G.: Troubles de la réception auditive du langage lors des lésions du cortex cérébral. Cortex, 12,3, 399-402 (1974).

2) Basso, A.; Casati, G. and Vignolo, L.A.: Phonemic identification defect in aphasia. Cortex, 13, 85-95 (1977).

3) Blumstein, S.E.; Baker, E. and Goodglass, H.: Phonological factors in auditory comprehension in aphasia. Neuropsychologia 15,1, 19-30 (1977).

4) Blumstein, S.; Cooper, W.E.; Zurif, E.B.; Caramazza, A.: The perception and production of voice onset time in aphasia. Neuropsychologia, 15, 371-383 (1977).

5) Dérouesné, J.; Beauvois, M.F. et Ranty, C.: Deux composantes dans l'articulation du langage oral: preuve expérimentale de leur indépendance. Neuropsychologia, 15, 143-153 (1977).

6) Jakobson, R.: Towards a linguistic typology of aphasic impairments. In: Disorders of Language. A CIBA Foundation Symposium, Churchill, London (1964).

7) Luria, A.R.: Higher cortical functions in man. Tavistock publications, London (1966).

Comprehension of Natural Sounds in Aphasia

R. COHEN and W. H. EHRENSTEIN, Sonderforschungsbereich 99 (Linguistik), University of Konstanz, W. Germany

Vignolo and his coworkers (3,5) have shown aphasics to be impaired not only in language performance but also on tasks requiring the matching of natural sounds to pictures of the corresponding sound sources. Aphasics appear to be exceptionally prone to "semantic" errors, i.e. to choose pictures belonging to the same semantic category as the correct source of sound, e.g. cock instead of canary. They performed as well as controls on a "Meaningless Sounds Discrimination Test" but failed in a "Meanfingful Sounds Identification Test".

Experiment I In order to further investigate the relative proprotion of semantic and acoustic errors a test was constructed (6) comprising 21 items corresponding to the items from the studies mentioned above (3,5) and 25 new items. The new items differed from the others with regard to the semantic distractors: though still belonging to the same semantic category as the sound source they were selected not as producers of acoustically different sounds (e.g. canary - cock) but as being characteristically silent (e.g. alarm clock - sundial). Thus confusion amongst these items could not be attributed to difficulties in auditory processing. To correct for differences in attention the number of "odd" responses (i.e. choice of a sound source which is neither acoustically nor semantically similar to the correct one, e.g. train - sheep) was taken as the best estimate, and subtracted from the number of semantic and acoustic errors.

Subjects were 20 Broca's and 19 Wernicke's aphasics, 20 brain-damaged patients without aphasia, and 20 chronic schizophrenics; all were right-handed male German speakers. Groups were matched for age ($47.2 \leq M \leq 48.2$) and an index combining educational level and occupation. To control for severity of brain damage, the two aphasic groups and the control group of brain-damaged patients were also matched with regard to their performance on Form A of the Trail Making Test.

Procedure. Patients were instructed to match one of four pictures on a given card to the sound delivered simultaneously by a tape recorder. Several practice trials were given to ensure that the task has been understood. On each trial the experimenter named the 4 depicted objects and then started the tape recorder.

Results. Considering all types of errors together, Broca's as well as Wernicke's aphasics made significantly ($z = 2.55$ resp. $z = 2.49$; $p < .05$) more errors than the brain-damaged controls without aphasia. The same was true ($z = 2.24$; $p < .05$) for the semantic errors from the 21 items adapted from (3,5). All other differences between groups remained nonsignificant ($z \leq 1.41$; $p > .10$). There was no evidence for a bias towards more "semantic" than "acoustic" errors, whether or not the error scores were corrected with respect to "odd" errors. For all groups, both acoustic and semantic errors exceeded the number of odd errors. In contrast to the items adapted from (3) and (5), aphasics did not make more "semantic" errors than the two other groups on the 25 newly constructed items with semantic distractors that were not associated with any characteristic sound. Aphasics took into account the muteness of the distractor, stressing the possible relevance of acoustic discriminations. Perhaps, paradoxically, the preponderance of "semantic" over "acoustic" errors in (5) should be reinterpreted: the "acoustic" distractors might have been easier for the aphasics to discriminate semantically than the "semantic" distractors were to discriminate with respect to their acoustic features.

Experiment II The cross-modal nature of the sound-to-picture matching task in Experiment I led us to carry out a second experiment matching sounds to words, presented in the same, auditory, modality (2).

Patients were the same as in Experiment I. The order in which Experiments I and II were carried out was balanced across patients.

Procedure. Stimuli were sounds produced by objects, animals and humans, ten for each category. The words were either nouns denoting the source (e.g. "dog") or verbs referring to the production of sound (e.g. "barking"). This differentiation between nouns and verbs was not possible for "human" sounds (laughing, coughing, crying). Each sound-word combination was presented twice in immediate succession. Fifty percent of the combinations were incorrect with the word denoting a semantically similar object or activity. The patient was instructed to listen to the presentation and to indicate by yes-no answers whether or not the combination was appropriate.

Results. Both groups of aphasics made significantly more errors than the brain-damaged controls and chronic schizophrenics for sounds produced by either animals or objects ($3.07 \leqq z \leqq 3.83$; $p < .01$). All other differences between groups were nonsignificant ($0.31 \leqq z \leqq 1.60$; $p > .10$). In contrast to the conditions using animal or object sounds aphasics performed as well as the control groups with respect to human sounds. Comparing performance in the three sound conditions within groups by means of the Friedman test showed significant effects only in the aphasics (Broca's $x^2 = 12.70$; $p < .01$); Wernicke's $x^2 = 6.32$; $p < .05$).

This difference between human and other sounds can hardly be reduced to the fact that only for human sounds the same words could be accepted as either verbs or nouns; for animal and object sounds aphasic patients made less errors with nouns than with verbs ($z = 2.51$; $p < .05$). Neither can it be reduced to differences in word frequencies (as estimated by a group of students): differences between human and object sounds were nonsignificant; only animal sounds showed a somewhat lower word frequency.

One might consider the possibility that word frequencies are different for different groups; aphasics might more often hear words referring to human activities as compared to sounds produced by animals or objects. Another factor might be that only for the human sounds the listeners could also be the "speakers" even if they were aphasic. Proprioceptive and/or innervatory cues stimulated by the acoustic patterns, as suggested by the motor theory of speech perception (cf. 4,7), could compensate for deficiencies in acoustic discrimination of aphasics. Here, we are generalizing from speech to other human-produced sounds. Total error scores from both experiments are highly correlated in both Broca's and Wernicke's aphasics with the Peabody Picture Vocabulary Test as a measure of verbal comprehension, $.58 \leq \text{rho} \leq .68$, with performance in picture naming, $.62 \leq \text{rho} \leq .82$, and with the Token Test, $.51 \leq \text{rho} \leq .69$. The deficiencies encountered in the two sound-matching tasks thus appear closely related to a more general impairment, characteristic of both fluent and non-fluent aphasics. This impairment cannot be reduced to semantic confusions but might be related to specific deficits (as shown elsewhere: 1,8) of aphasic patients in discriminating both verbal and non-verbal complex acoustic stimuli.

References:

1) Blumstein, S.E.; Baker, E. & Goodglass, H.: Phonological factors in auditory comprehension in aphasia. Neuropsychologia 15, 19-30 (1977).

2) Cohen, R.; Fries, P.; Woll, G.: Das Erkennen natürlicher Geräusche bei aphasischen Patienten. In preparation

3) Faglioni, P.; Spinnler, H. & Vignolo, L.A.: Contrasting behavior of right and left hemisphere-damaged patients on a discriminative and a semantic task of auditory recognition. Cortex 5, 366-389 (1969).

4) Liberman, A.M.; Cooper, F.S.; Shankweiler, D.P. & Studdert-Kennedy, M.: Perception of the speech code. Psychological Review 74, 431-461 (1967).

5) Spinnler, H. & Vignolo, L.A.: Impaired recognition of meaningful sounds in aphasia. Cortex 2, 337-348 (1966).

6) Strohner, H.; Cohen, R.; Kelter, S. & Woll, G.: "Semantic" and "acoustic" errors of aphasic and schizophrenic patients in a sound-to-picture matching task. Cortex 14, 391-403 (1978).

7) Studdert-Kennedy, M.: Speech perception. In: N.J. Lass (ed.), Contemporary issues in experimental phonetics. New York, Academic Press, 243-293 (1976).

8) Tallal, P. & Newcombe, F.: Impairment of auditory perception and language comprehension in dysphasia. Brain and Language 5, 13-24 (1978).

Lexical and Syntactic Factors in Language Comprehension of Aphasic Patients

W. HUBER, Department of Neurology, RWTH Aachen, West Germany

Introduction:

Most assumptions on the nature of aphasic disorders are based on language production. However, recent investigations of language comprehension (Pizzamiglio and Parisi, 1970; Lesser, 1974; Gainotti et al., 1975; Stachowiak et al., 1975) render many of these assumptions less justified. Is it also the case that all groups of aphasic patients are inferior to brain damaged and normal controls at least in some aspect of language comprehension? Is it also possible to delineate aphasic syndromes in terms of specific symptoms of impaired language comprehension? Is it at all possible to detect linguistic factors that influence language comprehension specifically and seperately in condition of aphasia? Are aphasic disorders of language comprehension supramodal in the sense that they occur in both the auditory-phonetic and in the visual-graphemic mode of presentation? Are aphasic disorders in language comprehension comparable in extent and range to those in language production?

In order to assess the influence of specific linguistic factors on language comprehension of aphasic patients we designed two types of word-picture and sentence-picture matching tasks.

Methods and Material:

In each task there was a multiple choice set of four pictures, one depicting the meaning of the verbal stimulus, one having a close and two having a remote linguistic relationship to the target picture. The verbal stimuli, words or sentences, were given in both the auditory and the visual mode of presentation. The four types of tasks were designed along the following linguistic parameters:

1. Semantic similarity between complex words. - The target picture referred to a stimulus word like hochziehen 'heaving up' in contrast to hochheben 'lifting up', literally 'picking up', the meaning of which was likewise depicted.

2. Homonymy of words. - The nondominant meaning was taken as verbal stimulus e.g. Pfeife meaning either 'whistle' (nondominant) or 'tobacco pipe' (dominant). The target picture of a whistle had to be discriminated from a picture of a cigarette which exhibits a contrast-coordinate relation to the dominant meaning of the homonym. (cf. Stachowiak, 1979).

3. Situational similarity between the meanings of sentences. - Similarity was based on differences in time reference between two pragmatically related situations. With a stimulus sentence like he'll certainly end up in jail we had a target picture of a man getting arrested, and a contrasting picture of a man already in jail.

4. Pronominalization of sentences. - Stimulus sentences were questions like which picture shows what she is doing requiring the semantic discrimination between personal pronouns. The

target picture was that of a girl cleaning up in contrast to that of a boy doing garden work.

Exactly the same linguistic parameters were observed in the auditory and the visual version of each type of task. All reactions were scored as follows: 3 for pointing to the correct picture, 2 for demanding a repetition of oral or visual representation and pointing to the correct picture, 1 for pointing to the picture with a close linguistic relationship to the stimulus, 0 for pointing to one of the two pictures with a remote linguistic relationship to the stimulus.

Subjects:

We examined 5 groups of 15 patients each, 3 groups of patients with global, Wernicke's and Broca's aphasia and 2 control groups of patients with and without damage of the non-dominant right hemisphere. All subjects, including the normal non-brain-damaged controls, were taken from a clinical population that was seen in our wards during the course of about half a year. The groups were matched as well as possible for sex, age, etiology, duration of brain damage and education. The classification of aphasic syndromes was based on the evaluation of spontaneous speech by four independent raters.

Results and Discussion:

The mean scores for auditory as well as for reading comprehension are given in figure 1. In both modes the overall pattern is rather similar.

Homonymous words and pronominalized sentences proved to be most difficult. Numerically, this holds true for all aphasic

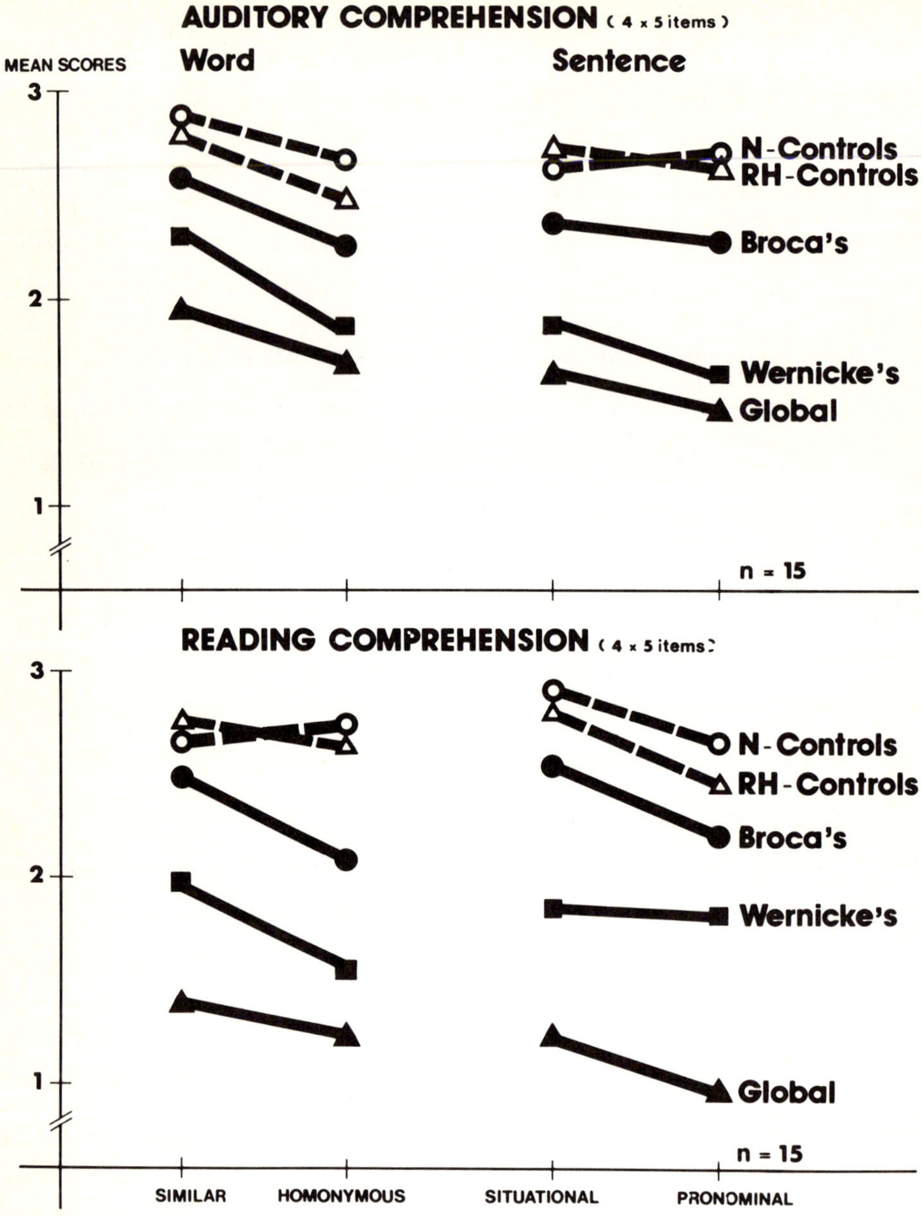

Fig. 1.

subgroups. The purely linguistic interpretation of this finding is that homonymy and pronominalization are language specific to a higher degree than semantic and situational similarity and therefore seem to be more sensitive to aphasia impairment. Thus the data would indicate that language comprehension in aphasia is indeed influenced by specific linguistic factors. However, the data certainly do not indicate that there are clear interactions between aphasic subgroups, neither with respect to the overall processing of words versus sentences nor with respect to the two lexical and the two syntactic parameters of each task. In all eight experimental conditions we found rather similar gradations: Broca's aphasics were least and global aphasics were most affected.

We applied analysis of variance separately to the data obtained from auditory and reading comprehension using a split-split-plot design (Kirk, 1968). There were significant main and simple effects, but no significant interactions with respect to the groups. Significant differences with respect to the two types of words were found in both the auditory and the reading condition, with respect to the two types of sentences, however, only in the reading condition. These were overall effects which could not be established for any of the individual groups, presumably because of the rather small sample sizes of 15 subjects only.

In order to compare the two modes of presentation we applied a third analysis of variance, again using a split-split-plot design with modes of presentation as the one split-factor and words versus sentences as the other one. Reading was found to be significantly more difficult only for patients with global aphasia on both the word and sentence level. For them, comprehension of written sentences was such a demanding task that only under this particular condition they were significantly poorer than patients with Wernicke's aphasia. Obviously, with extended damage to the dominant hemisphere purely graphemic difficulties are combined with the more basic lexical and syntactic impairment. With respect to differences among groups, comparisons yielded the following pattern in both modes of presentation: No differences were found between the Brocas and each of the control groups. Only Wernickes and globals were - as expected - significantly poorer than the two control groups. Furthermore, globals and Brocas, but not Wernickes and Brocas differed significantly under both the auditory and the reading condition.

From these results one certainly cannot conclude that the difficulties of aphasic patients to comprehend words and sentences are primarily caused by an impairment in acoustic and phonetic processing. Such a view could hardly explain the same or even higher amount of comprehension difficulties in the visual-graphemic mode of presentation. As in production, the aphasic impairment in comprehension is not restricted to just one mode of performance but is supramodal in nature. This latter assumption can also explain the rather parallel influence of specific lexical and syntactic features we found in both modes of performance.

Control experiment:

Our results are rather disappointing if one had hoped to find a differentiation between aphasic subgroups. Reliable differences were only found between patients with global and Broca's aphasia. This is in contrast to the results from a production task which was part of the same investigation. In this production task the

patients were shown pictures of situations and asked to describe the situation by a whole sentence. The range of verbal reactions adequate in form and content to be scored as correct was assessed in a pilot stüdy with normal subjects. Compatible reactions were given a score of 3. Deviations in form - score of 2 - were mainly expected from Broca's aphasics and deviations in content plus optional deviation in form - score of 1 - mainly from Wernicke's aphasics. No reaction, perseveration, automatism, jargon - all given a score of 0 - should be characteristic for global aphasics. The results - as seen on figure 2 - were in suprisingly good agreement with these expectations.
Again we applied an analysis of variance. Because of heterogeneous variances (assessed by Hartley's F_{max}-Test) we made a correction for the degrees of freedom (Brown and Forsythe, 1974).

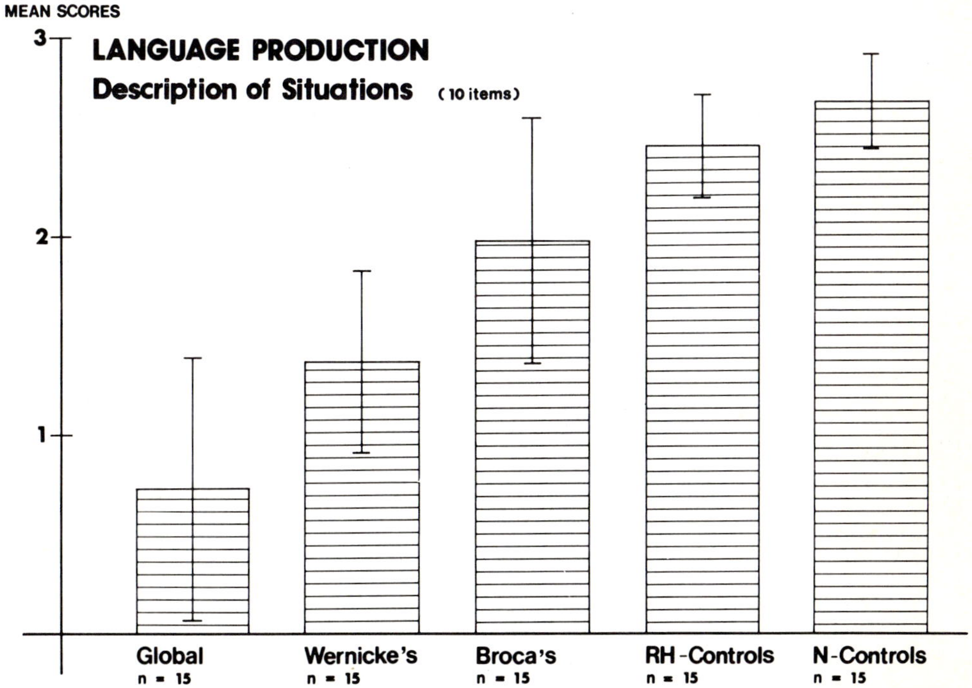

Fig. 2.

Succeeding pairwise comparisons yielded significant differences not only between each aphasic subgroup and each control group, but also between any two of the aphasic subgroups. The two control groups, however, did not differ significantly. The results of this control experiment make it quite clear that the degree and the range of aphasic impairment in language production differs quite remarkably from language comprehension. It seems reasonable to conclude that the linguistic strategies underlying comprehension are either less specialized and have a less limited representation in the brain or are functionally different from the strategies underlying language production. On the other hand, if one holds the view of many linguists that production and comprehension of language have organizational factors in common, one is led to conclude, that the impairment of these basic linguistic factors is more easily compensated for in comprehension than in production.

Acknowledgement: I would like to thank Dorothea Weniger, Klaus Poeck, Rainald Schuldes and Andrea Kleinmanns for their help in carrying out this study and Klaus Willmes (Medizinische Statistik, RWTH Aachen) for the statistical evaluation of the data.

References:

1) Brown, M.B.; A.B. Forsythe: The ANOVA and multiple comparisons for data with heterogeneous variances. Biometrics 30, 719-724 (1974).
2) Kirk, R.E.: Experimental design procedures for the behavioral sciences. Belmont, Cal.: Brooks and Cole (1968).
3) Lesser, R.: Verbal comprehension in aphasia: An English version of three Italian tests. Cortex 10, 278-284 (1974).
4) Pizzamiglio, L., D. Parisi: Studies on verbal comprehension in aphasia. In: G.B. Flores d'Arcais and W.J.M. Levelt (eds.), Advances in psycholinguistics. Amsterdam/London: North Holland.
5) Stachowiak, F.-J.: Die semantische Struktur des Lexikons. München, Fink (1979).
6) Stachowiak, F.-J.; W. Huber; K. Poeck; M. Kerschensteiner: Text comprehension in aphasia. Brain and Language 4, 177-195 (1977).

Interaural Integration in the Perception of Complete and Truncated Words by Brain Damaged and Control Subjects

E. PERRET and A. WYDLER, Neuropsychological Division, Dept. of Neurology, University of Zurich, Switzerland

The integration of acoustic information reaching the two ears of man has been investigated primarily at the functional level of sound localization, which appears to involve mainly brain stem structures of the central nervous system. When the binaural integration of meaningful stimuli, mostly verbal, is considered, however, the experimental data become more scanty. They are based almost exclusively on dichotic listening studies, according to the technique published by Broadbent (1954) and first applied to brain damaged patients by Kimura (1961). This author showed that of different verbal stimuli (digits) applied simultaneously to both ears through earphones, those to the right ear were usually better reproduced than those to the left ear. Kimura interpreted her results in terms of the contralateral auditory pathways from the right ear to the left hemisphere (dominant for speech) being functionally and structurally more efficient than the ipsilateral pathways from the left ear, and even having an inhibitory effect upon them. According to this interpretation, the perceptual difference between the two ears has its origin in deep brain structures, without involving the two cerebral hemispheres. In commissurotomized patients, Milner et al. (1968) and Sparks and Geschwind (1968) observed an almost total suppression of digits to the left ear in dichotic listening but not in the simple monaural condition. These findings point to the participation of both hemispheres in the dichotic perceptual process: The verbal stimuli to the left ear would predominantly project to the auditory cortex of the contralateral right hemisphere, and be transferred from there to the other hemisphere dominant for speech. Thus it appears that the simultaneous stimulation of both ears in man may involve either subcortical, or hemispheric and interhemispheric structures, or both.

In contrast to dichotic listening, the application of one part of a word to one ear and the other part to the second ear requires the binaural integration of two meaningless auditory stimuli (parts of a word) into one single, meaningful stimulus (the word). Matzker (1959) filtered words into low and high frequency components and applied these separately to the two ears. Calearo (1962) segmented the words in time, and delivered every second segment to one, the other to the other ear. Matzker as well as Calearo found a perceptual deficit in patients with a lesion in the brain stem, but no effect of lesions in the temporal lobe, pointing to an interaural integration of partial verbal information at the subcortical level.

In view of the discrepancy in the possible cerebral mechanisms involved in dichotic listening and of the few studies in which the effect of lesions at hemispheric level and in the brain stem can be compared in the perception of auditory verbal stimuli, the present study was carried out, aiming at a better understanding of the interaural integration mechanisms in different cerebral structures and in different conditions of auditory verbal perception.

Method:

Subjects: Five patients with left temporal (LT) and five patients with right temporal (RT) lesions verified neuroradiologically and neurosurgically were tested postoperatively. Eleven patients with a brainstem (BS) lesion assessed neurologically also participated in the study. Twelve subjects without known brain damage volunteered as control subjects. All subjects were clearly righthanded. The mean ages in the four groups did not differ significantly ($p=0.12$), but the control subjects were younger than the brain damaged patients.

Control Tests: In an abridged version of the *Token Test* (De Renzi and Vignolo, 1962) the LT group performed at a significant lower level than the control, RT and BS groups (multiple t-Tests, all $p < 0.01$). A similar difference to the disadvantage of the LT group was found in the multiple-choice vocabulary test of Lehrl et al. (1971), (multiple t-Tests, all $p < 0.001$), and in the attention span for digit sequences (multiple t-Tests, p-values equal to and smaller than 0.01). In the latter test, however, the BS group also proved inferior to the control and RT groups ($p = 0.02$ and $p < 0.01$ respectively).

Thus, although overtly aphasic patients had been eliminated, those with lesions in the left hemisphere (the LT group) did clearly show a language disturbance.

Dichotic Listening: Twelve series of three dichotic pairs of digits were first presented through earphones, and then repeated after inversion of the earphones to compensate for possible channel differences in the acoustic equipment.

Interaurally segmented words: Five lists of 18 monosyllabic nouns each from the Freiburg series for speech audiometry (Hahlbrock, 1970) proved to be of equal auditory perceptual difficulty in preliminary tests with 18 non-brain damaged subjects. There were 64 to 66 phonemes in each list. The presentation of each word lasted for 600 to 700 ms. The five lists were used repeatedly for each subject, and always in the same succession.

Complete words were presented either completely to one ear, or the initial 150 to 450 ms of each word were given to one ear, while their complementary final part was given to the other ear. Furthermore the words were *truncated*, in that only their initial 150 to 450 ms were delivered through the earphones, either monaurally (150, 350 and 450 ms), or partially to each ear (150 and 350 ms to one ear, then respectively 200 and 100 ms to the other ear). Both left and right ears experienced the same stimulus conditions in complete and truncated words, and in the durations of initial and final parts of the words. The stimulus initiations and terminations lasted for 7 ms and followed a Gaussian curve, in order to avoid acoustic click-effects in the earphones.

The subjects were instructed to repeat exactly what they heard, even though they might not recognize meaningful words. As a matter of fact, the errors of reproduction were almost exclusively in terms of missing phonemes, and so few false phonemes were given by the patients that this type of error has been discarded here.

Results:

Dichotic Listening: The analysis of variance on 4 groups of subjects by 2 ears yields significant main effects (groups, $p = 0.02$; ears, $p < 0.01$), but the interaction is not significant ($p = 0.7$). Overall, the performance of the control and RT groups is similarly high, whereas it is definitely lower in the BS and LT groups. In all groups, the digits to the right ear are better reproduced than to the left ear. In spite of the non-significant groups by ears interaction, the interaural laterality indices $(R - L) \times 100/(R + L)$ are similar in the control and BS groups (7.8 and 7.2 respectively), whereas they point to an effect of the side of the lesions in the temporal groups, relatively less digits to the ear contralateral to the lesions being reproduced: 11.2 in the RT group and 3.8 in the LT group.

Interaurally segmented words: The role of "aphasia", as measured by the Token Test, in this perceptual task is not evident: The patient of the LT group with the worst score in the Token Test (8 correct out of 22; the next lowest score being 15 correct out of 22) yields the lowest performance only in the reproduction of the final phonemes of complete words, but not of the related initial phonemes, and neither of the initial nor of the final phonemes of truncated words.

The general results in this task are analysed on the basis of the outcome of three factor analyses of variance: 4 groups of subjects (Controls - BS - RT - LT) by 5 conditions of stimulation (as described above) by the two ears (first) stimulated. For the sake of brevity, only the main effect of the groups and the interactions in which they are involved will be considered. Comparisons of single means are by the multiple t-Test.

Complete words (see first Figure). Significantly different numbers of *initial phonemes* are missed by the four groups of subjects ($p < 0.001$). Whereas the BS group is not strongly different from the control group ($p = 0.07$), the latter misses significantly less phonemes than both RT ($p = 0.003$) and LT ($p < 0.001$) groups. Relatively to the stimulus condition (interaction of groups by conditions, $p = 0.04$), both groups

COMPLETE WORDS

(missing phonemes)

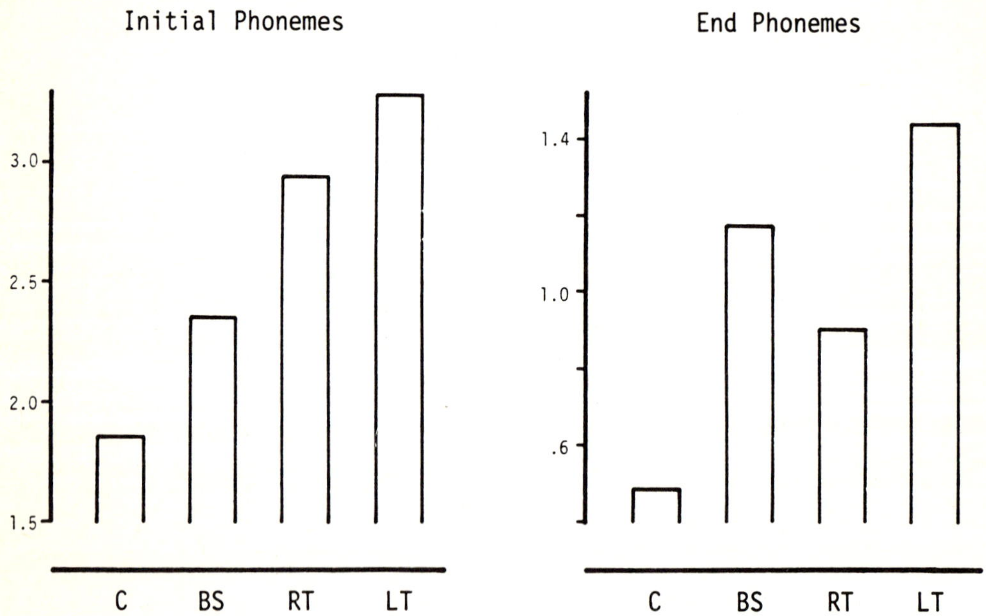

with temporal lesions perform worse than the control and BS groups, and the *temporal deficit* reaches its climax in the combination of 150 ms to one ear, then 500 ms to the other ear (all p smaller than or equal to 0.01).

The four groups of subjects also miss *final phonemes* differentially ($p < 0.001$). This is mainly shown by the inferior performance of the BS and LT groups compared to the controls (both $p < 0.001$), whereas the performance difference between control and RT groups lies only close to a significant value ($p = 0.053$). In this instance, therefore, the main performance deficit is found in the *BS and LT groups*.

Truncated words (see second Figure). As *initial phonemes* are concerned, the four groups of subjects differ significantly

TRUNCATED WORDS

(missing phonemes)

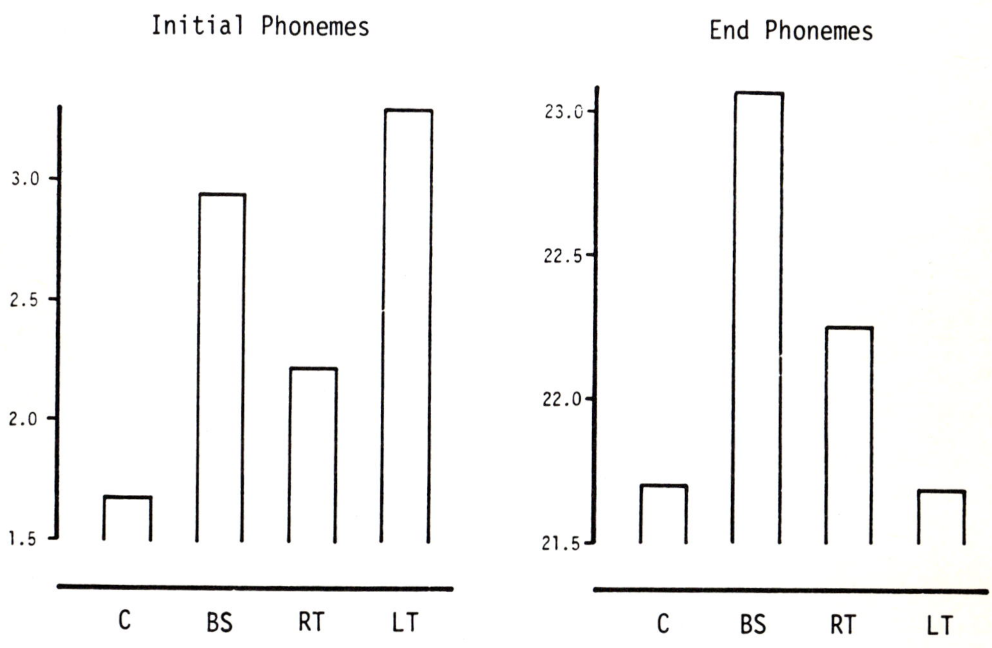

($p < 0.001$). Whereas the controls and RT do not differ significantly ($p = 0.08$), they are definitely superior to both BS and LT groups (p - values from 0.03 to smaller than 0.001), which in fact do not differ strongly ($p > 0.2$). The groups-by-stimulus-conditions interaction is significant ($p < 0.04$), which results mainly from the large superiority of controls over the three patient groups when 150 ms of the stimuli are delivered to one ear and the following 200 ms to the other ear (all $p < 0.001$). Besides the striking overall *BS and LT deficit*, the groups-by-ear-interaction differ significantly ($p = 0.04$), a finding which will be described later.

When the numbers of missed *final phonemes* is considered, the results are striking: the main effects of the groups of subjects is significant ($p = 0.01$). But the LT group performs as well as the controls (mean numbers of final phonemes missed, LT = 21.68, Controls = 21.71), and both are strongly superior to the BS group ($p = 0.004$ and $p < 0.001$). The RT group differs significantly neither from the LT and control groups (both $p \geq 0.2$) nor from the BS group ($p = 0.08$).

Ear differences. Generally, more of the phonemes to the right ear were correctly reported than to the left ear. Relatively to the groups of subjects, however, the ear differences for reported phonemes reaches significance only for the inital phonemes of the truncated words. This originates mainly in the differential effects of left and right *temporal lesions*, for which performance ranks as follows from the worst to the best: Right, then left ear in LT; left then right ear in RT.

In other words, temporal lesions hamper performance in the contralateral ear mainly.

Discussion:

Lesions in the brain stem (BS) entail a low overall performance in *dichotic listening* to verbal stimuli (digits). Although the mere neurological diagnosis of these lesions and of their localization does not allow strong inferences about the precise central nervous structures which have been destroyed, it may be assumed that those concerned in audition may have been involved in the pathological process - at least in part. This finding, then, would support the subcortical hypothesis of Kimura (1961). The fact, however, that the BS group had a poor attention span for digits must be taken into account here, as it may have basically impeded the reproduction of numerous digits, independently of the dichotic perceptual ability per se of the patients. While performing at an overall level almost as high as the controls, the right temporal (RT) group shows the largest ear difference to the disadvantage of the left, contralateral ear. This argues in favour of an involvement of the right hemisphere in verbal dichotic listening, in agreement with the results of Milner et al. (1968) and Sparks and Geschwind (1968). The deficit in the left temporal (LT) group was expected, as the cerebral structure involved is commonly assumed to play a major role in the perception of auditory verbal stimuli. Furthermore, the LT group had yielded poor results in all verbal control tests, so that its deficit in dichotic listening may partly be considered just another instance of generally lowered - mainly receptive - verbal abilities.

In the task of *auditory perception of words*, the interaural segmentation has not brought much new information. The binaural integration of word fragments into one single word is made more difficult by switching from one ear to the other after 150 ms, which may simply point to the difficulty for the auditory system of man to make use of such short-lived information, a difficulty which is enhanced by a brain lesion, especially when more information is delivered to the other perceptual channel of the same sense modality immediately thereafter (interaural masking effect?).

In complete words, i.e., in meaningful stimuli, the initial phonemes orient the search of similar, or identical phonemic information in the patient's corresponding repertoire, and the final phonemes may then be used as a confirmation of overlapping of the word heard and the element found in the repertoire. In truncated words, on the contrary, no word meaning can be reached because of the absence of the final phonemes. The initial phonemes, however, may well trigger the search in the phonemic repertoire, even though the subject knows that no confirmation of correspondence will be made available to him.

The LT deficit in reporting initial phonemes of both complete and truncated words and only final phonemes of complete words could result from a disturbance in the mechanism of searching for correspondence between a perceived word and its image in the phonemic repertoire. This would leave the perception of the final phonemes of truncated words unaffected, as the immediately preceding information has not permitted sufficient initial searching or even access to the repertoire. Such findings remind of some aphasic patients who repeat neologisms better than words.

The isolated clear weakness of RT patients to reproduce the initial phonemes of complete words, in the absence of other verbal deficits in the other tasks reported here cannot be explained in satisfactory terms. Neither a sensory or perceptual deficit in audition, nor the language abilities of the right hemisphere demonstrated in studies with commissurotomized patients can meaningfully account for the results of the RT group. The role of this cerebral structure in the task under scrutiny must be left open, hoping that further research may help to clarify it.

The BS group misses phonemes at the end of complete words, and both at the beginning and end of the truncated words. Nothing has been published as yet to show a specific ability of brain stem structures to process verbal information. Moreover, the low attention span for digits observed in this group cannot be made responsible for the low reproduction of words, which are clearly of shorter duration than the sequences of over four digits repeated correctly in the test of attention span. Hence it appears reasonable to assume a corticofugal action on the auditory structures of the brain stem. Within an intact central nervous system this might produce some gating effect, protecting the auditory system from an overflow of arriving information. A pathological process in the brain stem, however, would prevent the adequate interpretation of the corticofugal gating signals and hence the correct transmission of (mainly late) acoustic information to the cortical processing structures. If this assumption is correct, similar effects of brain stem lesions should be demonstrated for other, nonverbal types of auditory stimuli, and possibly even in other sense modalities than audition. This opens the way to further research on the role of brain stem structures in human behavior.

Supported in part by the Swiss National Science Foundation, Grants 6.182-0.76 and 6.183-0.76 to E. Perret.

References:

1) Broadbent, D.E.: The role of auditory localisation in attention and memory span. J.exp.Psychol. 47, 191-196 (1954).
2) Calearo, C.: "Binaural-Test": Periodically switched speech. Int.J.Audiol. 1, 212-217 (1962).
3) De Renzi, E. and Vignolo, L.A.: The Token Test: A sensitive test to detect receptive disturbances in aphasics. Brain 85, 665-678 (1962).
4) Hahlbrock, K.H.: Sprachaudiometrie. Stuttgart, Georg Thieme (1970).
5) Kimura, D.: Some effects of temporal-lobe damage on auditory perception. Canad.J.Psychol. 15, 156-165 (1961).
6) Lehrl, S.; Daun, H. and Schmidt, R.: Eine Abwandlung des HAWIE Wortschatztests als Kurztest zur Messung der Intelligenz. Arch.Psychiat.Nervenkr. 214, 353-364 (1971).
7) Matzker, J.: Two new methods for the assessment of central auditory functions in cases of brain disease. Ann.Otol.Rhinol. Laryngol. 68, 1185-1197 (1959).
8) Milner, B.; Taylor, L. and Sperry, R.W.: Lateralized suppression of dichotically presented digits after commissural section in man. Science 161, 184-186 (1968).
9) Sparks, R. and Geschwind, N.: Dichotic listening in man after section of neocortical commissures. Cortex 4, 3-16 (1968).

Auditory Analogue of Deep Dyslexia

M. C. GOLDBLUM, Unité 111, INSERM, Paris, France

The presence of semantic errors in the reading performance of patients who were eventually labeled "Deep Dyslexics" was specifically underlined by Marshall and Newcombe in 1966. Since this report a number of similar cases have been described and investigated in detail and it has emerged that several other phenomena are also regularly associated with this condition. In attempt to summarize the deficits in deep dyslexia, Morton and Patterson (In Press) have proposed that the four following aspects are fundamental:

1. Occurence of semantic, derivational and visual paralexias in reading single words aloud; also omissions.
2. Severe if not total impairment in any task (such as reading nonsense words) which requires a non-lexical route from graphemic to phonological code.
3. Part-of-speech effects in word reading such that function words are most impaired and nouns least impaired.
4. Abstractness effect in word reading such that imageable and concrete words are read better than abstract words.

Morton and Patterson go on to examine these four defining characteristics of deep dyslexia in the context of Morton's (1977) Logogen System. Considered in terms of this model, the inability to read nonsense words must be attributed to a breakdown of grapheme-phoneme correspondance. Word reading is therefore effected by the lexical (Logogen) pathway and the presence of semantic errors is taken to indicate that the information categorized at the level of the Input Logogen does not pass directly to the Output Logogen but rather passes by the intermediary cognitive system where this information receives a semantic definition (see Figure 1).

It is evident from Figure 1 that the Logogen System permits seperate inputs for visual and auditory modalities. These distinct inputs notwithstanding, the system nevertheless supposes that the treatment of information in both modalities is identical. Consequently, it should be possible to find the same de-

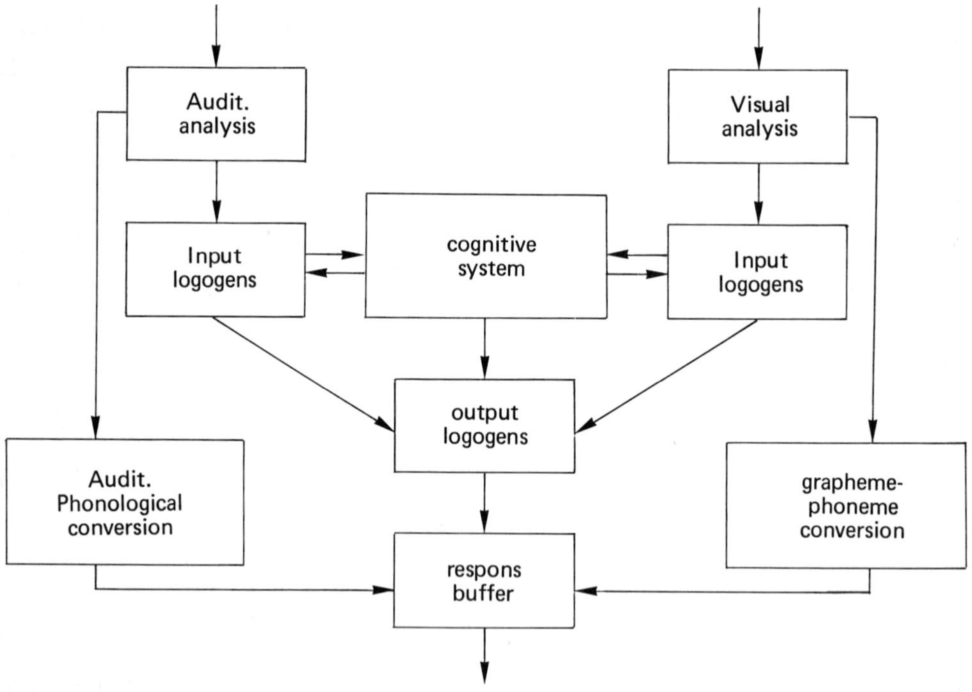

Fig 1. The 1977 version of the Logogen Model (Morton, 1977)

ficits in the auditory modality as those which have been described in the visual modality for deep dyslexics. This report bears on two cases that show such auditory deficits.

Description of Cases:

The first case is that of a right handed, 32 year-old woman who had a cerebro-vascular accident during childbirth. A neurological examination showed no evidence of motor or sensory deficits though she had a right inferior quadrantanopsia. A CAT Scan revealed the presence of an irregular zone of hypodensity that interested the left tempero-parieto-occipital region. Audiometry was normal. Her language was mostly fluent though sometimes interrupted by paraphasias. These included substitutions of phonologically similar words and phonemic paraphasias. Her comprehension of simple commands was preserved, however, some difficulties were noted in her execution of commands like "put the pen in the cup".

The second case is that of a 68 year-old, right handed woman who was brought to our attention because she had an almost total agraphia of five years duration which had initially been accompanied by a now resolved aphasia. Just prior to our assessment she suffered a left hemiplegia that regressed rapidly. An EEG performed after this most recent episode was globally perturbed reflecting the effects of a diffuse vascular lesion. In addition, focal slowing accompanied by occasional irregular discharges was noted over the left centro-parieto-temporal area. A Radioactive Isotope Scan showed evidence in favor of a vascular insufficiency of the posterior left hemisphere and, finally, a CAT Scan revealed the presence of a large vascular lesion involving the territory of the right Sylvian artery as well as a more limited, and probably older, vascular lesion of the left occipital region. The patient's oral language was normal and her comprehension was relatively good though some difficulties were noted in her execution of complex commands. Phonemic discrimination was normal.

In both these cases repetition performance was examined under a variety of conditions designed to illustrate the possible effect on repetition performance of the major factors described as affecting the word reading performance of deep dyslexics. In addition, the errors produced under these conditions were analysed in terms of the various categories identified as characteristic in deep dyslexia.

Repetition Performance

The scores obtained by these patients were clearly superior for meaningful (words) than for non-meaningful material (see Table 1). There was an effect on performance of the syllabic length of the stimulus to be repeated and high frequency word lists promoted slightly better performance (83% Correct) than low frequency word lists (71%) in the one case where this effect

Table 1. Number of Items correctly repeated represented as a percentage of the total number of items presented

Case	1		2	
	Words	N-Words	Words	N-Words
%	68	17	79	32

Table 2. Error Analysis: types of errors as a function of stimulus meaningfulness. Numbers are the percentage of errors for each stimulus category

Case	1			2		
Response Stimulus	Word	N-Word	Omission	Word	N-Word	Omission
Word	36	51	12	33	35	32
N-Word	28	69	3	29	63	8

was examined. Similarly, concrete word lists were better repeated by both patients (68% and 97%) than abstract word lists (58% and 83%).

Table 2 illustrates the proportion of error responses that were either words, nonsense words or omissions, as a function of the type of stimulus (words vs nonsense words).
Most striking is the proportion of nonsense word responses produced by these patients, a proportion which is extremely high where the stimulus was also a nonsense word. It is also notable that there were very few errors of omission.

Where the target stimuli were words and the errors committed were also words, a large proportion of these were semantic errors (see Table 3). For example, when the word synagogue was

Table 3. Error Analysis: Percentage of errors in each category for each patient for Word Repetition, all responses/errors were words

Error Category	Semantic	Derivational	Acoustic	Other
Case 1	25	0	58	17
Case 2	60	9	19	12

given, the patient was likey to reply church, for hurt she said bad and for diamond she said saphire.

Where the errors committed for word stimuli were nonsense words, a large proportion of these errors (Case 1: 65%, Case 2: 91%) bore an acoustic resemblance to the stimulus words. Similarly, where the stimuli were nonsense words and the errors produced were words, a strong proportion of these words were phonologically similar to the nonsense word stimuli (Case 1: 75%, Case 2: 88%). In contrast, when nonsense word errors in nonsense word repetition are considered, the proportion of acoustically similar errors drops considerably (Case 1: 53%, Case 2: 68%).

The influence of semantic factors on repetition was investigated under a variety of experimental conditions. For example, both patients had superior repetition performances for lists of words belonging to the same category (Case 1: 72%, Case 2: 88%), of which they were aware, than for lists of unrelated words (Case 1: 33%, Case 2: 80%). When one of these patients was asked to attend to the meaning of the stimuli, meanwhile, there was only a slight improvement in her repetition score (from 68% to 73%), however, a notable increase occurred in the number of both word errors (from 36% to 54%) and semantic errors (from 25% to 39%). For the other patient, presenting lists of words with high frequency synonyms led to a poorer repetition performance (72%) than that obtained with a control, no-synonym list (84%), and the frequency of semantic errors increased under this condition also. The same phenomenon was noted for sentence repetition but the effect of high frequency synonyms was even more marked in this context. Thus, the patient correctly repeated 6 out of

10 sentences composed of words which had no obvious synonyms and she did not produce any semantic errors on these sentences. In contrast, when she was asked to repeat sentences composed of words having near synonyms, such as "The tempest uprooted three large cedars", the patient was unable to correctly repeat a single sentence. She also produced a considerable number of semantic errors under this condition such that the preceding sentence, for example, was transformed into "The storm uprooted three big oaks".

A certain amount of agrammatism was noted in both these cases during verbal comprehension tasks. More specifically, both patients seemed unable to correctly interpret the meaning of prepositions.

Conclusion:

These patients are directly comparable to deep dyslexics on two of the four defining characteristics enumerated by Morton and Patterson:

1. Word repetition was relatively preserved and semantic and acoustic errors predominated, though derivational errors and errors of omission were also noted.
2. Nonsense word repetition was severely impaired.

With respect to the other two criteria the analogy is less clear. Although both patients demonstrated considerable evidence of agrammatism on non-repetition tasks and function words were less well repeated than lexical words, this effect was not as pronounced as the effect for nonsense words. It should be noted, however, that the difference between lexical and function words is difficult to investigate in a repetition task as many function words are ambiguous in the auditory modality because they have a direct lexical equivalent (i.e. Quand and Camp in French). Similarly, the effect of abstractness on word repetition was relatively minor though this also was in the same direction as the effect described for word reading in deep dyslexia.

Given these findings, the conclusion in terms of the Logogen Model is that the Acoustic to Phonologic Correspondance System is no longer functioning. Repetition then takes place by means of the lexical pathway. The presence of semantic errors indicates that the direct Input-Output Logogen connection is also dysfunctional and that repetition is therefore being carried out by means of the intermediary Cognitive System. A certain number of phenomena, however, are at variance both with deep dyslexia and the model proposed to account for it. In the first instance, the fact that some nonsense words were well repeated and that length was observed to effect repetition performance suggests that Acoustic to Phonologic correspondance was not totally disrupted, a finding which may be taken to indicate that this system is perhaps more robust in the auditory than in the visual modality.

Secondly, the occurrence of nonsense word errors during word repetition a) indicates that these patients are not identical to deep dyslexics and b) is contradictory with repetition by means of the lexical pathway which does not allow for the production of nonsense words.

The fact that these errors were phonologically similar to the target stimuli, meanwhile, suggests that perhaps repetition was being carried out by the Acoustic pathway. However, the finding that the nonsense word errors in nonsense word repetition were not acoustically similar to the target stimuli mitigates against such an interpretation. In addition, the observation that this phonological resemblance increased when semantic processing was encouraged demonstrates that repetition was, in fact, being carried out by the lexical pathway. Consequently, as this is an unforeseen type of error for the Logogen System, it seems likely that these patients have some additional deficit and that many of these "acoustic" errors are probably due to an articulatory deficit. Such errors were noted in the spontaneous speech of one of these patients and they are similar to the type of errors described in conduction aphasia.

It is, of course, impossible to decide on the basis of only two cases whether the phenomena and discrepancies observed here are due to specific properties of the auditory system or to factors particular to these two patients. The study of such dissociations in greater detail and larger numbers of cases, however, is necessary if we are to arrive at a better understanding of the various components associated with language processing in the auditory modality.

References:

Marshall, J.C. and Newcombe, F.: Syntactic and semantic errors in paralexia. Neuropsychologia 4, 169-176 (1966).
Morton, J.: Perception and Memory Course Unit D303. Open University Press (1977).
Morton, J. and Patterson, K.E.: A new attempt at an interpretation or an attempt at a new interpretation. In: M. Coltheart, K. Patterson and J. Marshall (eds.), Deep Dyslexia. London, Routledge ad Kegan Paul, in press.

The Influence of Prosodic Features in Language Comprehension in Aphasic Patients

DOROTHEA WENIGER, Department of Neurology, RWTH Aachen, West Germany

Introduction:

Prosodic features are an integral part of spoken language for the differences of meaning which they convey are signalled by means of variations in pitch, stress, and length. A main difference between prosodic features and other elements of the language system is that not all of their functions are rule-governed; some are situationally conditioned and thus linguistically not predictable. We have rules telling us which syllable to stress in some given word or sentence in normal speech. But depending on the situational context in which some given sentence is uttered the speaker will ignore the rules and place the main stress on the constituent which marks the center of information.

As numerous studies have shown, whenever a particular task involves linguistic abilities aphasic patients perform significantly poorer than other brain damaged patients and normal controls. One would therefore expect aphasic patients to differ in their ability to use variations of pitch and stress as cues in comprehending language depending on whether the function of these cues is a rule-governed one or not. The two experiments to be reported here investigate this hypothesis.

Experiment 1

A perception task was designed in which the emotional tone of a verbal stimulus must be identified in a multiple choice set of three photographs of facial expressions. The verbal stimuli are 10 declarative German sentences, each of 6 syllables' length and containing no lexical material which might suggest a particular emotional tone (e.g. she buys a new dress). Tape recordings were made of these 10 sentences, each sentence being spoken with 12 different intonation contours - variations of pitch conveying the affective state of the speaker (e.g. happiness, surprise, doubt, fear, etc.). Subjects must thus identify the emotional tone of 120 verbal stimuli.

A facial expression corresponding to the emotional mode of each intonation contour was selected from Ekman and Friesen (1975). These photographs were used because they are based on a detailed analysis of the physiological features constituting a particular facial expression. One facial expression in the multiple choice set always corresponds to the emotional tone of the presented verbal stimulus. The other two facial expressions serve as distractors and are taken from the remaining 11 photographs. On each presentation of a particular intonation contour the same two facial expressions are used as distractors. A pilot study showed that the target picture can be identified correctly more often when there is little similarity between the 3 facial expressions. To control this influence of similarity the emotional tone of the 12 intonation contours had to be identified in half of the presentations in a multiple choice set in which there is a pronounced similarity between the 3 facial expressions; in the other half there is little similarity between the 3 expressions.

It has often been argued that severely impaired aphasic patients rely on intonation contours in their comprehension of conversation as a compensatory strategy; evidence is usually taken from these patients' language production. If aphasic patients depend on intonation contours in their perception of language one would expect them to identify the emotional tone of a verbal stimulus better if it is presented in the absence of distracting linguistic cues. A copy of the recorded verbal stimuli was therefore low-pass filtered with an upper cutoff frequency of 510 Hz - a cutoff frequency which preserved the intonation contours but rendered the verbal stimuli unintell-igible.

To sum up - the test material consists of 10 sentences spoken with 12 different intonation contours and 2 x 12 multiple choice sets of facial expressions. The verbal stimuli are presented under two conditions, namely filtered and non-filtered; the former condition is presented first.

The subjects are aphasic patients with global, Wernicke's and Broca's aphasia. There is a control group of normal subjects and one of right brain damaged patients with no aphasia. In each of these 5 groups there are 15 subjects; the groups were matched as well as possible for sex, age, etiology, duration, and education.

A three factorial analysis of variance with repeated measure-ments on the factors condition of presentation and similarity of facial expression was performed. A significant interaction between the three factors was found. Figure 1 illustrates some of the main findings. As hypothesized, the absence of a similarity between the facial expressions leads to more correct identifications, at least numerically.

It is only under the non-filtered condition of presentation that this increase in correct responses is significant. The condition of presentation had an influence on the performance of all groups except the group of global aphasics. This group identified the emotional tone of the two sets of verbal stimuli equally poor. The identification of the emotional tone of the non-filtered verbal stimuli in a multiple choice set of dissimilar

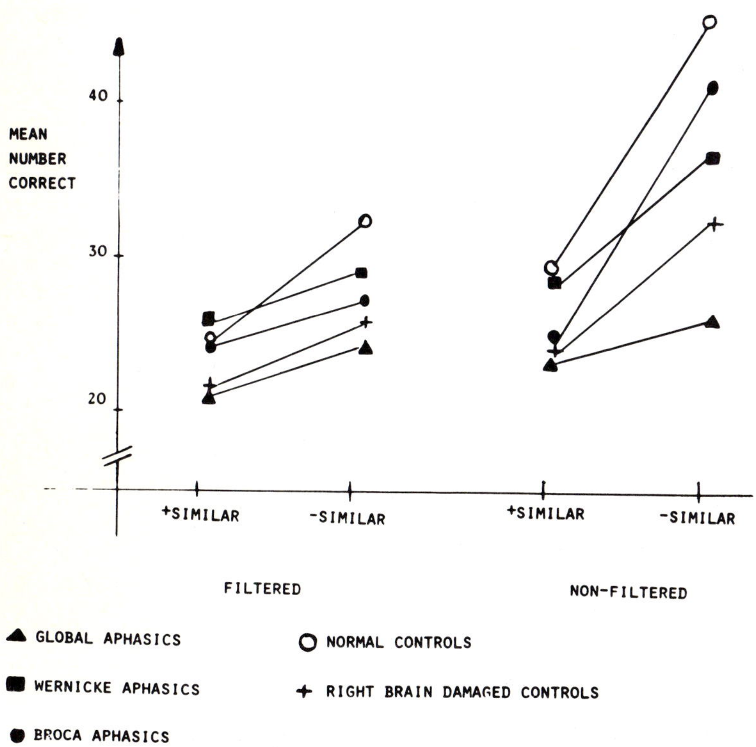

Fig. 1.

facial expressions is of particular interest with regards to the hypothesis made: the group of global aphasics differs from all groups except the group of right brain damaged patients with no aphasia; in addition, the group of right brain damaged patients differs from that of normal controls - a result one does not obtain when these two groups of subjects function as control groups in linguistic tasks. One might argue that the poor performance of the global aphasics is due to severe language impairment. But since the verbal stimuli contained no semantic cues regarding the emotional tone with which it is spoken it cannot be for mainly linguistic reasons that global aphasics performed as they did. The performance of the group of global aphasics and the group of right brain damaged patients must be due to a common disorder - which appears to be the processing of intonation contours. This finding does not exclude, however, a particicipation of the left hemisphere in processing intonation contours (Blumstein and Cooper, 1974; Zurif, 1974).

Experiment 2

This experiment is concerned with the perception of stress as a distinctive cue for discriminating phonemically similar but semantically different words - this being a rule-governed use of stress. Depending on whether the first or the second syllable is stressed in the word convict it means either 'prisoner' or 'to find guilty'. In German it is usually the first syllable of a word that is stressed. But by pairing compound nouns and verbs with noun phrases or prepositional phrases (e.g. Éingriff, 'operation' / ein Gríff, 'a handle'; áufbäumen, 'to rear' / auf Bä́umen, 'on trees') stress contrasts may be obtained. Twenty-six pairs of such contrastively stressed sequences of syllables were collected: 13 nouns were paired with noun phrases and 13 verbs with noun or prepositional phrases. The items of a contrast pair were presented consecutively to subjects whose task it was to identify the meaning of the acoustically presented stimulus item in a multiple choice set of pictures. To limit the number of chance responses the meaning of each stimulus item is to be identified in an array of 8 pictures: the meaning of each stimulus item being represented by 2 visually dissimilar pictures; 2 additional pictures are semantically related to each of the 2 stimulus items. In accordance with this set-up of pictures 3 types of errors were distinguished: stress errors (the selection of one of the 2 pictures presenting the meaning of the contrastively stressed stimulus item) semantic confusion errors (the selection of one of the 2 pictures which are semantically related to the meaning of the presented stimulus item) and the combination of these two errors (the selection of one of the 2 pictures which are semantically related to the contrastively stressed stimulus item).

The task was given to six experimental groups: a group of global, Wernicke's, Broca's and amnesic aphasics. The two control groups are right brain damaged patients with no aphasia and normal subjects. There are 16 subjects in each group and the groups were matched as well as possible for sex, age, etiology, duration, and education.

The distribution of the error types is the same for all groups. More stress errors are made (Fig. 2). One of the factors that was expected to have an influence on performance is the syntac-

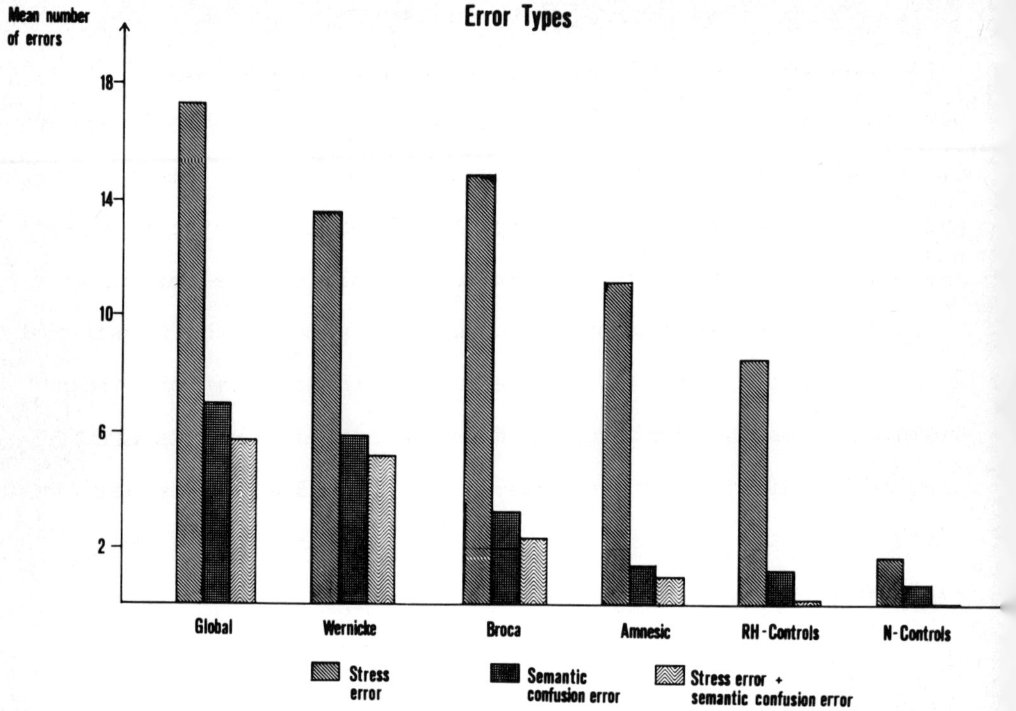

Fig. 2.

tic structure of the stimulus item. Regardless of the syntactic structure of the stimulus item the aphasic subjects always differ in their performance from normal controls. Depending on the syntactic complexity of the stimulus item there are differences of performance between the groups of aphasic patients and the group of right brain damaged patients.

One could argue that the stress errors made by aphasic subjects result from an impaired ability to discriminate stress differences. A discrimination test was therefore given to the four groups of aphasic subjects. Three different types of word pairs were to be judged as being either same or different (e.g. <u>éinhaken</u> - <u>éinhaken</u>, 'to fasten' / <u>éinhaken</u> - <u>ein Háken</u>, 'a hook'/ <u>éinhaken</u> - <u>ein Hámmer</u>, 'a hammer'). Hardly any errors were made in this task. It is apparently not an inability to discriminate stress patterns per se which affects the performance of aphasic patients. It is rather the ability to use stress differences in identifying the syntactic structure and lexical meaning of the stimulus items which appears to be impaired. On hearing a stimulus item aphasic subjects tend to point to the meaning of that item of a contrastively stressed pair which is more familiar and which is syntactically less complex. They do not appear to check whether the stress pattern of the identified meaning corresponds to the one of the presented stimulus item.

As the two experiments show prosodic features are processed differently depending on their linguistic function.

References:

1) Ekman, P.; Friesen, W.: Unmasking the Human Face. Englewood Cliffs Prentice-Hall (1975).
2) Blumstein, S.; Cooper, W.: Hemishperic processing of intonation contours. Cortex 10, 146-158 (1974).
3) Zurif, E.: Auditory lateralization: Prosodic and syntactic factors. Brain and Language 1, 391-404 (1974).